Malaria - Recent Advances and New Perspectives

Edited by Pier Paolo Piccaluga

Published in London, United Kingdom

Malaria - Recent Advances and New Perspectives
http://dx.doi.org/10.5772/intechopen.100821
Edited by Pier Paolo Piccaluga

Contributors
Urja Joshi, Dhara Jani, Hyacinth Highland, Linz-Buoy George, Pier Paolo Piccaluga, Erica Diani, Davide Gibellini, Wanyonyi Ignatius, Nikiwe Mhlanga, Hendriëtte Van der Walt, Vern L. Schramm, Yacoba V.T. Minnow, Kwame Kumi Asare, Samuel Uzondu, Anthony Attama, Richa Goel, Ezihe K. Ebuka, Emmanuel Obi, Nwangwu C. Udoka, Ukonze B. Chikaodili, Nwankwo N. Edith, Udezue Nkemakonam, Egbuche M. Chukwudi, Okeke C. Peter, Andrew Macnab, Carol Yovana Rosero-Galindo, Gloria Isabel Jaramillo-Ramirez, Franco Andres Montenegro-Coral, Cesar Garcia-Balaguera, Sepiribo Lucky Braide, Adaeze Echezona, Chinekwu Nwagwu, Adaeze Onugwu, Lydia Ugorji, Chinazom Agbo, Franklin Kenechukwu, John Ogbonna, Paul Akpa, Petra Nnamani, Audu Momoh

First published in London, United Kingdom, 2023 by IntechOpen
IntechOpen is the global imprint of INTECHOPEN LIMITED, registered in England and Wales, registration number: 11086078, 5 Princes Gate Court, London, SW7 2QJ, United Kingdom
Printed in Croatia

British Library Cataloguing-in-Publication Data
A catalogue record for this book is available from the British Library

Additional hard and PDF copies can be obtained from orders@intechopen.com

Malaria - Recent Advances and New Perspectives
Edited by Pier Paolo Piccaluga
p. cm.

This title is part of the Infectious Diseases Book Series, Volume 20
Topic: Parasitic Infectious Diseases
Series Editor: Alfonso J. Rodriguez-Morales
Topic Editor: Amidou Samie

Print ISBN 978-1-80356-791-4
Online ISBN 978-1-80356-792-1
eBook (PDF) ISBN 978-1-80356-793-8
ISSN 2631-6188

For EU product safety concerns:
IN TECH d.o.o., Prolaz Marije Krucifikse Kozulić 3, 51000 Rijeka, Croatia,
info@intechopen.com or visit our website at intechopen.com.

IntechOpen Book Series

Infectious Diseases

Volume 20

Aims and Scope of the Series

This series will provide a comprehensive overview of recent research trends in various Infectious Diseases (as per the most recent Baltimore classification). Topics will include general overviews of infections, immunopathology, diagnosis, treatment, epidemiology, etiology, and current clinical recommendations for managing infectious diseases. Ongoing issues, recent advances, and future diagnostic approaches and therapeutic strategies will also be discussed. This book series will focus on various aspects and properties of infectious diseases whose deep understanding is essential for safeguarding the human race from losing resources and economies due to pathogens.

Meet the Series Editor

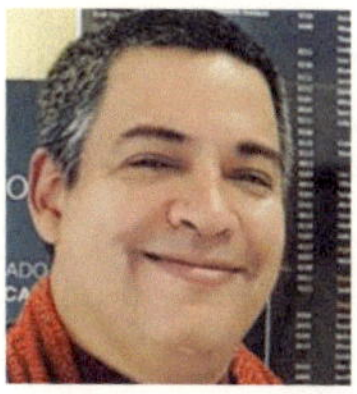

Dr. Rodriguez-Morales is an expert in tropical and emerging diseases, particularly zoonotic and vector-borne diseases (notably arboviral diseases), and more recently COVID-19 and Monkeypox. He is the president of the Publications and Research Committee of the Pan-American Infectious Diseases Association (API), as well as the president of the Colombian Association of Infectious Diseases (ACIN). He is a member of the Committee on Tropical Medicine, Zoonoses, and Travel Medicine of ACIN. Dr. Rodriguez-Morales is a vice-president of the Latin American Society for Travel Medicine (SLAMVI) and a member of the Council of the International Society for Infectious Diseases (ISID). Since 2014, he has been recognized as a senior researcher at the Ministry of Science of Colombia. He is a professor at the Faculty of Medicine of the Fundacion Universitaria Autonoma de las Americas, in Pereira, Risaralda, Colombia, and a professor, Master in Clinical Epidemiology and Biostatistics, at Universidad Científica del Sur, Lima, Peru. He is also a non-resident adjunct faculty member at the Gilbert and Rose-Marie Chagoury School of Medicine, Lebanese American University, Beirut, Lebanon, and an external professor, Master in Research on Tropical Medicine and International Health, at Universitat de Barcelona, Spain. Additionally, an invited professor, Master in Biomedicine, at Universidad Internacional SEK, Quito, Ecuador, and a visiting professor, Master Program of Epidemiology, at Diponegoro University, Indonesia. In 2021 he was awarded the "Raul Isturiz Award" Medal of the API and, the same year, the "Jose Felix Patiño" Asclepius Staff Medal of the Colombian Medical College due to his scientific contributions to the topic of COVID-19 during the pandemic. He is currently the Editor in Chief of the journal Travel Medicine and Infectious Diseases. His Scopus H index is 55 (Google Scholar H index 77) with a total of 725 publications indexed in Scopus.

Meet the Volume Editor

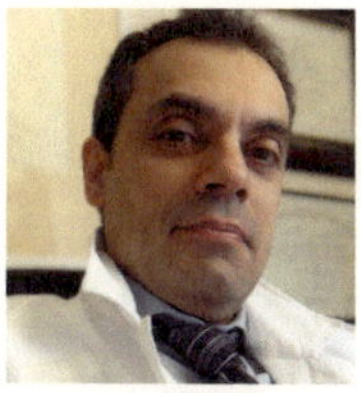

Pier Paolo Piccaluga, MD, Ph.D. is currently an Associate Professor of Pathology at the Department of Experimental, Diagnostic and Specialty Medicine, Bologna University School of Medicine—Institute of Hematology and Medical Oncology, and executive physician at The Biobank of Research, IRCCS S. Orsola-Malpighi Hospital. In 2018, he was appointed to teaching posts at the Queen Mary University of London and Jomo Kenyatta University of Agriculture and Technology, Nairobi, Kenya. He is the author of several international publications in journals such as *Nature Medicine, Journal of Clinical Investigation, Journal of Experimental Medicine, Journal of Clinical Oncology, Blood, Lancet Oncology*, and *Lancet Infectious Diseases*. Dr. Piccaluga is ranked a Top Italian Scientist (TIS) by VIA-Academy.

Contents

Preface

Malaria is an ancient disease, and references to what was almost certainly malaria can be found in a Chinese document from about 2700 BCE, in Mesopotamian clay tablets from 2000 BCE, in Egyptian papyri from 1570 BCE and in Hindu texts as far back as the sixth century BCE. While these historical records should be regarded with caution, more recent observations are certainly stronger. The early Greeks, including Homer in about 850 BCE, Empedocles of Agrigentum in about 550 BCE and Hippocrates in about 400 BCE, were aware of the characteristic poor health, malarial fevers and enlarged spleens seen in people living in marshy places. For over 2500 years the idea that malarial fevers were caused by miasmas rising from swamps persisted, and it is widely held that the word malaria comes from the Italian malaria, meaning spoiled air, although this has been disputed. With the discovery of bacteria by Antonie van Leeuwenhoek in 1676, the recognition of microorganisms as causes of infectious diseases, and the development of the germ theory of infection by Louis Pasteur and Robert Koch in 1878–1879, the search for the cause of malaria intensified. Scientific studies only became possible after the discovery of the parasites themselves by Charles Louis Alphonse Laveran in 1880 and the identification of mosquitoes as the vectors, first for avian malaria by Ronald Ross in 1897 and then for human malaria by the Italian scientists Giovanni Battista Grassi, Amico Bignami, Giuseppe Bastianelli, Angelo Celli, Camillo Golgi and Ettore Marchiafava between 1898 and 1900.

Since then, progress has been made in malaria knowledge, prevention, and treatment. Quinine alone has probably saved millions of lives since its formal introduction in the 20th century. Nonetheless, in that time frame, malaria has claimed between 150 million and 300 million lives, accounting for 2 to 5 percent of all deaths. Although its chief sufferers today are the poor of Sub-Saharan Africa, Asia, the Amazon Basin, and other tropical regions, 40 percent of the world's population still lives in areas where malaria is transmitted (**Figure 1**).

This book presents a brief overview of the pathobiology of malaria and the current standards of diagnosis and treatments, and provides some insights into novel preventive and therapeutic approaches.

While the primary responsibility for malaria prevention and treatment lies with medicine and pharmacology, political as well as social initiatives are no less important. Most countries where malaria was endemic at the beginning of the 20th century are now totally malaria free. It is conceivable that investments in those areas where malaria is still deadly would lead not only to obvious global health benefits, but also to economic benefits, given that malaria, HIV and other infective diseases represent major obstacles to the development of such countries.

This book is intended for all health professionals, particularly those involved in THE diagnosis and treatment of tropical and infectious diseases, as well as medical students and researchers.

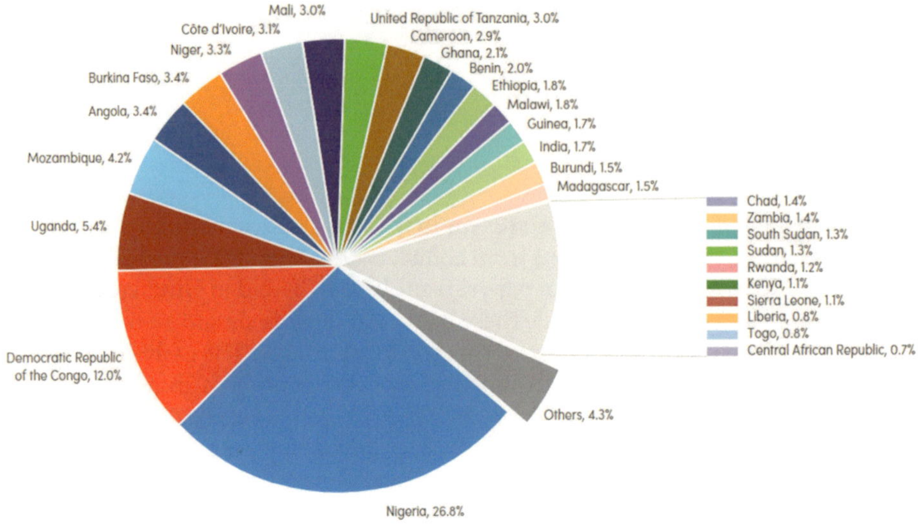

Figure 1.
Malaria cases worldwide in 2020 (data from WHO). Nigeria (26.8%), the Democratic Republic of the Congo (12.0%), Uganda (5.4%), Mozambique (4.2%), Angola (3.4%) and Burkina Faso (3.4%) accounted for 55% of all cases.

I am grateful to IntechOpen for the opportunity to edit this volume. I would like to thank Ms. Marica Novaković and Mr. Josip Knapic for their help and support, as well as all the contributors who have dedicated their time and effort to bringing this book to publication.

Pier Paolo Piccaluga, MD, Ph.D.
Professor,
Biobank of Research and Institute of Hematology
and Medical Oncology "Seràgnoli", IRCCS Azienda Ospedaliero
Universitaria di Bologna S. Orsola-Malpighi,
Department of Experimental, Diagnostic and Specialty Medicine,
Bologna University School of Medicine,
Bologna, Italy

Section 1

Introduction

Chapter 1

Introductory Chapter: Malaria in 2022 – Promises and Unmet Needs

Erica Diani, Davide Gibellini and Pier Paolo Piccaluga

1. Introduction

Malaria represents one of the most ancient and diffuse infective illnesses in the World. It was first described in a Chinese paper, dated 2700 before Christ, in which a patient with recurrent fever was described. Many records on papyri and clay tablets report similar cases, but the definition of causative agent of malaria had to wait for the germ theory and the first discovery of *Plasmodium* in human blood sample [1, 2]. After almost 5000 years, malaria continues to be frightening: in 2020, the WHO estimated 241 million cases and 627,000 deaths in the 85 countries in which malaria is endemic (WHO), and about of 75% of infected patients are children. In recent decades, various programs have been implemented in order to contain and reduce the transmission of malaria through prevention, diagnosis, and surveillance strategies. Unfortunately, the SARS-CoV-2 pandemic has caused an increase in the number of cases and deaths due to the interruption of malaria prevention and a sort of black out in the surveillance and case reports. Now, after 2 years of SARS-CoV-2 pandemic, the number of malaria cases and death has not been even updated; the last officially released data were in 2019, but it is absolutely necessary to maintain open the attention on this plague [3].

2. The biological cycle of *Plasmodia*

Malaria is a life-threatening disease characterized by recurrent periodically fever accompanied by nausea, vomiting and abdominal discomfort, fatigue, and headaches [4]. Infection is caused by five protozoan parasites of the genus *Plasmodium*: *P. falciparum, P. vivax, P. ovale, P. malariae,* and *P. knowlesi,* which are characterized by different periodicity and different severity of illness (see **Table 1**). In particular, *P. falciparum* is responsible for malignant tertian, which, in the more severe cases, can lead to the death of patients in 24 hours after the symptoms appear (WHO).

Transmission occurs through an arthropod vector, which can acquire the *Plasmodium* through the bite of an infected person. *Plasmodium* maturation proceeds in the Anopheles stomach and midgut, and the sporozoites (infective form) are released in another person by mosquito bite, starting new infection cycle [6, 7]. Rarely, the transmission can occur among persons through blood transfusion or organ transplants.

The biological cycle of *Plasmodia* takes place in two obligated hosts (**Figure 1**): a vertebrate and a female of mosquito Anopheles. In brief, the infection of a female

Plasmodium species	Incubation period	Periodicity of fever increase	Sign and Symptoms for severe disease
P. falciparum	9–14 days	3 days	Impaired consciousness: Glasgow Coma Scale score < 11;
			Multiple convulsion: > 2 seizures/days;
			Prostration: unable to sit, stand or walk alone;
			Significant bleeding: recurrent or prolonged bleeding from the nose, gum, venipuncture sites, hematemesis, or melena;
			Shock: circulatory collapse/shock.
P. vivax	12–17 days	3 days	Defined as falciparum malaria but w/o parasite density threshold.
P. ovale	16–18 days	3 days	Rarely occur.
			No parasite density threshold.
P. malariae	18–40 days	4 days	Rarely occur.
			No parasite density threshold.
P. knowlesi	9–12 days	2 days	Defined as for falciparum malaria except for parasite density (>100.000/mL) and for Jaundice and parasite density (>20.000/mL)

Modified by Daily et al. [5].

Table 1.
Characteristics of Plasmodium species infection and diagnosis criteria.

Anopheles occurs after a blood meal carried out on an infected human subject carrying the gametocytes, the sexual forms of the parasite, which are the only ones that can proceed with the development in the Anopheles body. The sporozoites are the final stage of development cycle and are also the human infective form of *Plasmodium*. At the end of the development cycle, the sporozoites, the forms of *Plasmodium* infecting humans, migrate into the salivary glands of the mosquito, from where they will be inoculated into another human subject through the bite. The development of the *Plasmodium* continues also inside the human host. Sporozoites can reach the liver, establishing a silent infection in the hepatocytes and undergoing a strong proliferation with the formation of the schizont within which maturation takes place in the form of merozoites. When the merozoites are mature, the schizont ruptures release them into the bloodstream where they invade the erythrocytes causing disease. Within the erythrocytes, the merozoites pass through another developmental stage, starting from ring form, to trophozoites, and ending to multinucleated schizonts (erythrocytic stage). This final step in the red blood can undergo a cycle (the intraerythrocytic developmental cycle, IDC) activated by the rupture of the schizont continuing the infectious phase where they reproduce again by schizogony, giving rise to new generations of parasites every 48 (tertian) or 72 (quartana) hours.

Some merozoites can further differentiate into female and male gametocytes, which, being present in the bloodstream of the infected patient for several weeks, can be ingested during a mosquito's meal, thus initiating a new transmission. Only for *P. vivax* and *P. ovale*, the liver stage infection is also characterized by a dormant phase also called hypnozoite, which causes a prolonged infection [8].

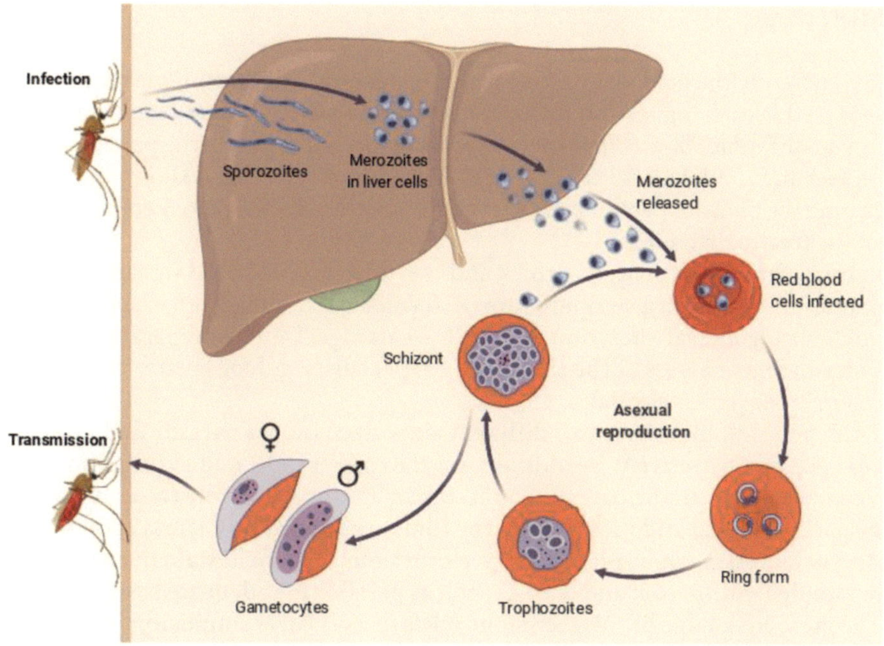

Figure 1.
Biological cycle of Plasmodium in human host. Reprinted from "Malaria Transmission Cycle", by BioRender, May 2019—https://app.biorender.com/biorender-templates/t-5e629f969501410088a0156b-malaria-transmission-cycle.

3. Malaria diagnosis

The first steps to try to reduce malaria cases and death are obvious: protective clothing, mosquito repellants, bed nets, screened accommodations, chemoprophylaxis (only for travelers in the endemic areas), avoid visiting friends infected, which is the cause of about 50% of new infections [3].

In October 2021, WHO approved the use of the malaria vaccine, RTS,S/ASO1 (GSK Belgium), in children from 5 months of age. This vaccine is based on a recombinant subunit protein of P. falciparum that is expressed during sporozoite stage. This new strategy is leading to reduced new malaria cases worldwide [9]. Recent study on the vaccination campaign impact reports that in a population of children from 5 months age, who received all four doses of malaria vaccine, in a follow-up time of 4 years, they observed a reduction in both clinical and severe malaria cases of 39% and 29%, respectively [10].

The second important step to eradicate and contain malaria contagion in endemic areas (including cases derived from traveling) is a correct and tempestive diagnosis of malaria with specific indication of which species of malaria is or are present in the sample, in order to use the most appropriate drug treatment.

Following the indication of WHO and of the British Society of Hematology [3, 11], the diagnostic assays for malaria are: microscopic examination in thin and thick film, Rapid Diagnostic Test (RDT) based on antigen, Indirect Fluorescent Antibody Test (IFA test), and also, recently introduced and accepted, the nucleic-acid detection method by PCR or LAMP technologies.

3.1 Microscopy

It is currently the gold standard to diagnose malaria. This technique requires experienced hematologists and technicians to prepare and observe blood smears, discriminate different *Plasmodium* species, and correctly quantitate the parasite density in the specimen. When *P. falciparum* or *P. knowlesi* are detected, it is very important to determine the parasite percentage because the species and the parasitemia level may affect the treatment choice.

In brief, for each patient, two thick and two thin films of blood smears should be prepared, starting from a venipuncture performed maximum 2–4 h earlier, in order to avoid morphological alteration due to EDTA storage. Double preparation is needed for independent analyses of the slides by two specialists and for greater control and precision in the parasite count.

Thick and thin films have two different aims: detection of parasite and identification of species, respectively. In addition, for the species indicated in thin film, it can be possible to perform the parasite count, taking into account only the asexual stage of the parasites (ring and merozoite). The films are colored by Giemsa stain at pH 7.2. For severe illness, it can be possible to perform a modified field stain in order to detect more rapidly *P. falciparum* and start as soon as possible the adequate treatment.

The great advantage of this technique relies in its relative simplicity; in fact, it can be performed in any laboratory that performs hematology tests, requiring no additional equipment. In addition, microscopy can provide three important data to start the patient treatment: presence of *Plasmodium*, its specie, and count. The main disadvantage is that morphological analysis requires experienced staff.

3.2 Rapid diagnostic test

Rapid diagnostic test is a faster alternative to microscopy detection. This immunochromatographic test is performed starting from some small drops of blood, and in about 15 minutes, the physician can visualize the presence of specific bands in the window of the test card. This immunochromatographic test, based on antigen or antibody, makes it possible to identify four out of five *Plasmodium* species, *P. knowlesi* being excluded.

This approach allows a faster but less sensitive diagnosis and might be not sufficient. The main advantage is that it does not require expert personnel and can even be self-performed, facilitating diagnosis where the doctor cannot reach the patients. On the other hand, as a limitation, we can only obtain information about the presence of one or more species of *Plasmodium*, but the amount of parasites is unveiled.

3.3 Indirect fluorescent antibody test

Indirect Fluorescent Antibody (IFA) test is based on the detection of antibodies in the patient serum. Due to the long time needed to carry out the procedure, it cannot be adopted as a routine test for malaria detection. However, IFA test is useful to screen the blood donors in malaria cases suspected to be transmitted by hemo-transfusions, when a donor is negative at microscopy test. The use of specific antibody allows to detect *Plasmodium* also in infected patient with very low parasitemia. In addition, IFA test is a good tool for the test of patient with chronic or repeated malaria infection and for patient whose diagnosis is unsure after starting drug therapy.

IFA test is available for all *Plasmodium* with exception of *P. knowlesi*, due to the availability of specific antibodies.

Another serology test employed is an immune-enzymatic assay, used principally for blood donors screening. The limit of this test is its sensitivity due to the possibility to detect only *P. falciparum vs "non-falciparum spp."*

3.4 Nucleic acid detection methods

To date, only a few referral laboratories use molecular methods to detect, define, and quantify *Plasmodium* infections, while these tests are principally used for research and epidemiologic scopes [12]. Only for a suspect of *P. knowlesi* infection, polymerase chain reaction (PCR) is becoming a standard to confirm the diagnosis before treatment initiation.

PCR-based techniques could be useful to detect malaria in case of infection at low-density parasitemia, which is difficult to detect also at microscopy or in the absence of an expert technician. Of note, the specific oligonucleotides used for the amplification allow, at the same time, detection, species definition and quantitation, even for low amounts of *Plasmodia* [13–17]. Prospectively, PCR-based tools are expected to be the gold standard in malaria diagnosis, as already happened in most infectious diseases. In fact, PCR is currently cheap, easy to perform even in low resources settings, fast, and absolutely accurate.

Loop-mediated isothermal amplification test (LMPA) can detect parasite DNA in a simpler way with respect to PCR [18–22]. The advantages of LMPA tests, compared with PCR, are that thermocyclers are not required. Conversely, sensitivity and specificity are variable, making this test not always reliable [23–26].

Author details

Erica Diani[1], Davide Gibellini[1] and Pier Paolo Piccaluga[2,3,4*]

1 Microbiology Section, Department of Diagnostic and Public Health, Verona University, Italy

2 Biobank of Research and Institute of Hematology and Medical Oncology Seràgnoli, IRCCS Azienda Ospedaliera-Universitaria S. Orsola-Malpighi, Bologna, Italy

3 Department of Experimental, Diagnostic, and Experimental Medicine, Bologna University School of Medicine, Bologna, Italy

4 Jomo Kenyatta University of Agriculture and Technology and University of Nairobi, Kenya

*Address all correspondence to: pierpaolo.piccaluga@unibo.it

References

[1] Cox FE. History of human parasitology. Clinical Microbiology Reviews. 2002;**15**(4):595-612. DOI: 10.1128/CMR.15.4.595-612.2002. Erratum in: Clinical Microbiology Reviews. 2003 Jan;**16**(1):174. PMID: 12364371; PMCID: PMC126866

[2] Cox FE. History of the discovery of the malaria parasites and their vectors. Parasites & Vectors. 2010;**3**(1):5

[3] World Health Organization. WHO Guidelines for Malaria. Geneva: World Health Organization; 2022. Available from: http://apps.who.int/bookorders

[4] White NJ, Pukrittayakamee S, Hien TT, Faiz MA, Mokuolu OA, Dondorp AM. Malaria. The Lancet. 2014;**383**(9918):723-735

[5] Daily JP, Minuti A, Khan N. Diagnosis, treatment, and prevention of malaria in the US. Journal of the American Medical Association. 2022;**328**(5):460

[6] Aly ASI, Vaughan AM, Kappe SHI. Malaria parasite development in the mosquito and infection of the mammalian host. Annual Review of Microbiology. 2009;**63**(1):195-221

[7] Frischknecht F, Matuschewski K. *Plasmodium* sporozoite biology. Cold Spring Harbor Perspectives in Medicine. 2017;7(5):a025478

[8] Josling GA, Williamson KC, Llinás M. Regulation of sexual commitment and Gametocytogenesis in malaria parasites. Annual Review of Microbiology. 2018;**72**(1):501-519

[9] World Health Organization. WHO Recommends Groundbreaking Malaria Vaccine for Children at Risk. 2021

[10] Praet N, Asante KP, Bozonnat MC, Akité EJ, Ansah PO, Baril L, et al. Assessing the safety, impact and effectiveness of RTS,S/AS01E malaria vaccine following its introduction in three sub-Saharan African countries: Methodological approaches and study set-up. Malaria Journal. 2022;**21**(1):132

[11] Rogers CL, Bain BJ, Garg M, Fernandes S, Mooney C, Chiodini PL. British Society for Haematology guidelines for the laboratory diagnosis of malaria. British Journal of Haematology. 2022;**197**(3):271-282

[12] Proux S, Suwanarusk R, Barends M, et al. Considerations on the use of nucleic acid-based amplification for malaria parasite detection. Malaria Journal. 2011;**10**:323. DOI: 10.1186/1475-2875-10-323

[13] Vafa Homann M, Emami SN, Yman V, Stenström C, Sondén K, Ramström H, et al. Detection of malaria parasites after treatment in travelers: A 12-months longitudinal study and statistical modelling analysis. eBioMedicine. 2017;**25**:66-72

[14] Steenkeste N, Incardona S, Chy S, Duval L, Ekala MT, Lim P, et al. Towards high-throughput molecular detection of *Plasmodium*: New approaches and molecular markers. Malaria Journal. 2009;**8**(1):86

[15] Okell LC, Ghani AC, Lyons E, Drakeley CJ. Submicroscopic infection in *Plasmodium falciparum* – endemic populations: A systematic review and meta-analysis. The Journal of Infectious Diseases. 2009;**200**(10):1509-1517

[16] Giha H, Hviid L, Richardson W, Elhassan IM, Arnot DE, Theander TG,

et al. Detection of very low level *Plasmodium falciparum* infections using the nested polymerase chain reaction and a reassessment of the epidemiology of unstable malaria in Sudan. The American Journal of Tropical Medicine and Hygiene. 1996;**54**(4):325-331

[17] Vannachone B, Kobayashi J, Toma H, Inthakone S, Manivong K, Nambanya S, et al. A field study on malaria prevalence in southeastern Laos by polymerase chain reaction assay. The American Journal of Tropical Medicine and Hygiene. 2001;**64**(5):257-261

[18] Notomi T. Loop-mediated isothermal amplification of DNA. Nucleic Acids Research. 2000;**28**(12):63e-663e

[19] Poon LL, Wong BW, Ma EH, Chan KH, Chow LM, Abeyewickreme W, et al. Sensitive and inexpensive molecular test for falciparum malaria: Detecting *Plasmodium falciparum* DNA directly from heat-treated blood by loop-mediated isothermal amplification. Clinical Chemistry. 2006;**52**(2):303-306

[20] Hopkins H, González IJ, Polley SD, Angutoko P, Ategeka J, Asiimwe C, et al. Highly sensitive detection of malaria parasitemia in a malaria-endemic setting: Performance of a new loop-mediated isothermal amplification kit in a remote clinic in Uganda. The Journal of Infectious Diseases. 2013;**208**(4):645-652

[21] Patel JC, Lucchi NW, Srivastava P, Lin JT, Sug-aram R, Aruncharus S, et al. Field evaluation of a real-time fluorescence loop-mediated isothermal amplification assay, RealAmp, for the diagnosis of malaria in Thailand and India. Journal of Infectious Diseases. 2014;**210**(8):1180-1187

[22] Perera RS, Ding XC, Tully F, Oliver J, Bright N, Bell D, et al. Development and clinical performance of high throughput loop-mediated isothermal amplification for detection of malaria. PLoS One. 2017;**12**(2):e0171126

[23] Thekisoe O, Pöschl B, Chutipongvivate S, Panagiotis K, Waneesorn J. Comparative diagnosis of malaria infections by microscopy, nested PCR, and LAMP in Northern Thailand. The American Journal of Tropical Medicine and Hygiene. 2010;**83**(1):56-60

[24] Piera KA, Aziz A, William T, Bell D, González IJ, Barber BE, et al. Detection of *Plasmodium knowlesi*, *Plasmodium falciparum* and *Plasmodium vivax* using loop-mediated isothermal amplification (LAMP) in a co-endemic area in Malaysia. Malaria Journal. 2017;**16**(1):29

[25] Katrak S, Murphy M, Nayebare P, Rek J, Smith M, Arinaitwe E, et al. Performance of loop-mediated isothermal amplification for the identification of submicroscopic *Plasmodium falciparum* infection in Uganda. The American Journal of Tropical Medicine and Hygiene. 2017;**97**(6):1777-1781

[26] Morris U, Aydin-Schmidt B. Performance and application of commercially available loop-mediated isothermal amplification (LAMP) kits in malaria endemic and non-endemic settings. Diagnostics. 2021;**11**(2):336

Section 2

Malaria Diagnosis

Chapter 2

Malaria Diagnostics

Nikiwe Mhlanga and Hendriëtte Van der Walt

Abstract

The imminent scenario of malaria burden on endemic regions burdens healthcare and is a threat to non-endemic regions. Microscopy and rapid diagnostic tests (RDTs) remain the gold standard for malaria detection in resource-constrained regions. They still present low sensitivity at low parasite density, however, with microscopy also requiring trained personnel, expensive and time consuming. Affordable, rapid, specific, sensitive and simple malaria diagnostics remain elusive. Molecular-based diagnostics, polymerase chain reaction and loop-mediated isothermal amplification, although highly sensitive even at low parasitemia, still have challenges hindering their use in resource-constrained regions. This chapter discusses the conventional microscopy, spectroscopy, RDTs and molecular platforms in malaria detection. It also highlights current interventions on mitigations of their existing hurdles and adaptability to developing regions. Such inventions include the amalgamation of different techniques, nanotechnology and artificial intelligence.

Keywords: microscopy, SERS, RDTs, LAMP, PCR

1. Introduction

The malaria protozoan continues to yield despondency in third World Health Organisation (WHO) regions. In 2019, 227 million global cases were estimated, and in 2020, it increased to 241 million cases [1]. **Figure 1** gives an approximation of endemic WHO regions where malaria transmission still occurs. The continuous battle is prevailing even with the availability of state-of-the-art malaria detection techniques, which have evolved from the gold standard microscopy to rapid diagnostics, nucleic-based polymerase chain reaction (PCR) and loop-mediated isothermal amplification (LAMP). Heightening the infections in these regions is the inaccessibility of the existing techniques. Some of them are too expensive and not readily available, yet even with rapid diagnostic tests (RDTs), which are readily available and simpler, and low sensitivity especially for low parasite density and asymptomatic infections remains a hurdle. A controlled disease and prevention plan including early, sensitive, accessible, affordable, user-friendly and rapid detection tools is mandatory in these regions [3].

Malaria is caused by a protozoan parasite of the *Plasmodium* genus with five species *viz.falciparum*, *vivax*, *malariae*, *ovale* and *knowlesi*. The *P. falciparum* is the most prevalent, infectious and fatal of the five. Malaria infection is detrimental in young children and pregnant women due to underdeveloped and temporal loss of immunity, respectively. The parasite is transmitted from a female anopheles mosquito to a human *via* feeding when the latter bites the host [4–7].

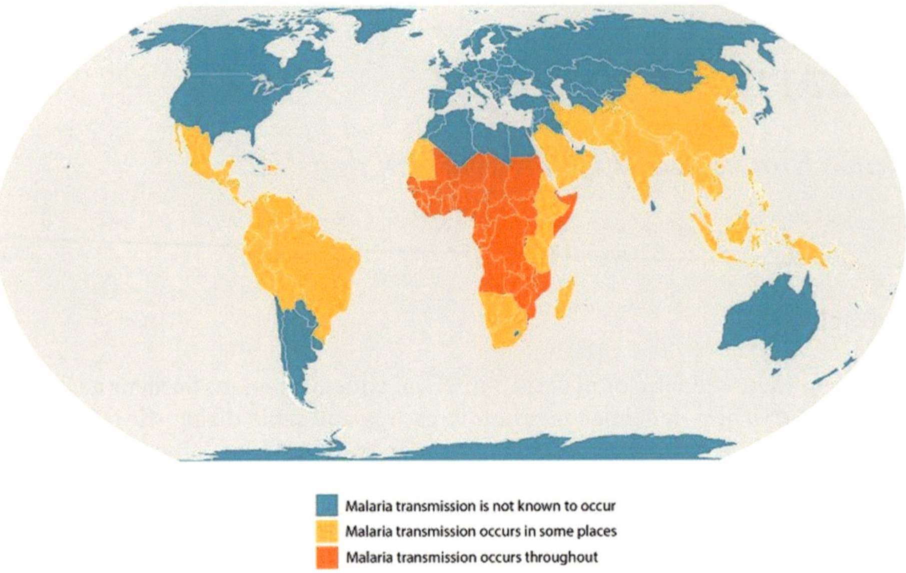

Figure 1.
An approximation of malaria-endemic WHO regions [2].

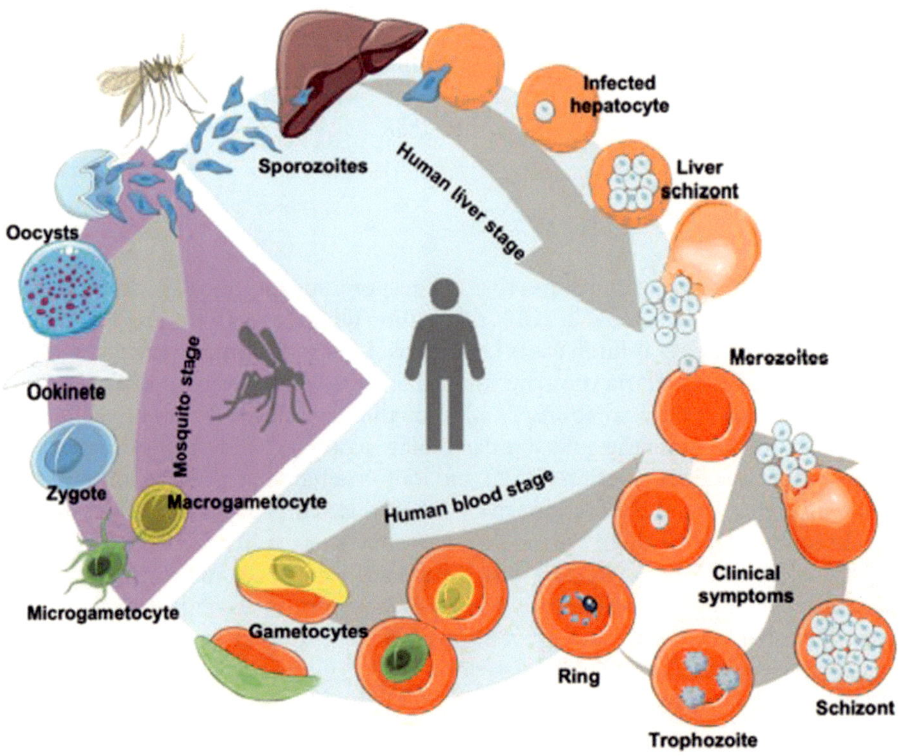

Figure 2.
A malaria parasite life cycle. Reprinted with permission from ACS [3].

The parasites target the lungs and red blood cells (RBCs) and the former has a latent phase that can reoccur after years of initial infection [5]. Sporozoites are transferred from the mosquitoes' salivary glands into the human bloodstream, where after they migrate to the human liver. In the liver, an exoerythrocytic infection stage initiates, that is, asexual reproduction in the liver hepatocyte of sporozoites transformation and multiplication into thousands of schizonts/merozoites. Within a couple of days (6–8), the matured merozoites rapture the host hepatocyte and are released into the bloodstream, where they invade the RBCs. Internalised in the RBCs, they undergo asexual reproduction. This infection stage is named the erythrocytic cycle [4]. The erythrocytic stage is initiated with tiny ring forms that turn into a larger amoeboid forms (trophozoite) and finally merozoites. The host RCBs rupture to release the matured merozoites, which will invade new RBCs. The continuous invasion of the RBCs burdens the RCBs and triggers severe pathological and patient sicknesses such as anaemia [4]. **Figure 2** illustrates the lifecycle of the *Plasmodium* species. Some of the merozoites develop into female and male gametocytes that circulate in the bloodstream to be re-ingested by a mosquito where they start a new cycle. Male and female gametocytes are fertilised into zygotes that transform into sporozoites that flow in the mosquito's salivary glands [4].

2. Microscopic detection of malaria

2.1 Conventional microscopy

Light microscopy, a gold standard conventional malaria diagnostic, uses Giemsa-stained thick and thin blood smears of peripheral blood from the intraerythrocytic malaria cycle to detect the *Plasmodium* species [3, 4, 7, 8]. The thick and thin blood smears are used to deduce the parasite and parasite species, respectively. **Figure 3** shows the *P. falciparum* light microscopy morphology from the smears. Microscopy, however, also presents challenges: low sensitivity at low parasitemia is laborious and costly, and requires a trained microscopist and it is not standardised; uses a bulky visual/light microscope and is not suitable for point-of-care testing (POCT) [3–5]. Also because microscopy is a morphological diagnostic tool, misdiagnosis is possible between species with close morphological resemblance [4]. It has an average detection limit of about 50 parasites/μL.

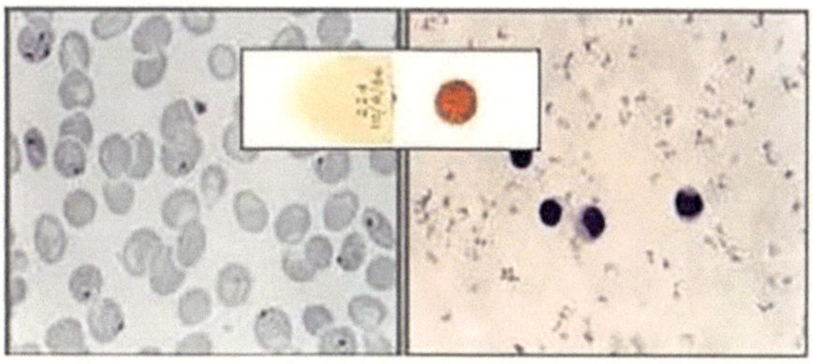

Figure 3.
Microscopy images of P. falciparum *from thick (right) and thin (left) blood smear [9].*

2.2 Modern microscopic interventions

As alluded to in the previous section, although microscopy is the malaria diagnosis gold standard, its bulkiness, expense and lab basis are some of the challenges that require mitigation. The automated microscopy platform is merited by improved and standardised malaria detection. It inherits the benefits of a light microscope and also mitigates its challenges and hence yields rapidity, improved scanning area and enhanced consistency [10]. Human microscopists are eliminated by the automated system. It inherits three reliant elements: sample preparation, digital microscopy with automated scanning and a computer vision algorithm that analyses captured images [10].

Faizullah et al. [11] proposed an automated convolutional neutral network (CNN) model for malaria detection from microscopy blood smear images. Knowledge distillation, data augmentation, autoencoder, feature extraction CNN model and classification support vector machine or K-nearest neighbours (KNN) were used to develop the CNN algorithm. The algorithm detected malaria from images with 99.23% accuracy. To enable both clinical and field use, it was integrated into a smartphone and backed up on server-back-up web, to support offline and online applications. Hasan et al. [12] tried different models: Adaboost, KNN, decision tree, random forest, support vector machine and multinomial naive Bayes on a database of 27,558 cell images. Adaboost, random forest, support vector machine and multinomial naive Bayes achieved good results (91%). Yoon et al. [8] developed a fully automated microscopic system characterised by a plastic chip, fluorescent dye for malarial staining and an image analysing program for detection and parasitemia determination. Use of the fluorescent dye as opposed to the Giemsa stain afforded rapidity, sensitivity and accuracy. The automated system showed a higher degree of linearity and precision in the detection of *P. falciparum* culture with a limit of detection of 0.00066112% (30 parasites/μL) [8].

The bulkiness of the traditional microscopy also negates its field application. Cybolоki et al. [13] combined optical principles with origami and fabricated two-dimensional microscopy, a cheaper alternative to the bulky light microscope. The foldscope is assembled from a flat sheet in a few minutes and provides over 2000 x magnification with submicron resolution. It alleviates conventional microscopy and can be used in the field since it does not use external power.

Microscopy under polarised light is also used to diagnose malaria *via* hemozoin (Hz). Hz is an end product of the malaria proliferation stage. Owing to its interesting properties of magnetism and acoustic and optical nature, it is explored as a biomarker [3]. Due to its birefringent nature, it is viewed with polarised light microscopy. This approach detects 30 parasites/ μ L but is negated by the use of an expensive polarised light, complexity and bulkiness [3]. An affordable alternative invention by Pirnstill et al. [14] uses optical smartphone-based transmission polarised light microscopy.

3. Spectroscopic malaria detection

3.1 Ultraviolet visible spectrometer

An ultraviolet-visible (UV-Vis) spectrometer is used in the detection of malaria, that is, confirming malaria cases *via* changes in excitation peaks. This system utilises nanoparticles such as gold (Au) and silver (Ag) that inherently have strong optical absorption, which signal aggregation by red-shift. The nanoparticles in the vicinity

DOI: http://dx.doi.org/10.5772/intechopen.106631

of the biomolecules aggregate and hence trigger a measurable change in the optical signal [5]. Recently, Adegoke et al. [15] advanced this platform by coupling UV-Vis with near-infrared spectroscopy to detect and quantify low parasitemia (1-1x10^{-6}%) of ring-stage malaria-infected blood under physiological conditions using a multiclass classification.

3.2 Vibrational optical spectroscopies

Vibrational optical spectroscopies study the characteristic vibrational modes of molecules. The vibrational modes have specific vibrational frequencies, which are a molecule's characteristic fingerprint. These systems are used to study the molecular attributes of biological molecules in biosensing. Fourier transform infrared (FTIR) and Raman spectroscopy are complementary vibrational spectroscopic systems [16]. Raman spectroscopy has been tried in the detection of malaria focused on plasma [17].

An advanced variant of Raman, surface-enhanced Raman spectroscopy (SERS), uses plasmonic metallic nanoparticles such as Au and Ag as substrates to enhance traditionally weak vibrational peaks. Funing et al. [17] applied SERS to differentiate between healthy and *P. falciparum*-infected RBCs. Ag nanorod arrays were used for the SERS effect and direct detection of the parasite was confirmed *via* SERS spectra. The ring stage characteristic peak was at 1599 cm^{-1}, while trophozoite and schizoid stages had the same peak and an additional stretching vibration peak at 723 cm^{-1}. Thus, the Ag-based SERS platform effectively detected *P. falciparum* from three stages: ring, trophozoite and schizoid.

Mhlanga et al. [18] also explored the SERS platform for the detection and quantification of *P. falciparum*. A labelled SERS detection system that mimics the ELISA sandwich was used and it entailed the following elements: a solid SERS substrate alloyed with plasmonic Ag and Au, a capture P. *falciparum* antibody immobilised on the solid substrate and detection SERS probe conjugate. The detection conjugate was a plasmonic nanoparticle (Au/Ag), conjugated to a SERS tag/label and a detection antibody. The system was tested on the P. *falciparum* antigen and WHO malaria non-infectious blood specimens with varying levels of parasite density. The SERS immunoassays are investigated to be coupled with RDTs [19, 20] and lab-on-chip [21], in preparation for field-based application readiness.

Khoshmanesh et al. [22] explored optical attenuated total reflectance Fourier transform infrared spectroscopy for detection and quantification of the malaria parasite ring and gametocyte forms. A detection limit of 0.00001% parasitemia (1 parasite µL of blood; p 0.008) was reported.

Machine learning algorithms are also the future of spectroscopic malaria detection. Although their application is still in its infancy, it will solve a lot of challenges. Machine learning algorithms could improve SERS data processing for example through calibration multicomponent samples and the identification of interferences in complex biochemical samples, identifying SERS hotspots and analysing complex SERS spectra [23]. Irreproducibility of the SERS substrate is the bottleneck for their commercialisation or clinical application. Artificial intelligence algorithms are envisioned to mitigate this challenge and yield reproducibility and ultimately commercialization.

Nanotechnology is also a platform envisaged to revolutionise diagnostics and alleviate some of the challenges. For instance, the SERS prototype suffers from a lack of reproducibility. Expansion of SERS substrates from traditional plasmonic nanoparticles to two-dimensional graphitic nanostructures has the potential to mitigate irreproducibility and attain uniformity of the SERS hotspots.

Mwanga et al. [24] mobilised both experimental FTIR and machine learning algorithms to differentiate malaria positive and negative filter papers containing dried blood spots (DBS). For machine learning, the algorithm was trained using a PCR data set of 296 patients with 123 positive results and 173 negative PCR results. The trained model was evaluated *via P. falciparum* detection on the DBS. The logistic regression yielded 92% accuracy on *P. falciparum* and 85% on mixed strains.

4. Nuclei-based malaria diagnostics

The nuclei-acid amplification-based test (NAATs) application in malaria detection surges in high-resourced, clinical care regions. The resourced regions use NAATs in epidemiological studies, and in clinical trials for malaria treatment and vaccine, as a reference standard in the evaluation of malaria diagnostics and general malaria disease management [25]. NAATs in diagnostics offer several advantages: enhanced sensitivity (1–20 parasite/μl), multiplexing potential, parasite quantification, species differentiation and early detection of the parasite [25, 26]. NAATs excellent sensitivity, especially for low parasite density, surpasses those of the gold standards, microscopy and RDTs, although WHO still recommends parasite-based tests for resource-constrained regions due to affordability [25].

4.1 Polymerase chain reaction (PCR) diagnostics

PCR is focused on the amplification of a small quantity of DNA, into manageable and detectable quantities. Performed over three steps, in multiples of 20–40, DNA or RNA is replicated to millions of copies. The steps involve the initial denaturation of the double-stranded DNA at temperatures around 90–96°C, annealing of primers (one each for the 3′ and 5′ ends), specific to the DNA sequence to be replicated, at reduced temperatures of around 50–65°C and the final elongation/extension to complete the DNA strand. The elongation is performed by specialised, high-temperature functioning DNA polymerase. The most commonly used polymerase is extracted from *Thermus aquaticus* (Taq), with optimum elongation performed at 72°C [27–31].

Although highly sensitive and specific, PCR is seldom used for malaria detection in endemic areas due to its high cost and need for skilled personnel. This makes it impractical for use in remote or rural settings [24]. PCR is also able to detect low parasitemia values, undetectable through other methods, and can identify the different species. In addition, real-time PCR can quantify and track infection load [24]. Due to the sensitive nature of PCR, non-invasive testing in other bodily fluids, such as sweat, urine, saliva and faeces, has become possible [24].

Homann et al. [32] used the 18S rRNA gene for quantitative PCR (qPCR) towards tracking traveller infections over 12 months. In addition, they employed nested PCR towards the genotype of the *msp2* gene of *P. falciparum*. They found a limit of detection of 0.12 and 5 parasites/μl for the qPCR and nested PCR, respectively. Qualitative PCR allows for the quantification of a PCR product, usually through the use of a dye or fluorophore attached to a common piece of DNA sequence. Nested PCR employs two sets of primers, with the first set producing the product to be amplified by the second set of primers. This has greatly improved the sensitivity of PCR [33].

In addition, the use of multiple primers, for various targets, in the form of multiplex PCR, has allowed for the simultaneous amplification of a variety of target DNA strands, making the process quicker, but also allowing for the detection of various species of a *Plasmodium* for example [34]. Allowing this technique is the preference for the diagnosis of multiple malaria species within a single sample [33]. Fitri et al. [33] summarised some of the primers used in nested, semi-nested, hemi-nested, multiplex PCR and LAMP towards the detection of various *Plasmodium* species.

Costa et al. [35] developed a droplet digital PCR (ddPCR) method for the detection of malaria DNA in saliva. They employed a similar technique to qPCR, using the same probes and primers and a droplet generator. When compared with other sample types (blood and mouth swabs), the ddPCR showed a sensitivity of 73% for saliva samples and 99 and 59% for blood and swabs, respectively. Although these results show promise, the authors warn that this might be misleading due to the small number of DNA samples tested.

4.2 Loop-mediated isothermal amplification

Loop-mediated isothermal amplification (LAMP) is a variant of NAATs that proffers simplicity and rapidity as opposed to PCR [26]. It uses the *Plasmodium* species DNA from blood samples to diagnose malaria. The LAMP DNA amplification set-up uses four primers: inner (forward and backward), forward and backward outer primers that bind on six unique sequences on the target sense and antisense strands. The reaction can be catalysed by additional primers, looping forward and backward [36]. A loopam™ malaria Pan/pf kit pioneered in Europe, Uganda and Zanzibar showed higher sensitivity to infections compared with PCR. Although the loopam™ malaria Pan/pf is simple and user-friendly in addition to enhanced sensitivity, it is currently expensive and not as simple as RDTs [37].

LAMP can potentially be extended to field testing because its reagents are stable at 25 and 37°C [26]. For field applications, LAMP is coupled with other diagnostic platforms such as lab-on-a-chip. Safavich et al. [38] comprehensively reviewed the techniques towards the development of LAMP-microchip/microdevice.

5. Malaria rapid diagnostic testing

To decrease the burden on traditional diagnostic techniques, the use of rapid diagnostic tests (RDTs) for the detection of Malaria (predominantly *P. falciparum*) has become increasingly popular. Its popularity stems from its ease of use, short turnaround time and no need for electricity or specialised equipment [39].

Most RDTs function on the same base, where malaria antigen is detected in a blood sample that flows through a membrane, to be captured by specific anti-malaria antibodies [39], depicted by coloured lines on the membrane surface [40]. These products mainly target *P.falciparum*-specific proteins, such as lactase dehydrogenase (LDH), aldolase or histidine-rich protein II (HRP-II) [39]. The *pHRP-II* protein is specific towards the detection of *P. falciparum*, while the pLDH and *Plasmodium* aldolase are found in all species [40].

Histidine-rich protein II of *P. falciparum* is water-soluble and produced by *P.falciparum* gametocytes and the asexual stages. It is expressed on the membrane surface of red blood cells and remains in the blood after the treatment onset. *Plasmodium* aldolase is an enzyme expressed during the parasite glycolytic pathway of the blood stages of *P. falciparum* and non-falciparum malaria parasites. Monoclonal antibodies produced against *P. aldolase* are pan-specific. They have been used in conjunction with *pfHRP-II*, for the detection of pan malarial antigen (PMA) in combined immunochromatographic assays [41].

The soluble, glycolytic parasite lactate dehydrogenase enzyme (pLDH) is produced by both sexual and asexual stages of the living parasite. The enzyme is present and gets released from the erythrocytes infected by the parasite. The enzyme is present in all four species of human malaria, with different pLDH isomers for each [41].

Although various reports have mentioned the excellent performance of these RDTs, reports of large variation in sensitivity and reliability in malaria-endemic countries have led to guidelines developed by the WHO for establishing lot-to-lot quality control measures [39]. Although this rapid diagnostic tool seems to be of great use to the healthcare worker, it still relies on other methods for disease confirmation, infection characterisation and treatment monitoring [39].

As RDTs are immune-chromatographic lateral flow antigen-detection tests, they rely on capturing antibodies labelled with a dye to visualise the detection and control lines on a nitrocellulose membrane encased in a plastic casing, cassette. For the detection of malaria, the dye-labelled antibodies detect the *Plasmodium* antigen in the testing sample. The formed complex is captured by a secondary antibody immobilised on the membrane, resulting in a visible test line. The control line confirms the dye-labelled antibody's integrity, although not its ability to detect the parasitic antigen [42].

The test is usually conducted from a finger prick with only around 5–15 μl of blood and a total test time of only 5–20 min. As HRP II persists for up to 30 days post-eradication of parasitic infection, it is not suggested for monitoring disease progression. Disease progression is best monitored by pLDH or aldolase that is eliminated quickly, although plasmodial gametocytes also produce pLDH that may result in false positives [43, 44].

As the pHRP-II protein detects *P. falciparum*, pLDH specifically detects either *P. falciparum* or *P. vivax* or is pan-specific (common to all species). *P. aldolase* is pan-specific. The development of an RDT with all these variants allows for the detection of only *P. falciparum*, only *P. vivax* or any combination [45].

The RDTs do have various diagnostic limitations: 1) the before mentioned proteins cannot distinguish or detect *P. ovale*, *P. malariae* or *Pheidole knowlesi*, 2) some *P. falciparum* species (South America) do not produce the common HRP-II proteins, excluding the use of RDTs based on these proteins in those areas, 3) assays containing *P. falciparum HRP-II* (*pfHRP-II*) proteins, but not pHRP-II, show cross-reactivity with *Schistosoma mekongi* infections, 4) rheumatoid factor and other circulating auto-antibodies can cross-react with some assays, 5) high parasitemia for *P. falciparum* could give false-positive results for a *pHRP-II* assay meant to detect *P. vivax*, 6) the RDTs cannot determine parasitemia magnitude, while microscopy can, and 7) as *HRP-II* is not cleared from the blood, it cannot be used to monitor therapy effectiveness [45]. A list of the commercially available RDTs is available from The Global Fund [46].

To combat these limitations, various groups are working towards the inclusion of nanomaterials into the RDTs. Here, the nanomaterials with tuneable size, shape and plasmonics increase the selectivity and sensitivity of these point-of-care devices. The incorporation of metallic gold, silver, copper and platinum-palladium nanoparticles, as well as magnetic iron oxide, silica, ceria nanoparticles and luminescent quantum dots, is summarised by Nishat et al. [47]. Au nanoparticles (40 nm) were coupled with *pfHRP-II* towards the development of a biosensor for malaria detection.

In another study, Ag nanoparticles were catalysed by Au nanoparticles to enhance *HRP-II* detection [47].

As previously mentioned, the paramagnetic nanoparticle, Hemozoin, is a by-product and biomarker for the malaria parasite, similar chemically and structurally to β-hematin. As hemozoin is more stable, available and cheaper than *pfHRP-II*, it is recommended for use in the RDT development [48].

An ideal RDT should be able to detect a minimum of 100 parasites/μL. Armani et al. [49] utilised β-hematin and reported a limit of detection at <8.1 ng/mL in 500 μL blood (26 parasites/μL) [48]. Electrochemical sensors employing β-hematin incorporated CuO, Fe_2O_3 and Al_2O_3 nanoparticles. The catalytic activity with Au electrodes was shown, with CuO affording consistently low levels of detection (0.83 μg/mL) [48]. As mentioned by Noah et al., biosensors have seen little attention, with vast potential in not only detecting malaria parasites but also quantifying parasitemia, allowing for infection tracking [48].

Ditombi et al. [50] compared four RDTs for malaria and found that all RDTs had a sensitivity >95%, with only two tests showing specificity above 85%. With the inclusion of the WHO Methods Manual for product testing of malaria rapid diagnostic tests [51], the quality and trust in RDTs improved. Aidoo et al. [52] reported an increase in the RDT testing rate for malaria from 36 (2010) to 84% (2018) in sub-Saharan Africa, with an increase from 100 million supplied malaria RDTs in 2010 to 348 million in 2019. RDTs have also allowed for increased availability of testing for malaria in remote and rural areas [52].

Feleke et al. [53] conducted an immense study on the mutation of *P. falciparum* to evade detection by *pfHRP-II* RDTs. They found that 28.9% of the samples, positive

	Microscopy	**RDT**	**PCR**
Principle technique	Morphological interpretation	Antibody and antigen-binding	Amplification of DNA
Target diagnostic	All parasite stages (early trophozoite, mature trophozoite, schizont and gametocyte)	*Pf*-HRP-II, *Pf*-pLDH, pan-p-LDH, aldolase and *Pf*-GAPDH	rRNA/ssrRNA small subunits, SCIAvar gene
Sensitivity	≥5 parasites/μl (Expert), 50–100 parasites/μl (Average)	50–250 parasites/μl	< 5 parasites/μl
Specificity	High (difficult to diagnose *Pheidole knowlesi* from single and mixed infection)	Moderate (Can only identify *P. falciparum* and *P. vivax*	High, specie differentiation and identification
Time consumption	≤ 60 minutes	10–20 minutes	2–8 hours
Interpretation	Quantitative	Qualitative	Qualitative and quantitative
Advantages	Direct cost is low, and samples can be stored	Fast, simple, applicable and practical	Requires a tiny sample
Disadvantages	Specialised equipment, well-trained staff	Expensive, cannot perform drug monitoring	Large cost towards supplies, machinery and staff training

Table 1.
Comparison of diagnostic methods for Plasmodium species: microscopy, PCR and RDTs [33].

for *P. falciparum*, had discordant profiles within the RDT. This links to a pfHRP2/3 deletion for *P. falciparum*, making them only detectable through LDH-based RDTs.

6. Conclusion

Malaria remains problematic for both endemic and non-endemic WHO regions. Non-endemics regions due to globalisation and travelling are at risk of importing malaria cases. Malaria disease management is mandatory in the endemic regions and include efficient diagnostics and treatment. The detection assays for malaria should inherently be affordable, rapid, specific, sensitive and simple for low-resourced regions. **Table 1** comprehensively compares the available malaria detection platforms: microscopy, RDTs and PCR. PCR remains superior in its ability to detect sub-5 μL parasite values, with differentiation between all known *Plasmodium* species. It takes longer than microscopy, where 5 μL parasitemia can still be detected by advanced microscopists, but both still require highly skilled personnel and laboratory equipment. Currently, RDT, although with low sensitivity, remains a better option for low-resourced regions merited by detection limit at least 10x higher than microscopy and PCR, and simplicity and POCT usability without specialised equipment [33]. Artificial intelligence, nanotechnology and multimodal systems are envisioned to transform malaria diagnostics, especially in the mitigation of challenges associated with the different diagnostics.

Acknowledgements

Authors acknowledge the Department of Science and Innovation, South Africa and Mintek for funding.

Author details

Nikiwe Mhlanga[1*] and Hendriëtte Van der Walt[1,2]

1 DSI/Mintek Nanotechnology Innovation Centre, Randburg, South Africa

2 Life Sciences Department, UNISA, Roodepoort, South Africa

*Address all correspondence to: nikiwem@mintek.co.za

References

[1] World Health Organisation. World Malaria Report. Geneva: World Health Organisation; 2021. p. 2021

[2] Baptista V, Costa MS, Calçada C, Silva M, Gil JP, Veiga MI, et al. The future in sensing technologies for malaria surveillance: A review of hemozoin-based diagnosis. ACS Sensors. 2021;**6**(11):3898-3911

[3] Centre for controlled disease control and prevention, when malaria occurs. 2020. Available from: https://www.cdc.gov/malaria/about/distribution.html [Accessed: 10 July 2022]

[4] Kasetsirikul S, Buranapong J, Srituravanich W, Kaewthamasorn M, Pimpin A. The development of malaria diagnostic techniques: A review of the approaches with focus on dielectrophoretic and magnetophoretic methods. Malaria Journal. 2016;**15**(1):1-14

[5] Hauck TS, Giri S, Gao Y, Chan WC. Nanotechnology diagnostics for infectious diseases prevalent in developing countries. Advanced Drug Delivery Reviews. 2010;**62**(4-5):438-448

[6] Varela-Aramburu S, Ghosh C, Goerdeler F, Priegue P, Moscovitz O, Seeberger PH. Targeting and inhibiting *Plasmodium falciparum* using ultra-small gold nanoparticles. ACS Applied Materials & Interfaces. 2020;**12**(39):43380-43387

[7] Poostchi M, Silamut K, Maude RJ, Jaeger S, Thoma G. Image analysis and machine learning for detecting malaria. Translational Research. 2018;**194**:36-55

[8] Yoon J, Jang WS, Nam J, Mihn D-C, Lim CS. An automated microscopic malaria parasite detection system using digital image analysis. Diagnostics. 2021;**11**(3):527

[9] Microbe online, thick and thin blood smear for malaria diagnosis. 2021. Available from: https://microbeonline.com/microscopic-diagnosis-of-malaria/ [Accessed: 10 July 2022]

[10] Pollak JJ, Houri-Yafin A, Salpeter SJ. Computer vision malaria diagnostic systems—Progress and prospects. Frontiers in Public Health. 2017;**5**:219

[11] Fuhad KF, Tuba JF, Sarker MRA, Momen S, Mohammed N, Rahman T. Deep learning based automatic malaria parasite detection from blood smear and its smartphone based application. Diagnostics. 2020;**10**(5):329

[12] Hasan M, Islam S, Dey A, Das A, Tista SC. Detection of malaria disease using image processing and machine learning. In: International Conference on Intelligent Computing & Optimization. Thailand: Springer; 2021

[13] Cybulski JS, Clements J, Prakash M. Foldscope: Origami-based paper microscope. PLoS One. 2014;**9**(6):e98781

[14] Pirnstill CW, Coté GL. Malaria diagnosis using a mobile phone polarized microscope. Scientific Reports. 2015;**5**(1):1-13

[15] Adegoke JA, De Paoli A, Afara IO, Kochan K, Creek DJ, Heraud P, et al. Ultraviolet/visible and near-infrared dual spectroscopic method for detection and quantification of low-level malaria Parasitemia in whole blood. Analytical Chemistry. 2021;**93**(39):13302-13310

[16] Richards O, Jenkins C, Griffiths H, Paczkowska E, Dunstan PR, Jones S, et al.

Vibrational spectroscopy: A valuable screening and diagnostic tool for obstetric disorders? Frontiers in Global Women's Health. 2021;**1**:610582

[17] Chen F, Flaherty BR, Cohen CE, Peterson DS, Zhao Y. Direct detection of malaria infected red blood cells by surface enhanced Raman spectroscopy. Nanomedicine: Nanotechnology, Biology and Medicine. 2016;**12**(6):1445-1451

[18] Mhlanga N, Domfe T, Skepu A, Ntho TA. Sandwich-based surface-enhanced Raman scattering probes for detection and quantification of malaria. Journal of Raman Spectroscopy. 2020;**51**(12):2416-2424

[19] Yadav S, Sadique MA, Ranjan P, Kumar N, Singhal A, Srivastava AK, et al. SERS based lateral flow immunoassay for point-of-care detection of SARS-CoV-2 in clinical samples. ACS Applied Bio Materials. 2021;**4**(4):2974-2995

[20] Li G, Niu P, Ge S, Cao D, Sun A. SERS based lateral flow assay for rapid and ultrasensitive quantification of dual laryngeal squamous cell carcinoma-related miRNA biomarkers in human serum using Pd-Au core-shell nanorods and catalytic hairpin assembly. Frontiers in Molecular Biosciences. 2021;**8**:1354

[21] Ochoa-Vazquez G, Kharisov B, Arizmendi-Morquecho A, Cario A, Aymonier C, Marre S, et al. Microfluidics and surface-enhanced Raman spectroscopy: A perfect match for new analytical tools. IEEE Transactions on NanoBioscience. 2019;**18**(4):558-566

[22] Khoshmanesh A, Dixon MW, Kenny S, Tilley L, McNaughton D, Wood BR. Detection and quantification of early-stage malaria parasites in laboratory infected erythrocytes by attenuated total reflectance infrared spectroscopy and multivariate analysis. Analytical Chemistry. 2014;**86**(9):4379-4386

[23] Plou J, Valera PS, García I, de Albuquerque CD, Carracedo A, Liz-Marzán LM. Prospects of surface-enhanced Raman spectroscopy for biomarker monitoring toward precision medicine. ACS Photonics. 2022;**9**(2):333-350

[24] Mwanga EP, Minja EG, Mrimi E, Jiménez MG, Swai JK, Abbasi S, et al. Detection of malaria parasites in dried human blood spots using mid-infrared spectroscopy and logistic regression analysis. Malaria Journal. 2019;**18**(1):1-13

[25] Cunningham JA, Thomson RM, Murphy SC, de la, Paz Ade M, Ding XC, Incardona S, et al. WHO malaria nucleic acid amplification test external quality assessment scheme: Results of distribution programmes one to three. Malaria Journal. 2020;**19**(1):1-12

[26] Ocker R, Prompunjai Y, Chutipongvivate S, Karanis P. Malaria diagnosis by loop-mediated isothermal amplification (LAMP) in Thailand. Revista do Instituto de Medicina Tropical de São Paulo. 2016;**58**:1-6

[27] Rahalakshmi S. Different types of PCR techniques and its applications. International Journal of Pharmaceutical, Chemical and Biological Sciences. 2017;**7**(3):285-292

[28] Kralik P, Ricchi M. A basic guide to real time PCR in microbial diagnostics: Definitions, parameters, and everything. Frontiers in Microbiology. 2017;**8**:108

[29] Garibyan L, Avashia N. Research techniques made simple: Polymerase chain reaction (PCR). The Journal of Investigative Dermatology. 2013;**133**(3):e6

[30] Wages J Jr. Polymerase chain reaction. Encyclopedia of Analytical Science. 2005:243

[31] Khalil MI. Different types of PCR. Global Scientific Journals. 2021;**9**(2):758-768

[32] Vafa Homann M, Emami SN, Yman V, Stenstrom C, Sonden K, Ramstrom H, et al. Detection of malaria parasites after treatment in travelers: A 12-months longitudinal study and statistical modelling analysis. eBioMedicine. 2017;**25**:66-72

[33] Fitri LE, Widaningrum T, Endharti AT, Prabowo MH, Winaris N, Nugraha RYB. Malaria diagnostic update: From conventional to advanced method. Journal of Clinical Laboratory Analysis. 2022;**36**(4):e24314

[34] Dormond L, Jaton-Ogay K, de Valliere S, Genton B, Bille J, Greub G. Multiplex real-time PCR for the diagnosis of malaria: Correlation with microscopy. Clinical Microbiology and Infection. 2011;**17**(3):469-475

[35] Costa GL, Alvarenga DAM, Aguiar ACC, Louzada J, Pereira DB, de Oliveira TF, et al. Improving the molecular diagnosis of malaria: Droplet digital PCR-based method using saliva as a DNA source. Frontiers in Microbiology. 2022;**13**:882530

[36] Suea-Ngam A, Bezinge L, Mateescu B, Howes PD, deMello AJ, Richards DA. Enzyme-assisted nucleic acid detection for infectious disease diagnostics: Moving toward the point-of-care. ACS Sensors. 2020;**5**(9):2701-2723

[37] Cook J, Aydin-Schmidt B, González IJ, Bell D, Edlund E, Nassor MH, et al. Loop-mediated isothermal amplification (LAMP) for point-of-care detection of asymptomatic low-density malaria parasite carriers in Zanzibar. Malaria Journal. 2015;**14**(1):1-6

[38] Safavieh M, Kanakasabapathy MK, Tarlan F, Ahmed MU, Zourob M, Asghar W, et al. Emerging loop-mediated isothermal amplification-based microchip and microdevice technologies for nucleic acid detection. ACS Biomaterials Science & Engineering. 2016;**2**(3):278-294

[39] Tangpukdee N, Duangdee C, Wilairatana P, Krudsood S. Malaria diagnosis: A brief review. The Korean Journal of Parasitology. 2009;**47**(2):93-102

[40] Mbanefo A, Kumar N. Evaluation of malaria diagnostic methods as a key for successful control and elimination programs. Tropical Medicine and Infectious Diseases. 2020;**5**(2):1-15

[41] Kakkilaya BS. Rapid diagnosis of malaria. Laboratory Medicine. 2003;**8**(34):602-608

[42] Kitutu FE, Wamani H, Selling KE, Katabazi FA, Kuteesa RB, Peterson S, et al. Can malaria rapid diagnostic tests by drug sellers under field conditions classify children 5 years old or less with or without plasmodium falciparum malaria? Comparison with nested PCR analysis. Malaria Journal. 2018;**17**(1):1-12

[43] Mukkala AN, Kwan J, Lau R, Harris D, Kain D, Boggild AK. An update on malaria rapid diagnostic tests. Current Infectious Disease Reports. 2018;**20**(12):1-8

[44] Wongsrichanalai C, Barcus MJ, Muth S, Sutamihardja A, Wernsdorfer WH. A review of malaria diagnostic tools: Microscopy and rapid diagnostic test (RDT). Defining and Defeating the Intolerable Burden of Malaria III: Progress and Perspectives: Supplement

to Volume 77 (6) of American Journal of Tropical Medicine and Hygiene. 2007:1-23

[45] Wilson ML. Malaria rapid diagnostic tests. Clinical Infectious Diseases. 2012;**54**(11):1637-1641

[46] The global fund, list of rapid diagnostics test (RDT) kits for malaria classified according to the Global Fund Quality Assurance Policy. 2022. pp. 1-13. Available from: https://www.theglobalfund.org/media/5891/psm_qadiagnosticsmalaria_list_en.pdf

[47] Nishat S, Awan FR, Bajwa SZ. Nanoparticle-based point of care immunoassays for in vitro biomedical diagnostics. Analytical Sciences. 2018:18R001

[48] Noah NM, Ndangili PM. Current trends of nanobiosensors for point-of-care diagnostics. Journal of Analytical Methods in Chemistry. 2019;**2019**:2179718

[49] Armani A, Chen D, McBirney S, Kaypaghian K, Huber H, Ameri H. Portable optical diagnostics for early malaria detection. In: Frontiers in Biological Detection: From Nanosensors to Systems XI. United States: SPIE; 2019

[50] Ditombi BCM, Minko JI, Tsamba RP, Ngomo JMN, Nymane T, Ognagosso FBB, et al. Comparative performance of four malaria rapid diagnostic tests, Vikia malaria pf/pan, Meriline-Meriscreen Pf/Pv/Pan, right sign malaria Pf/Pan, and right sign malaria Pf, among febrile patients in Gabon. Revista da Sociedade Brasileira de Medicina Tropical. 2020;**53**:e20190274

[51] World Health Organization. Methods manual for product testing of malaria rapid diagnostic tests. In: Manual of Standard Operating Procedures for Assessment of Malaria Rapid Diagnostic Tests within the Product Testing Programme of WHO Version 1. Geneva: World Health Organization; 2008

[52] Aidoo M, Incardona S. Ten years of universal testing: How the rapid diagnostic test became a game changer for malaria case management and improved disease reporting. The American Journal of Tropical Medicine and Hygiene. 2021;**106**(1):29-32

[53] Feleke SM, Reichert EN, Mohammed H, Brhane BG, Mekete K, Mamo H, et al. Plasmodium falciparum is evolving to escape malaria rapid diagnostic tests in Ethiopia. Nature Microbiology. 2021;**6**(10):1289-1299

Section 3

Pathophysiology and Clinics of Malaria

Chapter 3

Pathology of Malaria

Pier Paolo Piccaluga and Wanyonyi Ignatius

Abstract

Malaria is an acute febrile illness that is caused by infection with *Plasmodium spp*. parasites. Malaria is a serious illness and sometimes it may be fatal resulting in mortality and morbidity. The clinical picture painted in patients with malarial infection occurs following the release of the merozoites into the bloodstream following the rupture of infected red cells. In the infection with the *P. falciparum*, the commonest form affecting humans, all stages of red cells are infected making the infection quite severe as compared to infection with other species which infects the old and young red cells only which contributes to a small percentage of red cells. In this chapter, the Authors review the current knowledge about Malaria epidemiology, pathogenesis and anatomic pathology. The diverse clinical pictures as well as the association with genetic conditions and diseases are discussed.

Keywords: malaria, plasmodium malariae, pathology, histology, gross and microscopic pathology, cerabral malaria, pathogenesis

1. Introduction

Malaria is an acute febrile illness that is caused by infection with *Plasmodium spp*. parasites. Malaria is a serious illness and sometimes it may be fatal resulting in mortality and morbidity.

There were an estimated 241 million malarial cases in 2020 higher than malarial cases in 2019 (227 million cases), a difference of 14 million cases. The rise in malarial cases is thought to be associated with the COVID-19 pandemic, that led to service disruption. The case incidence of malaria from 2000 has declined from 81 per 1000 populations at risk to 56 per 1000 populations at risk. However, in 2020 the case incidence has increased to 59 per 1000 populations at risk. Globally, death due to malaria in 2020 is reported at 627000 which is a rise as compared to the trends in malaria death that has a seen a drop from 896,000 cases in 2000 to 558,000 cases in 2019. It is estimated that 68% (47,000 cases) of the additional deaths due to Malaria are attributed to disruption of services following COVID-19 pandemic. Globally, the malaria mortality rate as of 2020 is 15 per 100,000 population at risk which is higher compared to 2019 which was 14 per 100,000 population at risk. Among children under 5 years, the mortality rate in 2020 increased to 77% as compared to 76% in 2019. Globally, 96% of the malaria cases and deaths were from 29 out of 85 countries with malaria-endemic. Nigeria (26.8%), the Democratic Republic of Congo (12.0%), Uganda (5.4%), Mozambique (4.2%), Angola (3.4%), and Burkina Faso (3.4%) account for 55% of the cases globally. Half of the mortality cases were from

Nigeria (31.9%), the Democratic Republic of Congo (13.2%), The United Republic of Tanzania (4.1%), and Mozambique (3.8%). The WHO African region accounts for 95% of the malarial cases and 96% of the malarial deaths. In the African region, 80% of the cases are among children under 5 years. In Africa, the number of malaria cases in 2020 is 233 per 1000 populations at risk higher than in 2019 at cases per 1000 population cases. The South-east Asia region accounts for 2% of the malaria cases globally among the nine malaria-endemic countries in 2020. India accounts for 83% of malaria cases due to infection by *Plasmodium vivax*. The WHO Eastern Mediterranean Region accounted for 5.7 million cases in 2020 with the increase seen in Sudan, Somalia, and Djibouti. *P. vivax* accounted for about 18% of the cases mainly in Afghanistan and Pakistan. In WHO western Pacific region contributed to 1.7 million cases with an increase of 19% from 2019 cases. The malaria death increased to 3200 death in 2020 as compared to 2600 in 2019. WHO region of Americas registered a reduction in the case incidences by 58% between 2000 and 2020 with a resultant reduction in malaria death by 56% since 2000. Most of the cases in this region were due to *P. vivax*. In WHO European region, there has been free of malaria cases since 2015 with the last case reported in 2014 in Tajikistan with no malaria death from 2000 to 2020.

There are attempts globally to eliminate malaria in different countries. According to WHO a country is declared malaria-free following at least 3 consecutive years with zero indigenous cases. Islamic Republic of Iran and Malaysia reported zero indigenous malaria cases for the third consecutive year and while Belize and Cabo Verde for the second consecutive time. China and El Salvador were certified malaria-free in 2021 following 4 years of zero malaria cases [1].

1.1 Plasmodium

Plasmodium was first described in the late nineteenth century by Charles Laveran and over time, many species have been discovered. Plasmodium is a unicellular eukaryote that cannot survive outside the host (obligate parasite). The parasite affects different hosts such as reptiles, birds, and mammals and it requires an insect host of the genera Culex and Anopheles. In humans, *P. vivax, Plasmodium falciparum, P. malariae, P. ovale* and *Plasmodium knowlesi* are the most common species affecting humans. *P. falciparum* is the most lethal infection in humans resulting in thousands of deaths.

1.2 Lifecycle of palsmodium

The life cycle of plasmodium involves distinct stages in the mosquito and vertebrate host. The life cycle can be divided into the sexual phase that occurs in the insect and the asexual phase while inside the vertebrate host.

Upon taking the blood meal, the female anopheles mosquito releases the sporozoites into the bloodstream of an individual. The sporozoites enter the circulation and they attach and enter the hepatocytes through receptors for serum proteins thrombospondin and properdin. In the hepatocytes, sporozoites mature into schizonts. Schizonts are the multinucleated staged cells that form during asexual reproduction. The schizonts in the hepatocytes mature and enlarge which causes the hepatocytes to rupture and release thousands of merozoites into the circulation. For *P. vivax* and *P. ovale*, some schizonts remain in liver cells in the dormant stage called hypnozoites that are responsible for relapses by invading the bloodstream weeks or years later. Upon release of the merozoites into the bloodstream, they invade the erythrocytes for the formation of erythrocytic schizogony. The merozoites bind to sialic acid residue on the glycophorin molecule on the surface of the red cells and enter through active membrane penetration aided by a lectin-like molecule. The merozoites undergo asexual multiplication in the infected red cells to form trophozoites characterized by a single chromatin mass. The trophozoite develops into ring-shaped trophozoites and later on forms schizonts with multiple chromatin masses. Some trophozoites differentiate forming male and female gametocytes. The infected red cells rupture to release the merozoites into the bloodstream alongside the products of the red cells that are responsible for some of the clinical presentation. The female anopheles mosquito as it feeds on human blood to nourish its eggs, it ingests the merozoites and gametocytes from the infected host. The male and female gametocytes in the mosquito are known as the sporogonic cycle. In the mosquito stomach, the male and female gametocytes (microgamete and macrogametes) form the zygote. The zygote after some time becomes motile and elongated forming ookinetes. The ookinetes invade the midgut wall of the mosquito to transform it into an oocyst. The oocyst grows over time and ruptures to release sporozoites which migrate into the salivary gland awaiting inoculation into the new host following a blood meal.

2. Malaria pathogenesis and pathophysiology

The clinical picture painted in patients with malarial infection occurs following the release of the merozoites into the bloodstream following the rupture of infected red cells. The malaria parasite has a wide variety of symptoms which ranges from absent or very mild symptoms to severe cases and even death. Owing to this the infection is categorized into uncomplicated malaria and severe malaria. The incubation period varies depending on the individual factors and the species of plasmodium. The incubation period is the period of the introduction of the sporozoites to the development of the first symptoms. The incubation period varies from 7 to 30 days. However, *P. falciparum* has a short incubation period while *P. malariae* has a longer period.

The release of the merozoites from the rupture of the liver cells infects the red cells. In the infection with the *P. falciparum*, all stages of red cells are infected making the infection quite severe as compared to infection with other species which infects the old and young red cells only which contributes to a small percentage of red cells. The malarial parasites while in the red blood cells derive their energy primarily from the red cells. They can metabolize 70 times faster as compared to the red cells resulting in hypoglycemia and lactic acidosis. The rupture of the infected red cells releases the merozoites alongside the waste and toxic substances from the red cells. The released merozoites infect other healthy red cells in the circulation. Since the infected red cells are destroyed, and red cells are destroyed every time the merozoites infect new red cells, the patient experiences intravascular hemolysis. Intravascular hemolysis results in worsening anemia requiring immediate treatment and transfusion in a patient with very low hemoglobin levels (<5 g/dL). The intravascular hemolysis results in the production of hemoglobin that causes the urine to change and appear as dark colored in the patient. The intravascular hemolysis also causes an increased amount of yellow discoloration due to overloading the ability of the body to conjugate bilirubin causing jaundice on the sclera and mucous membrane and skin. The released products and toxic substances in ruptured red cells cause the body to release cytokines such as tumor necrosis factor (TNF) which contributes to fevers. An increase in body temperature results in sweating and chills. The merozoite surface antigen being foreign to the body as well evokes immune responses that lead to the production of the cytokines. These cytokines such as TNF, Interferon-gamma, and Interleukin-1 have the potential of suppressing the red blood cell production thus reducing the restoration of hemoglobin concentration, increasing fever, stimulating reactive nitrogen species production that causes tissue damage, and inducing endothelial receptor expression of *P. falciparum* erythrocyte membrane protein 1 (PfEMP1) which is responsible for sequestration. These cytokines as well irritate the vomiting centers resulting in the vomiting as part of clinical presentation.

The infected red cells appear sticky and adhered to the blood vessels causing obstruction of the blood flow and causing ischemia in the affected areas and organs. The sticky red cells as well clump together forming a rosette that if large enough have the potential to obstruct blood flow in major blood vessels. In addition, several proteins such as PfEMP1 contribute to the attachment of red cells on the endothelium leading to sequestration. The PfEMP1 bind to the endothelial cells through CD36, thrombospondin, VCAM1, ICAM1, and E-selectin. The sequestration of the red cells in the blood vessel endothelium and the ability of the body to take away damaged red cells mostly occur in the spleen contributing to splenomegaly in some patients. Sequestration of the red cells, and destruction of the red cells leading to anemia coupled with obstruction of blood flow results in the reduction of tissue perfusion causing fatigue, general body weakness, and ischemia.

2.1 *P. falciparum*

P. falciparum is responsible for most malarial cases, especially in the WHO African region. The parasite can infect red blood cells of all ages thus resulting in high parasitemia as compared to *P. ovale* and *P. vivax* which infect only young red cells. High parasitemia results in severe hemolysis that causes hemoglobinuria which has the potential of damaging the kidneys and causing renal failure worsening the prognosis. Infection with *P. falciparum* has the specific property of sequestration. The organisms exhibit adherence properties that result in sequestration of the parasites in small post-capillary vessels. Through sequestration of the parasite, the patient may develop an altered mental state and even a coma. Infection with *P. falciparum* is associated with a high burden of cytokines released by the body which in addition to high parasitemia resulting in end-organ failures. End organ disease specifically involves the central nervous system, lungs, and kidneys.

2.2 *P. vivax*

P. vivax infects the immature red blood cells only thus associated with limited parasitemia. However, due to the presence of hypnozoites in the liver lying dormant, 50% of the infected patients experience relapses within a few weeks to 5 years following the initial illness. The relapses decrease in periodicity and intensity over time.

2.3 *Plasmodium ovale*

P. ovale infects only the immature red cells and thus has limited parasitemia than *P. falciparum*. The infection is less severe as compared to *P. vivax* and often resolves without treatment. Due to the presence of hypnozoites in the liver, relapses may occur.

2.4 *Plasmodium malariae*

P. malariae species have a longer incubation period and therefore the patient may remain asymptomatic for a longer duration. Recrudescence is quite common in a patient infected with *P. malariae*. In addition, *P. malariae* is associated with the deposition of the antibody–antigen complexes on the glomeruli damaging the basement membrane to cause nephrotic syndrome.

2.5 *P. knowlesi*

The infection of *P. knowlesi* should be treated aggressively just as patients with *P. falciparum* as it causes fatal disease. It was identified in Malaysian Borneo, Thailand, Myanmar, Singapore, the Philippines, and neighboring countries.

3. Genetic factors and malaria

Genetic factors play a crucial role in influencing malaria infection. Two biological characteristics identified in protecting the certain type of malaria are sickle cell trait and negative for Duffy blood group [2].

Individuals with sickle cell traits are relatively protected from infection by *P. falciparum*. Sickle cell traits are individuals with heterozygous for abnormal hemoglobin gene S. The individuals have one copy of the abnormal hemoglobin gene HbS and a copy of normal hemoglobin gene HbA. *P. falciparum* cannot survive in the red cells with HbS conferring protection to individuals. The presence of sickle cell traits is mainly in areas with a high prevalence of *P. falciparum* in the WHO African region. According to the cohort study, the presence of the sickle cell trait confers 60% of the protection against overall mortality with the protection occurring between 2 and 16 months of life, before the development of the immunity.

People who are negative for the Duffy blood group have shown to be resistant to infection with *P. vivax*. The *P. vivax* infection is rare in West Africa because of the presence of Duffy-negative individuals that confer protection against the infection. *P. ovale* which can infect the Duffy negative red cells predominates in this setting.

Blood cell dyscrasias such as hemoglobin *C. thalassemia* and G6PD deficiency are prevalent in the malaria areas which confer protection against the infection.

4. Acquired immunity against malaria infection

Acquired immunity influences malaria infection in individuals and communities. Through repeated infection, an individual develops partially protective immunity. Despite the acquired immunity, the individuals may get infected by the malaria parasite but the severity of the illness will be less ad they may lack the typical symptoms. The acquired immunity allows the individual to mount the immune response to the presence of the parasite in the circulation leading to a reduction in the severity of the infection. The areas that have a high malarial infection such as *P. falciparum* in the south Saharan region in Africa have individuals with acquired immunity. The mother who has repeated infection with *P. falciparum* can confer protection to the newborn. While the newborn is in-utero, the maternal antibodies are transferred through the placenta to the fetus which confers protection to the newborn up to the first few months of life. After the reduction of the maternal antibodies in the circulation, the young children become susceptible to infection leading to an increase the infection. If the children survive the repeated infection to an older age of about 2–5 years, they attain acquired immunity. Owing to the acquired immunity in the areas of high transmission such as the WHO African region, there is increased mortality affecting the young population (90% of the mortalities were children in 2020 mortality cases) with less mortality affecting the adults. In areas where there is lower transmission such as Asia and Latin America, infection is minimal and few individuals are exposed to repeated infection. The individuals do not develop acquired immunity. Following the lack of acquired immunity, a larger proportion of the older children are as well affected by the epidemic of malaria infection.

5. Sickle cell disease and malaria

Despite the presence of sickle cell trait conferring protestation against malarial infection over the healthy population, the presence of sickle cell disease does not confer any protection. Sickle cell disease occurs when the individual has a mutation in both alleles resulting in homozygous HbS. Sickle cell disease carries the worst prognosis with infection by the malarial parasite, especially *P. falciparum*. The worst prognosis contributed to the reduced half-life of sickled red cells and increased ability to undergo sequestration. Coupled with hemolysis and reduced hemoglobin concentration among the sicklers, they easily undergo severe anemia and severe hypoxia which worsen sickling and obstruction of the blood vessel resulting in end-organ disease. Sickle cell disease does not tolerate infection with malaria infection requires immediate and aggressive management to improve the prognosis [2–4].

6. Clinical features of cerebral malaria

Cerebral malaria is the most severe neurological complication that arises following infection with *P. falciparum*. It is estimated that annually, 575,000 cases of children in the sub-Saharan region are affected by cerebral malaria. According to WHO, cerebral malaria refers to the clinical syndrome where there is coma at least 1 hour after termination of seizure or correction of hypoglycemia and presence of parasitemia for *P. falciparum* on the peripheral blood smear with other causes evident to causing coma. Loss of consciousness is the hallmark of cerebral malaria with coma being the most severe presentation. However, for a diagnosis of cerebral malaria to be made, the patient should have no other cause of coma such as viral encephalitis, metabolic disorder, and poisoning among others. Apart from the altered mental status, cerebral malaria may be followed by progressive weakness and prostration. In adults, cerebral malaria presents as one of the organ failures following end-organ disease with severe *P. falciparum* infection.

The development of cerebral malaria following infection with *P. falciparum* occurs in cases of high parasitemia. It is thought that infected red cells are sequestrated through the attachment on the endothelium that causes occlusion of the cerebral capillaries. This coupled with sequestration of the parasites cause reduction in blood circulation in the microvasculature resulting in a decreased supply of nutrients and oxygen. The obstruction of the blood flow shuts down energy production which is needed to maintain the blood–brain barrier. As a result, ischemia ensues and there is a neuronal alteration that causes cerebral swelling and increased the cerebral intracranial pressure. This leads to altered consciousness and retinal changes. The damage to the blood vessels as well leads to intracranial hemorrhage the leads to altered mental status. Cytokines and chemokine are also described as through a complex role in protecting and posing harmful effects in the pathogenesis of cerebral malaria. Schizogony triggers pro-inflammatory cytokines that may contribute to cerebral malaria while anti-inflammatory cytokine poses protective benefits. Unlike in bacterial and viral infections, altered mental status following *P. falciparum* infection does not result from the presence of the parasite in the brain parenchyma but due to cerebral occlusion that causes end ran tissue damage due to disruption of brain parenchyma.

Cerebral malaria is fatal and without treatment, the mortality rates increase exponentially. In children treated with intravenous antimalarial medication, the mortality is about 5–20%. However, despite the recovery, many children sustain significant brain injuries. About 11% have gross neurological deficits which may improve with time while 25% have long-term impairments, especially in cognition, motor, and behavior domain. About 10% develops epilepsy. The risk factors include seizures, deep and prolonged coma, intracranial hypertension, and hypoglycemia.

7. Congenital malaria

Congenital malaria refers to the infection with malaria parasite present in the peripheral smear of the newborn from 24 hours to 7 days of life. It is thought that the parasite can infect the placenta and gain access to fetal circulation. Congenital malaria is rare but it is fatal if not detected earlier in newborns. However, in areas where malaria is endemic, congenital malaria is rare as compared to other areas. This is because, in malaria-endemic areas, the maternal have had repeated attacks thus developing acquired immunity. The antibodies in the maternal circulation are therefore protected against the development of congenital malaria and protection in the early stages of life. The occurrence of congenital malaria is at 0.3% in the immune mothers and 7.4% in the non-immune mothers. The symptoms of congenital malaria occur within 10 to 30 days of life. They include fever, anemia, and splenomegaly in most cases. Other presentations may include hepatomegaly, jaundice, loose stool, and poor feeding among others. Since this presentation mimics most conditions in the neonates such as neonatal jaundice and neonatal sepsis, the diagnosis is often missed leading to mortality and morbidity [5, 6].

Congenital malaria is of concern among neonates. Given that the parasite is present in utero, the human body learns to recognize the parasite as self, contrary to the normal case where the parasite is considered an antigen to cause activation of immune responses. The parasite, therefore, can multiply and cause damage to red cells without evoking immune responses as in the case of a healthy individual. Therefore, the newborn experience excessive hemolysis and resultant organomegaly. Lack of the ability to recognize the parasite as an antigen coupled with an immature immune system allows the parasite to multiply necessitating immediate treatment to improve the outcome among the neonates. Owing to intravascular hemolysis, the neonates present with anemia and splenomegaly which are the most common forms of presentation. Intravenous antimalarial medication is essential in management [5, 6].

8. Gross and microscopic pathology

8.1 Bone marrow

P. falciparum infection demonstrates dyserythropoietic with iron sequestration and erythrophagocytosis, especially in the acute phase. The dysthrombopoeisis has large atypical megakaryocytes and giant platelets. The defect is present for up to 3 weeks after infection resolution.

8.2 Spleen

Splenic enlargement is one of the findings of all types of malaria. However, with *P. falciparum*, the spleen may not be palpable even though splenomegaly is one of the earliest signs of malaria. In the initial stage, grossly, the spleen enlarges, round and hard on palpation but tender. As the disease progresses, it becomes larger and harder but less tender. Splenic enlargement results from the engorgement of blood vessels initially, with oedema of the pulp in the initial cases. However, later there is lymphoid and reticuloendothelial hyperplasia and increased hemolytic and phagocytic function. Pulp sclerosis and dilated sinuses occur due to relapses. Splenic rupture occurs in some cases of malarial infection due to rapid and considerable enlargement, and it poses a serious complication, especially in primary malaria episodes. Splenic rupture has been found less likely in chronic splenomegaly due to fibrosis and peri splenitis.

Tropic splenomegaly syndrome is characterized by marked enlargement of the spleen with a spleen weighing 2–4.4 kgs. Usually seen among the adult population in Africa and India, presenting with a huge spleen. The spleen demonstrates marked hyperplasia of lymphoid with dilated sinuses. With splenomegaly, there is increased phagocytosis of red and white cells, and the patient has a picture of anemia, leucopenia and thrombocytopenia, though the general health is well maintained. There may be concomitant enlargement of the liver with lymphoreticular infiltration of sinusoids. The patients have high levels of IgG and M against malaria. However, the use of antimalarial medication reduces the splenic size [7, 8].

Treatment of malarial infection results in splenic regression, usually within weeks, but the duration may be protracted with large fibrotic spleen secondary to repeated malaria, though complete involution is common. The patient undergoing splenectomy has a risk of latent infection reactivation since the spleen plays a crucial role in the immune response against malaria.

8.3 Liver

In malarial infection, hepatomegaly also occurs in the early stages. The liver is enlarged, firm and tender. It may appear brown, gray or black following malaria pigment deposition. Microscopically, there is oedema and dilatation of hepatic sinusoids containing hypertrophied Kupffer cells and parasitized red cells. In severe malarial cases, shock and disseminated intravascular coagulation result in small areas of centrilobular necrosis. Prolonged infection results in stromal induration and diffuse proliferation of fibrous connective tissue, but changes of cirrhosis are absent [7, 8].

P. falciparum affects mesenchyma and hepatocytes, causing malarial hepatitis due to functional changes. Malarial hepatitis is characterized by conjugated hyperbilirubinemia, increased levels of transaminase and alkaline phosphatase. Severe infection with *P. falciparum* is due to hepatocellular damage due to impaired local microcirculation.

In repeated infection, there is significant hepatomegaly with associated splenomegaly, but no functional abnormality exists. Despite prolonged malarial infection having diffuse fibrous connective tissue proliferation, malaria is not a proven cause of liver cirrhosis.

8.4 Lungs

Acute pulmonary oedema may occur in a patient with *P. falciparum* infection, presenting as a rare but fatal complication. It occurs due to impairment in microcirculation, with capilarying showing endothelial lesions and perivascular oedema. The edematous endothelium results in the narrowing of the lumen. In addition, microscopically, pulmonary vascular, capillaries, and venule show diffuse inflammatory and parasitized red cells. Interstitial oedema and hyaline membrane formation may also be seen [7, 8].

8.5 Cardiovascular system

Cardiovascular functioning is deranged with malarial infection, especially during the paroxysmal episode. There is peripheral vasodilation causing decreased blood pressure and postural hypotension, tachycardia, transient systolic murmur, muffled heart sound and occasional cardiac dilatation. In the patient with pre-existing cardiac dysfunction, malarial infection aggravates the dysfunction leading to fatal cardiac failure. The microcirculation changes involve myocardial capillaries congestion with lymphocytes, plasma cells and parasitized red cells. Pigment-laden macrophages are also seen microscopically [7, 8].

8.6 Gastrointestinal system

Malaria may manifest with abdominal symptoms such as nausea, vomiting, anorexia, abdominal distension and epigastric pain in the acute phase. Nausea and vomiting are usually central in origin. In addition, the patient may have watery diarrhea, mimicking gastroenteritis or cholera. Some patients may experience severe abdominal colic mimicking appendicitis and acute abdomen.

P. falciparum infection results in impaired splanchnic microcirculation, causing bowel ischemia, necrosis and ulceration. In addition, there is mucosal oedema which hampers absorption. These changes may also lead to the absorption of toxins and precipitate septic shock [7, 8].

8.7 Kidneys

Kidneys may be affected during malarial infection. Acute diffuse malarial nephritis rarely occurs with patients exhibiting hypertension, oedema and albuminuria. However, albuminuria alone is common during an acute attack. *P. malariae* may lead to nephrotic syndrome, described as Quartan malaria nephropathy. It is an immune-mediated nephropathy characterized by oedema, hypertension and albuminuria, occurring weeks after infection [7, 8].

Severe disease with *P. falciparum* causes acute renal failure in 0.1–0.6% of the patients. Impairment in microcirculation associated with severe *P. falciparum* infection leads to anoxia, sebsequate glomeruli, and renal tubule necrosis. Disseminated intravascular coagulation may worsen acute renal failure.

8.8 Central nervous system

As mentioned, the CNS presentation is due to the dissemination of malarial parasites into the brain, paroxysmal fever and side effects of antimalarial drugs. The patient presents with headache, vomiting, delirium, anxiety and restlessness during fever paroxysms, with symptoms resolving once the fever normalizes. Chloroquine, quinine, mefloquine and halofantrine can lead to vertigo, restlessness, hallucinations, confusion, delirium, tinnitus, dizziness, convulsions and sometimes frank psychosis.

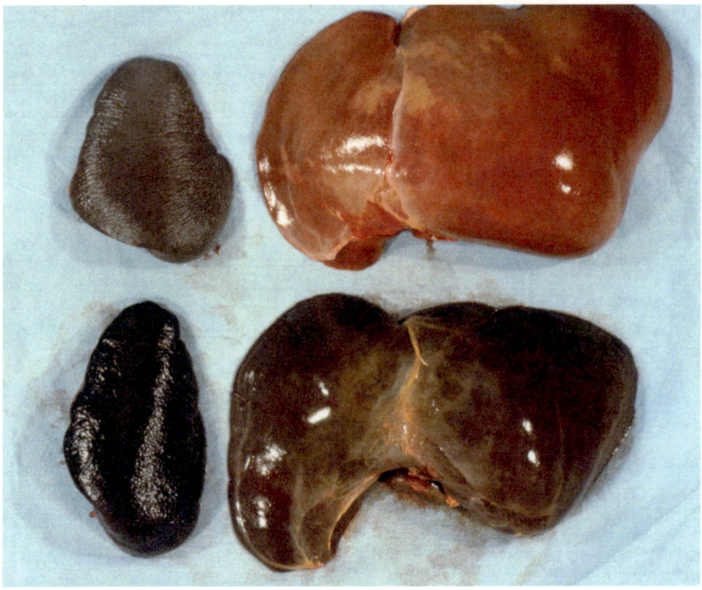

Figure 1.
Liver and Spleen Malaria. Gross pathology of the liver and spleen At the top of this picture are the spleen (left) and liver (right) from an autopsy of a child. They show a normal spleen and liver appearance. At the bottom of the picture are the spleen and liver from the autopsy of a child who died of malaria, which are a darker color than the normal organs. The dark color comes from extreme congestion and heavy deposition of haemozoin. (From: P. falciparum malaria: liver and spleen. Welcome Collection. CC0 1.0 Universal).

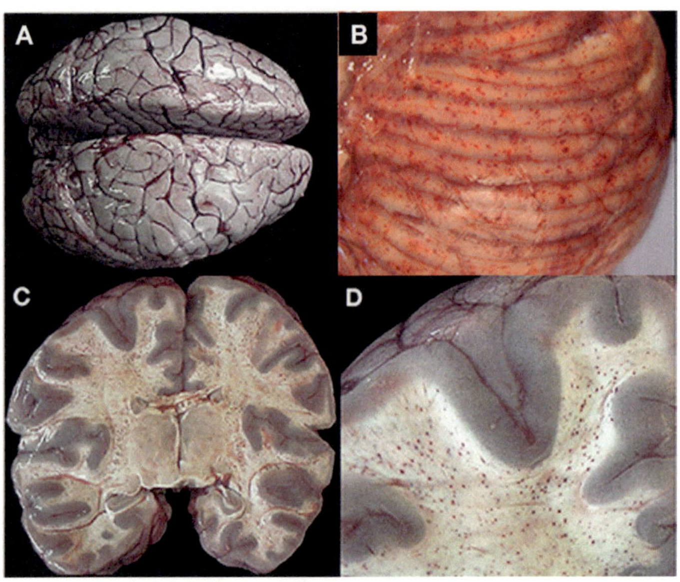

Figure 2.
Gross pathology of cerebral malaria. The vast majority of cases, regardless of diagnosis, showed brain swelling with flattened gyri and narrowed sulci (A). In this example, the brain has the classic "slate gray" to "purple" appearance of CM which is possibly due to malaria pigment within vessels (A). The cerebellum had petechial hemorrhages in both the gray and white matter and thus, visible on the surface grossly (B). In the classic CM2 appearance, petechial hemorrhages are seen diffusely in the white matter throughout the brain (C). A higher magnification demonstrates the abrupt transition from white to gray matter and the lack of hemorrhages in the gray (D). From Milner et al. [9].

Quinine is associated with hypoglycemic coma, while artemisinin cause brainstem dysfunction based on animal studies [7, 9].

P. falciparum in CNS causes cerebral hypoxia and anoxia through impairing microcirculation as the parasitized red cells have decreased deformability and increased cytoadherence, causing occlusion of microcirculation. Malarial encephalitis and meningoencephalitis arise due to cerebral anoxia, the development of malarial granulomas and punctate hemorrhages [9].

Macroscopically, the brain is usually edematous during the autopsy, appearing leaden or plum colored with a cut surface slatey gray hue. The sulci are narrowed, and the gyri flattened due to brain swelling. The small blood vessels are congested with parasitized red cells. Mature forms of parasites including schizonts are found in brain biopsies. The large vessels demonstrate evidence of margination, where the parasites are arranged in a layer along the endothelium. Despite this, the

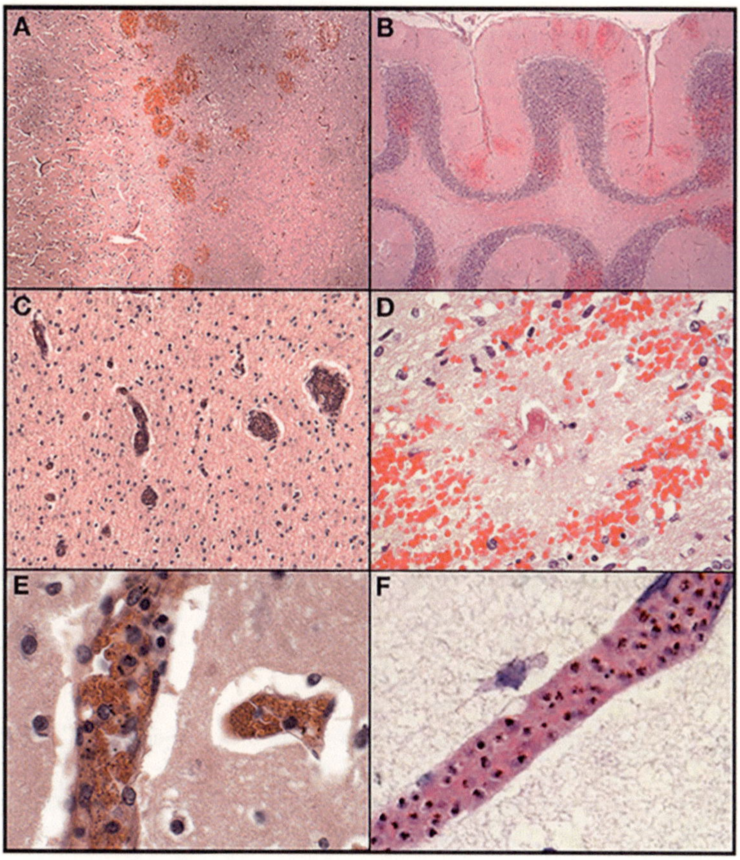

Figure 3.
Histological features of cerebral malaria. The abrupt transition from gray to white matter (A) and the presence of ring hemorrhages are demonstrated in this classic case of CM (CM2, 100X, H&E). The cerebellum (B) with ring hemorrhages in all levels including white and gray matter are shown (100x, H&E). Visibly congested blood vessels (C) even at low power may be the result of dense sequestration downstream; these vessels can contain both parasitized and uninfected red bloods (200X, H&E). The classic appearance of a ring hemorrhage with fibrin (D) is shown; these hemorrhages can also include pigmented parasites, free pigment, and admixed fibrin within the microvessel at the nexus of the lesion; uninfected erythrocytes constituting the surrounding hemorrhage are seen (400X, H&E). Two examples of sequestration showing predominantly early (less pigmented) parasites (E), and late stage (more pigmented) parasites (F) densely packing vessels (1000X, H&E). From Milner et al. [9].

endothelium also shows pseudopodial projections, which may be in close apposition to the knobs on the surface of parasitized red cells. There is numerous petechial hemorrhage proximal to the occlusive plug of end arterioles in the white matter. The ring hemorrhage is diffuse in the brain with hemorrhage containing fibrin, pigmented parasites, free pigments and admixed fibrin. The uninfected red cells are seen in surrounding hemorrhage. Diirck's granulomata may be seen in areas of hemorrhage characterized by a small collection of microglial cells surrounding an area of demyelination. In addition, the brain demonstrates the abrupt transition from gray to white matter which, together with ring hemorrhage, are classical findings of cerebral malaria (**Figures 1–3**) [9].

Author details

Pier Paolo Piccaluga[1,2,3,4*] and Wanyonyi Ignatius[4]

1 Biobank of Research, IRCCS S. Orsola-Malpighi Academic Hospital, Bologna, Italy

2 Department of Experimental, Diagnostic, and Specialty Medicine, University of Bologna School of Medicine, Bologna, Italy

3 Institute of Hematology and Medical Oncology "L. and A. Seràgnoli", Italy

4 Department of Pathology, Jomo Kenyatta University of Agriculture and Technology, Nairobi, Kenya

*Address all correspondence to: pierpaolo.piccaluga@unibo.it

References

[1] World Health Organization. World malaria report 2021. 2021

[2] Aidoo M, Terlouw DJ, Kolczak MS, McElroy PD, ter Kuile FO, Kariuki S, et al. Protective effects of the sickle cell gene against malaria morbidity and mortality. Lancet. 2002;**359**:1311-1312

[3] Balla G, Vercellotti GM, Muller-Eberhard U, Eaton J, Jacob HS. Exposure of endothelial cells to free heme potentiates damage mediated by granulocytes and toxic oxygen species. Laboratory Investigation; A Journal of Technical Methods and Pathology. 1991;**64**(5):648-655

[4] Rénia L, Howland SW, Claser C, Gruner AC, Suwanarusk R, Teo TH, et al. Cerebral malaria: Mysteries at the blood-brain barrier. Virulence. 2012;**3**(2):193-201

[5] Thapar RK, Saxena A, Devgan A. Congenital malaria. Medical Journal, Armed Forces India. 2008;**64**(2):185

[6] Lesko CR, Arguin PM, Newman RD. Congenital malaria in the United States: A review of cases from 1966 to 2005. Archives of Pediatrics & Adolescent Medicine. 2007;**161**(11):1062-1067

[7] Mackintosh CL, Beeson JG, Marsh K. Clinical features and pathogenesis of severe malaria. Trends Parasitol. Dec 2004;**20**(12):597-603. DOI: 10.1016/j.pt.2004.09.006. PMID: 15522670

[8] Rowe JA, Claessens A, Corrigan RA, Arman M. Adhesion of *Plasmodium falciparum*-infected erythrocytes to human cells: Molecular mechanisms and therapeutic implications. Expert Reviews in Molecular Medicine. 2009;**11**:e16. DOI: 10.1017/S1462399409001082

[9] Milner DA Jr, Whitten RO, Kamiza S, Carr R, Liomba G, Dzamalala C, et al. The systemic pathology of cerebral malaria in African children. Frontiers in Cellular and Infection Microbiology. 2014;**4**:104. DOI: 10.3389/fcimb.2014.00104

Chapter 4

The Submicroscopic *Plasmodium falciparum* Malaria in Sub-Saharan Africa – Current Understanding of the Host Immune System and New Perspectives

Kwame Kumi Asare

Abstract

The bottlenecks in malaria infections affect malaria control and eradication programs. The gaps in the relationships between stages specific parasites molecules and their effects in the various stages of malaria development are unknown. The challenge hampers the wholesome understanding of policies and programs implemented to control and eliminate malaria infections in the endemic areas. Submicroscopic malaria and its transmission dynamisms are of interest in malaria control programs. The role of various stages of natural protective immunity in submicroscopic malaria infections and the insight into the collaborative role of antibodies from antigens for maintaining lower and submicroscopic malaria could provide a relevant guideline for vaccine developments. The chapter discusses the roles of mosquito and malaria antibodies in maintaining submicroscopic *P. falciparum* infection and its transmission potentials in malaria-endemic areas and the new perspectives on the inter-relatedness of stage-specific antibodies to improve malaria control programs in Sub-Saharan Africa.

Keywords: Malaria, Plasmodium falciparum, Anopheles gambiae, stage specific immunity, Submicroscopic infection, gSG6-P1, PfCSP, PfEBA175, Pfs230

1. Introduction

Malaria is a protozoan disease of global health importance. Malaria affects about 241 million people with 627,000 deaths [1–3]. The majority of malaria cases and deaths occur in Sub-Saharan Africa [4]. The malaria eradication campaign has marked reductions in malaria morbidity and mortality [2, 5]. The eradication is challenged by the recent stall gains achieved in malaria control programs [6, 7].

Malaria infection is initiated and transmitted during a blood meal by an infected female Anopheles mosquito [8]. The mosquito injects saliva containing sporozoites for liver invasion and liver-stage merozoites development and subsequent rapturing and infection of the red blood cells (RBCs) [9, 10]. The blood-stage merozoites undergo several rounds of replication and reinvasion of RBCs; a small proportion of the merozoites form the sexual stage gametocytes (male and female gametocytes) are required for malaria transmission from humans to mosquitoes to complete the parasite life cycle (**Figure 1**) [11–15].

The malaria parasites employ several parasite antigens (parasite proteins) for initial recognition and reversible attachment, reorientation and irreversible attachment, and final tissue or cell invasion and development [16–18]. The circumsporozoite protein (CSP), erythrocyte membrane protein 1 (PfEMP-1), repetitive interspersed family proteins (RIFINs) and ookinete surface antigen (Pfs230) are exposed to the host immune system to induce complex immune response at each stage of the parasite development [19–21]. Other factors such as malaria control strategies (treatment, vector control strategies), malaria distribution, epidemiological factors and chronic malaria infections account for low parasite density and submicroscopic malaria infections in malaria-endemic populations [22–27].

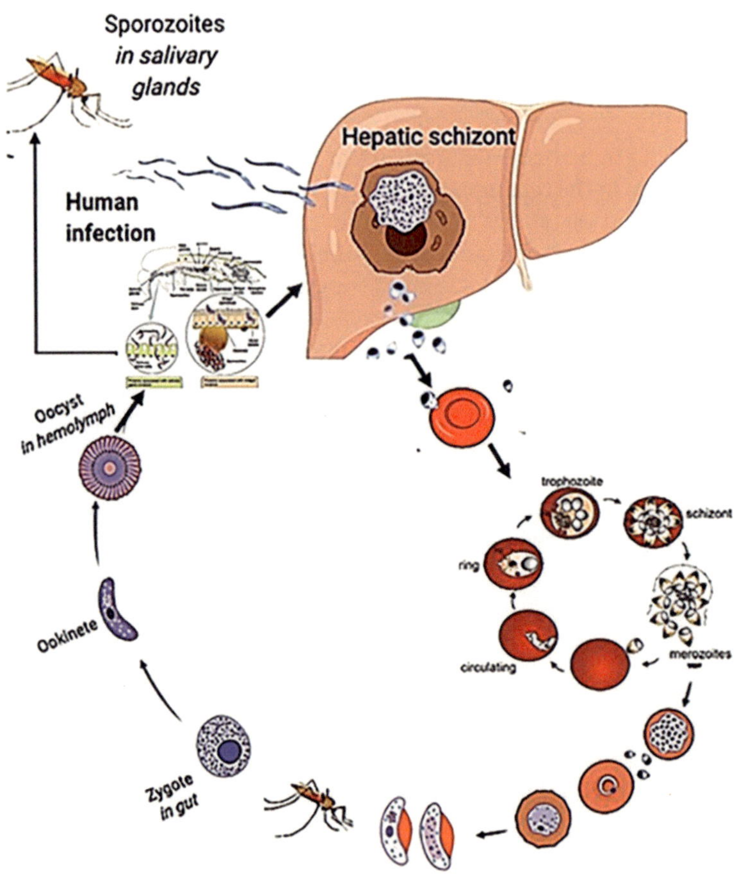

Figure 1.
Life cycle of malaria parasite. In the pre-erythrocytic stage: Plasmodium falciparum*-infected Anopheles mosquito bites a human and transmits sporozoites into the bloodstream. Sporozoites migrate through the dermis and bloodstream to invade hepatocytes; divide to form multinucleated schizonts. Erythrocytic phase: The liver stage schizonts rupture and release merozoites into the circulation and subsequent invasion into red blood cells. The merozoites mature from ring forms to trophozoites to multinucleated schizonts. Some merozoites differentiate into male or female gametocytes. Anopheles mosquito ingests gametocytes into the midgut, where it develops into sporozoites.*

2. The submicroscopic *Plasmodium falciparum* malaria

Submicroscopic malaria is *Plasmodium* parasite infections below the detection limit of microscopy [28]. Large numbers of falciparum malaria go undetected by the current point-of-care diagnostic (POC) techniques due to the low sensitivity of microscopy and rapid diagnostic test (RDTs) [28–30].

Human malaria, *Plasmodium falciparum*, *Plasmodium vivax*, *Plasmodium malariae*, *Plasmodium ovale* and *Plasmodium knowlesi*; *Plasmodium falciparum* malaria is the most virulent species that subvert the host physiology, results in severe complications such as cerebral malaria, severe anaemia, and respiratory distress and causes most deaths [31]. However, estimating the malaria burden and transmission intensity caused *by P. falciparum* in highly endemic Sub-Saharan Africa is essential for malaria control and eradication efforts [32, 33].

The undetected malaria infections serve as a reservoir and prominent contributor to malaria transmission [34, 35]. The underlying mechanisms for residual submicroscopic parasitaemia or gametocytaemia and its transmission dynamics are poorly understood. Thus, submicroscopic *P. falciparum* gametocyte densities could result in mosquito infections and maintain malaria transmission in the endemic communities [35]. A recent study showed that diagnosed and treated malaria-infected individuals had higher submicroscopic prevalence 30 days after treatment [36]. The low *P. falciparum* malaria infections in endemic Sub-Saharan Africa are associated with partial humoral immunity in the population [37–39].

3. Humoral antibody immunity to malaria

Acquisition of antibodies in *P. falciparum* malaria infection reduces parasitaemia and the risk of severe and mild malaria cases [40, 41]. The mechanisms such as antibody-dependent cellular inhibition (ADCI) and antibody-dependent cellular

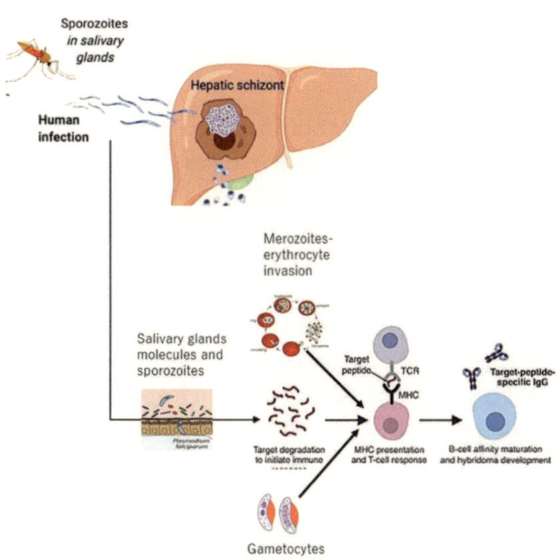

Stage	IgG antibodies	Function
Pre-erythrocytic	gSG6 P1	1. Biomarker for exposure to mosquito bites 2. Play a role in sporozoite liver invasion and development?
	PfCSP	1. Inhibits sporozoites liver invasion 2. First malaria vaccine ever rollout CSP (RTS, S vaccine)
Erythrocytic	PfEBA-175	1. Blocking PfEBA-GPA interaction 2. Inhibition of *P. falciparum* erythrocyte invasion
Sexual	Pfs230	1. Blocks oocyst production 2. Plays a critical role in the interaction between male exflagellation and oocyst production

Figure 2.
Stage-specific development of IgG antibodies in P. falciparum *malaria and their functional roles.*

cytotoxicity (ADCC) play a role in malaria infection [42]. The hyperimmune immunoglobulin G (IgG) and the predominant isotypes (IgG1, IgG2 and IgG3) in malaria-endemic areas have lower parasitaemia and lower risk of malaria attack [43–45]. The natural immunity to malaria develops gradually and is hyper-polymorphic [44]. The functionality of parasite antigen and antibodies interactions determines the quality of protection against malaria [46]. The robust immune response elicited at the various developmental stages of *P. falciparum* is poorly understood. Several of the parasite variant antigens are vaccine candidates. Thus, the IgG antibodies reduce parasitaemia and clinical symptoms in malaria-endemic communities. The insight into the collaborative role of antibodies from various antigens for maintaining lower and submicroscopic malaria could provide a relevant guideline for vaccine developments (**Figure 2**).

4. Pre-erythrocytic antibodies in *P. falciparum* endemic areas

4.1 *An. gambiae* salivary gland protein-6 peptide 1 (gSG6-P1) antibody

The active micro-components in Anopheles saliva prevent blood coagulation, induce complement activation, elicit and modify the immune response to influence the vector-malaria transmission [47]. *An. gambiae* salivary gland protein 6 (gSG6) has recently attracted scientific interest as a biomarker to estimate the intensity of exposure to mosquito bites and the risk of malaria infection [48–50]. The IgG immune antibody against gSG6-P1 has high sensitivity and specificity to determine the entomological inoculation rate (EIR) and overcome some of the challenges associated with EIR [51, 52]. The IgG antibody is an essential estimation of the risk of malaria transmission in the endemic areas [53]. Aside using gSG6-P1 IgG antibodies to estimate the risk of infection or vector-malaria transmission, does gSG6-P1 play any role in *Plasmodium falciparum* invasion and development? A question that will prove vital to the control efforts of malaria if rightly answered.

4.2 The circumsporozoite protein (CSP) antibody

The female Anopheles mosquito inoculates saliva containing sporozoites which migrate from the dermis into the hepatocytes [53, 54]. *P. falciparum* sporozoites are highly susceptible to the induced antibody against the most abundant sporozoite surface protein, the CSP [55–57]. The prolonged exposure of anti-CSP against sporozoites severely affects the development of the liver stage infections, thus reducing the chances of successful blood-stage of *P. falciparum* infections [56]. Currently, CSP based RTS, S anti-malaria vaccine is the only malaria vaccine that has been rolled out with efficacy of approximately 78% [58, 59]. These favourable safety profiles and protection-inducing immunity do not interfere with the general immune response mechanisms in a paediatric population. Although the RTS, S malaria vaccine has achieved a milestone, it is not without several concerns in high parasitaemia levels (>5000 parasites/ul) among subjects considered to be protected [60]. The inexplicable variations in the protection-induced immune response by CSP antibody in asymptomatic and symptomatic malaria require further understanding.

5. The erythrocytic stage antibodies in *P. falciparum* endemic areas

5.1 *P. falciparum* erythrocyte binding antigen-175

The merozoites invade red blood cells through parasite ligands-host receptors interactions to facilitate initial attachment, apical reorientation, tight junction formation and final entry into the red blood cells [61]. The exposed parasite ligands to the host immune system induce antibodies against parasite ligands [62–64]. Naturally acquired PfEBA-175 antibodies bind *P. falciparum* erythrocyte binding antigen-175 (PfEBA-175) to prevent red blood cell invasion [65, 66]. The PfEBA-175 engagement with Glycophorin A (GPA) remains one of the major pathways for red blood cells invasion and establishment of clinical disease in malaria [67, 68]. Therefore, blocking this critical pathway of parasite invasion into RBCs has become an approach to controlling malaria. The PfEBA-175-RII IgG-mediated antibody offers protection by binding to the functional R217 loop region of the PfEBA-175 inhibiting *P. falciparum* invasion of RBCs [69, 70]. Although the malaria parasite uses PfEBA-175-GPA invasion pathway, it can also adopt alternative ways to invade the PfEBA-175 antibody RBCs invasion blockage [71]. The high levels of PfEBA-175 antibody among the population in malaria-endemic areas and high-level submicroscopic malaria infection suggest a role of the PfEBA-175-GPA pathway in malaria infections [66, 72]. This is backed by the high relative avidity of IgG antibodies against EBA175RIII-V in low malaria-endemic communities [66, 73, 74].

5.2 Pfs230 gametocyte antibody

The sustained reservoirs of submicroscopic or asymptomatic malaria infections are not well understood [75–77]. The *P. falciparum* mature stage gametocytes could persist at submicroscopic levels for effective transmission to the mosquito [78, 79]. The exposure of gametocyte antigen Pfs230 expressed on the mature gametocyte surface and the gamete surface induces an antibody response in the human host [80–82]. There is a natural antibody response against the Pfs230 in malaria-endemic populations [83, 84]. The Pfs230 antibody blocks the fusion of gametes in the mosquito and prevents transmission [85, 86]. The anti-gametocytes IgG antibodies against Pfs230 reduce oocyst intensity by 55–70% and up to 44% reduction in proportions of infected mosquitoes [87]. The Pfs230 antibody has been associated with recent and concurrent high-density gametocyte exposure and impacts the dynamism of transmission by significantly reducing the infectiousness of high gametocyte density infections.

5.3 The missing links and the inter-relationships between stage-specific *P. falciparum* antibodies

There are several missing links in the association between the effects of various stage-specific antibodies and how they subsequently affect the development of the other parasites' stages [88]. For instance, there are several unknown points in the sexual stage immunity which could aid in the reduction of transmission to mosquitoes and elimination of malaria; such as how the Pfs230 antibody develops in either microscopic or submicroscopic gametocyte carriage, and the subsequent impacts on parasite development in mosquitoes and reinfection of the human host is still obscure. The current

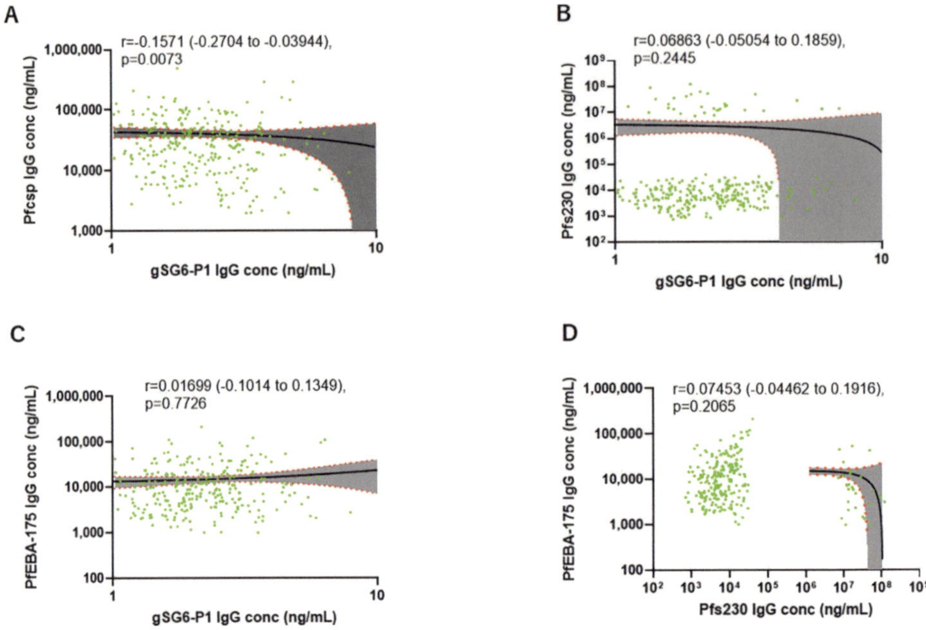

Figure 3.
A strong negative correlation between PfCSP IgG antibody and anopheles gSG6-P1 IgG antibody. A. Correlation between IgG antibodies concentration of PfCSP and gSG6-P1. B. Correlation between IgG antibodies concentration of Pfs230 and gSG6-P1. C. Correlation between IgG antibodies concentration of PfEBA-175 and gSG6-P1. D. Correlation between IgG antibodies concentration of PfEBA-175 and Pfs230. The statistical analysis was performed using spearman correlation. The IgG antibody concentration of PfCSP and IgG antibody concentration of anopheles gSG6-P1 showed a significant negative correction $r = -0.1571$ $(-0.2704$ *to* $-0.03944)$, $p = 0.0073$. *The observed strong negative correlation between IgG antibodies of PfCSP and gSG6-P1 is an indication that salivary gland proteins may play a role in the invasion and development of malaria sporozoites in the liver. Further studies are required to ascertain the specific role of gSG6-P1 in liver-stage malaria infection.*

knowledge of the functionality of the Pfs230 antibody has shown to be dependent on density [89–92]. Also, factors that reduce or prevent blood-stage parasitaemia development have the potential to reduce gametocyte development and reduce malaria transmission [93, 94]. Other immune factors such as antibodies against Anopheles salivary proteins and their relationship to the development of the liver-stage malaria parasites, erythrocytic phase development or sexual stage development are poorly understood.

However, current study has revealed a strong negative correlation between IgG antibodies of PfCSP and gSG6-P1. There is no evidence of an association between IgG antibodies of gSG6-P1, PfEBA175, Pfs230 or IgG antibodies of PfEBA175 and IgG antibodies of Pfs230 (**Figure 3**). Although the exact role of gSG6-P1 is unknown, this finding suggests either gSG6-P1 is involved in sporozoites invasion or the liver stage development.

6. The new perspectives

The salivary gland molecules may play a role in sporozoite survival and invasion of hepatocytes. However, there is no identified role of salivary gland molecules on sporozoite migration through the skin to the liver or development in the liver.

Previous studies have reported a putative mucin-like protein, the anti-platelet protein, the long-form D7 salivary protein, the putative gVAG protein precursor, the D7-related 3.2 protein, gSG7 salivary proteins, and the gSG6 protein may be involved in sporozoite maturation and transmission [95]. The authors of this study could not establish the direct association or role of the individual salivary gland proteins in the development of malaria parasites.

Also, the salivary gland molecules and underlying mechanisms for sporozoites recognition and invasion of the mosquito salivary gland are poorly understood. Until recently, the unique sporozoite ligand-salivary gland receptor interaction and molecules involved in triggering the mosquito salivary gland invasion were unknown. The discovery of *Anopheles* salivary gland protein, the CSP-binding protein (CSPBP) and its role in the mosquito salivary glands invasion has opened a new understanding of the invasion mechanism of sporozoites [96]. The antibodies raised against the CSPBP reduced sporozoites load by 25% and 90% in 14 and 18 days after the infected blood meal by mosquitoes, respectively [96].

In the hepatocyte invasion, region II of the C-terminal region of the sporozoite CSP attaches to the liver cells through the heparan sulfates proteoglycans (HSPG) [97, 98]. The conformations of CSP play a role in the sporozoite migration through different tissues in mosquito and human hosts [99]. However, factors involved in the sporozoite migration, invasion and development in hepatocytes remain largely unknown. The mosquitoes' gamma interferon-inducible thiol reductase (mosGILT) negatively influences sporozoite speed and cell traversal movement in the host [100–102]. Thus, the mosquito salivary gland proteins could either enhance or reduce the transmission of malaria parasites. The interaction of the PfCSP and gSG6-P1 proteins may play an essential role in sporozoites development in the human host. This finding is new information that requires further research into the role of gSG6-P1 in the development of pre-erythrocytic phase parasites.

In conclusion, submicroscopic malaria infection and transmission is one of the bottlenecks in malaria control and elimination strategy in malaria-endemic areas. The inoculation of the female Anopheles salivary gland content and sporozoites initiate the entire malaria human host developmental process. However, there are several missing links to how vector and parasite molecules influence the development and establishment of malaria infection. The observed strong negative correlation between IgG antibodies of PfCSP and gSG6-P1 is an indication that salivary gland proteins may play a role in the invasion and development of malaria sporozoites in the liver. Further studies are required to ascertain the specific role of gSG6-P1 in liver-stage malaria infection.

Author details

Kwame Kumi Asare
Department of Biomedical Science, University of Cape Coast, School of Allied Health Sciences, College of Allied Health Sciences, Cape Coast, Ghana

*Address all correspondence to: kwamsare@hotmail.com; kwame.asare@ucc.edu.gh

References

[1] Gómez-Díaz E, Ranford-Cartwright L. Evolutionary race: Malaria evolves to evade sickle cell protection. Cell Host & Microbe. 2022;**30**(2):139-141

[2] Sinnis P, Fidock DA. The RTS, S vaccine—A chance to regain the upper hand against malaria? Cell. 2022;**185**(5):750-754

[3] Negatu GA, Abebe GA, Yalew WG. Prevalence of malaria and associated factors among malaria-suspected patients attending Hamusit health center, Northwest Ethiopia: A cross-sectional study. Journal of Parasitology Research. 2022;**2022**

[4] World Health Organization. The potential impact of health service disruptions on the burden of malaria: a modelling analysis for countries in sub-Saharan Africa. World Health Organization; 2020. https://apps.who.int/iris/handle/10665/331845. License: CC BY-NC-SA 3.0 IGO

[5] Shretta R, Liu J, Cotter C, et al. Malaria Elimination and Eradication. In: Holmes KK, Bertozzi S, Bloom BR, et al., editors. Major Infectious Diseases. 3rd edition. Washington (DC): The International Bank for Reconstruction and Development / The World Bank; 2017 Nov 3. Chapter 12. Available from: https://www.ncbi.nlm.nih.gov/books/NBK525190/. DOI: 10.1596/978-1-4648-0524-0_ch12

[6] Manguin S, Dev V, editors. Towards Malaria Elimination: A Leap Forward. BoD–Books on Demand; 2018. https://www.intechopen.com/books/6339

[7] Strategic Advisory Group on Malaria Eradication. Malaria eradication: benefits, future scenarios and feasibility. A report of the Strategic Advisory Group on Malaria Eradication. Geneva: World Health Organization; 2020. Licence: CC BY-NC-SA 3.0 IGO

[8] Cox FE. History of the discovery of the malaria parasites and their vectors. Parasites & Vectors. 2010;**3**(1):1-9

[9] Kappe SH, Kaiser K, Matuschewski K. The plasmodium sporozoite journey: A rite of passage. Trends in Parasitology. 2003;**19**(3):135-143

[10] Kappe SH, Buscaglia CA, Nussenzweig V. Plasmodium sporozoite molecular cell biology. Annual Review of Cell and Developmental Biology. 2004;**20**:29-59

[11] Kumar H, Tolia NH. Getting in: The structural biology of malaria invasion. PLoS Pathogens. 2019;**15**(9):e1007943

[12] Perrin AJ, Bisson C, Faull PA, Renshaw MJ, Lees RA, Fleck RA, et al. Malaria parasite schizont egress antigen-1 plays an essential role in nuclear segregation during schizogony. mBio. 2021;**12**(2):e03377-e03320

[13] Smith TG, Lourenco P, Carter R, Walliker D, Ranford-Cartwright LC. Commitment to sexual differentiation in the human malaria parasite, plasmodium falciparum. Parasitology. 2000;**121**(2):127-133

[14] Venugopal K, Hentzschel F, Valkiūnas G, Marti M. Plasmodium asexual growth and sexual development in the haematopoietic niche of the host. Nature Reviews Microbiology. 2020;**18**(3):177-189

[15] Baker DA. Malaria gametocytogenesis. Molecular

and Biochemical Parasitology. 2010;**172**(2):57-65

[16] Fujioka H, Aikawa M. Structure and life cycle. Chemical Immunology. 2002;**80**(1):1-26

[17] Cowman AF, Crabb BS. Invasion of red blood cells by malaria parasites. Cell. 2006;**124**(4):755-766

[18] Carruthers VB, Blackman MJ. A new release on life: Emerging concepts in proteolysis and parasite invasion. Molecular Microbiology. 2005;**55**(6):1617-1630

[19] Kengne-Ouafo JA, Sutherland CJ, Binka FN, Awandare GA, Urban BC, Dinko B. Immune responses to the sexual stages of plasmodium falciparum parasites. Frontiers in Immunology. 2019;**136**

[20] Tan J, Piccoli L, Lanzavecchia A. The antibody response to plasmodium falciparum: Cues for vaccine design and the discovery of receptor-based antibodies. Annual review of Immunology. 2019;**37**:225-246

[21] Ismail HA. Functional Antibody Responses to the Plasmodium Falciparum Merozoite. Sweden: Karolinska Institutet; 2014

[22] Okell LC, Bousema T, Griffin JT, Ouédraogo AL, Ghani AC, Drakeley CJ. Factors determining the occurrence of submicroscopic malaria infections and their relevance for control. Nature Communications. 2012;**3**(1):1-9

[23] Nkumama IN, O'Meara WP, Osier FH. Changes in malaria epidemiology in Africa and new challenges for elimination. Trends in Parasitology. 2017;**33**(2):128-140

[24] Cotter C, Sturrock HJ, Hsiang MS, Liu J, Phillips AA, Hwang J, et al. The changing epidemiology of malaria elimination: New strategies for new challenges. The Lancet. 2013;**382**(9895):900-911

[25] Idris ZM, Chan CW, Kongere J, Gitaka J, Logedi J, Omar A, et al. High and heterogeneous prevalence of asymptomatic and sub-microscopic malaria infections on islands in Lake Victoria, Kenya. Scientific Reports. 2016;**6**(1):1-3

[26] Dobaño C, Santano R, Vidal M, Jiménez A, Jairoce C, Ubillos I, et al. Differential patterns of IgG subclass responses to plasmodium falciparum antigens in relation to malaria protection and RTS, S vaccination. Frontiers in Immunology. 2019;**10**:439

[27] Sturrock HJ, Hsiang MS, Cohen JM, Smith DL, Greenhouse B, Bousema T, et al. Targeting asymptomatic malaria infections: Active surveillance in control and elimination. PLoS Medicine. 2013;**10**(6):e1001467

[28] Ouédraogo AL, Bousema T, Schneider P, De Vlas SJ, Ilboudo-Sanogo E, Cuzin-Ouattara N, et al. Substantial contribution of submicroscopical plasmodium falciparum gametocyte carriage to the infectious reservoir in an area of seasonal transmission. PLoS One. 2009;**4**(12):e8410

[29] Britton S, Cheng Q, McCarthy JS. Novel molecular diagnostic tools for malaria elimination: A review of options from the point of view of high-throughput and applicability in resource limited settings. Malaria Journal. 2016;**15**(1):1-8

[30] Chadwick S, Townes DA, Perrone LA. Utility of point of care and rapid diagnostics in humanitarian emergencies. The Journal of Applied Laboratory Medicine. 2021;**6**(1):236-246

[31] Sena-dos-Santos C, Braga-da-Silva C, Marques D, dos Santos A, Pinheiro J, Ribeiro-dos-Santos Â, et al. Unraveling cell death pathways during malaria infection: What do we know so far? Cell. 2021;**10**(2):479

[32] Weiss DJ, Lucas TC, Nguyen M, Nandi AK, Bisanzio D, Battle KE, et al. Mapping the global prevalence, incidence, and mortality of plasmodium falciparum, 2000-17: A spatial and temporal modelling study. The Lancet. 2019;**394**(10195):322-331

[33] Alonso PL, Tanner M. Public health challenges and prospects for malaria control and elimination. Nature Medicine. 2013;**19**(2):150-155

[34] Karl S, Gurarie D, Zimmerman PA, King CH, St. Pierre TG, Davis TM. A sub-microscopic gametocyte reservoir can sustain malaria transmission. PLoS One. 2011;**6**(6):e20805

[35] Kaura T, Kaur J, Sharma A, Dhiman A, Pangotra M, Upadhyay AK, et al. Prevalence of submicroscopic malaria in low transmission state of Punjab: A potential threat to malaria elimination. Journal of Vector Borne Diseases. 2019;**56**(1):78

[36] Slater HC, Ross A, Felger I, Hofmann NE, Robinson L, Cook J, et al. The temporal dynamics and infectiousness of subpatent plasmodium falciparum infections in relation to parasite density. Nature Communications. 2019;**10**(1):1-6

[37] Aguzie IO. Pregnancy-associated malaria, challenges and prospects in sub-Saharan Africa. Clinics Mother Child Health. 2018;**15**(1):1-8

[38] Modiano D, Luoni G, Sirima BS, Lanfrancotti A, Petrarca V, Cruciani F, et al. The lower susceptibility to Plasmpdium falciparum malaria of Fulani of Burkina Faso (West Africa) is associated with low frequencies of classic malaria-resistance genes. Transactions of the Royal Society of Tropical Medicine and Hygiene. 2001;**95**(2):149-152

[39] Carneiro I, Roca-Feltrer A, Griffin JT, Smith L, Tanner M, Schellenberg JA, et al. Age-patterns of malaria vary with severity, transmission intensity and seasonality in sub-Saharan Africa: A systematic review and pooled analysis. PLoS One. 2010;**5**(2):e8988

[40] Rogerson SJ, Wijesinghe RS, Meshnick SR. Host immunity as a determinant of treatment outcome in plasmodium falciparum malaria. The Lancet Infectious Diseases. 2010;**10**(1):51-59

[41] Leoratti FM, Durlacher RR, Lacerda MV, Alecrim MG, Ferreira AW, Sanchez MC, et al. Pattern of humoral immune response to plasmodium falciparum blood stages in individuals presenting different clinical expressions of malaria. Malaria Journal. 2008;**7**(1):1-1

[42] Behr C, Dubois P. Evaluation of human T-cell response to malaria antigens in naturally acquired immunity. Research in Immunology. 1991;**142**(8):643-649

[43] Boyle MJ, Reiling L, Feng G, Langer C, Osier FH, Aspeling-Jones H, et al. Human antibodies fix complement to inhibit plasmodium falciparum invasion of erythrocytes and are associated with protection against malaria. Immunity. 2015;**42**(3):580-590

[44] Perlmann P, Troye-Blomberg M. Malaria and the immune system in humans. Malaria Immunol. 2002;**80**:229-242

[45] Rotman HL, Daly TM, Clynes R, Long CA. Fc receptors are not required for antibody-mediated protection against lethal malaria challenge in a mouse model. The Journal of Immunology. 1998;**161**(4):1908-1912

[46] Chaudhury S, Ockenhouse CF, Regules JA, Dutta S, Wallqvist A, Jongert E, et al. The biological function of antibodies induced by the RTS, S/AS01 malaria vaccine candidate is determined by their fine specificity. Malaria Journal. 2016;**15**(1):1-2

[47] Stone CM. Foraging Behavior and Reproductive Success of the Malaria Mosquito *Anopheles gambiae* ss *(Diptera: Culicidae)* (Doctoral dissertation, The Ohio State University); 2011. pp. 38-45. https://etd.ohiolink.edu/apexprod/rws_etd/send_file/send?accession=osu1312404297&disposition=inline

[48] Rizzo C, Ronca R, Fiorentino G, Verra F, Mangano V, Poinsignon A, et al. Humoral response to the Anopheles gambiae salivary protein gSG6: A serological indicator of exposure to Afrotropical malaria vectors. PLoS One. 2011;**6**(3):e17980

[49] Ali ZM, Bakli M, Fontaine A, Bakkali N, Hai VV, Audebert S, Boublik Y, Pagès F, Remoué F, Rogier C, Fraisier C. Assessment of anopheles salivary antigens as individual exposure biomarkers to species-specific malaria vector bites. Malaria Journal 2012;**11**(1):1-4

[50] Drame PM, Poinsignon A, Marie A, Noukpo H, Doucoure S, Cornelie S, et al. New salivary biomarkers of human exposure to malaria vector bites. In: Anopheles Mosquitoes-New Insights into Malaria Vectors. London, UK: IntechOpen; 2013

[51] Sagna A, Poinsignon A, Remoue F. Epidemiological applications of assessing mosquito exposure in a malaria-endemic area. In: Arthropod Vector: Controller of Disease Transmission. Vol. 2. Academic Press; 2017. pp. 209-229. https://www.sciencedirect.com/science/article/pii/B9780128053607000125

[52] Doucoure S, Drame PM. Salivary biomarkers in the control of mosquito-borne diseases. Insects. 2015;**6**(4):961-976

[53] Stone W, Bousema T, Jones S, Gesase S, Hashim R, Gosling R, et al. IgG responses to Anopheles gambiae salivary antigen gSG6 detect variation in exposure to malaria vectors and disease risk. PLoS One. 2012;**7**(6):e40170

[54] Douglas RG, Amino R, Sinnis P, Frischknecht F. Active migration and passive transport of malaria parasites. Trends in Parasitology. 2015;**31**(8):357-362

[55] Flores-Garcia Y, Nasir G, Hopp CS, Munoz C, Balaban AE, Zavala F, et al. Antibody-mediated protection against plasmodium sporozoites begins at the dermal inoculation site. mBio. 2018;**9**(6):e02194-e02118

[56] Kurtovic L, Behet MC, Feng G, Reiling L, Chelimo K, Dent AE, et al. Human antibodies activate complement against plasmodium falciparum sporozoites, and are associated with protection against malaria in children. BMC Medicine. 2018;**16**(1):1-7

[57] Livingstone MC, Bitzer AA, Giri A, Luo K, Sankhala RS, Choe M, et al. In vitro and in vivo inhibition of malaria parasite infection by monoclonal antibodies against plasmodium falciparum circumsporozoite protein (CSP). Scientific Reports. 2021;**11**(1):1-5

[58] Thompson HA, Hogan AB, Walker PG, White MT, Cunnington AJ,

Ockenhouse CF, et al. Modelling the roles of antibody titre and avidity in protection from plasmodium falciparum malaria infection following RTS, S/AS01 vaccination. Vaccine. 2020;**38**(47):7498-7507

[59] Kester KE, Cummings JF, Ockenhouse CF, Nielsen R, Hall BT, Gordon DM, et al. Phase 2a trial of 0, 1, and 3 month and 0, 7, and 28 day immunization schedules of malaria vaccine RTS, S/AS02 in malaria-naive adults at the Walter reed Army Institute of research. Vaccine. 2008;**26**(18):2191-2202

[60] Dodoo D, Atuguba F, Bosomprah S, Ansah NA, Ansah P, Lamptey H, et al. Antibody levels to multiple malaria vaccine candidate antigens in relation to clinical malaria episodes in children in the Kasena-Nankana district of northern Ghana. Malaria Journal. 2011;**10**(1):1-9

[61] Ghosh S. Dissecting the function of essential rhoptry genes of the malaria parasite (Doctoral dissertation, Deakin University); 2016. https://dro.deakin.edu.au/view/DU:30088998

[62] Wright GJ, Rayner JC. Plasmodium falciparum erythrocyte invasion: Combining function with immune evasion. PLoS Pathogens. 2014;**10**(3):e1003943

[63] Weiss GE, Crabb BS, Gilson PR. Overlaying molecular and temporal aspects of malaria parasite invasion. Trends in Parasitology. 2016;**32**(4):284-295

[64] Gaur D, Mayer DG, Miller LH. Parasite ligand–host receptor interactions during invasion of erythrocytes by plasmodium merozoites. International Journal for Parasitology. 2004;**34**(13-14):1413-1429

[65] Jaskiewicz E, Jodłowska M, Kaczmarek R, Zerka A. Erythrocyte glycophorins as receptors for plasmodium merozoites. Parasites & Vectors. 2019;**12**(1):1-1

[66] Amoah LE, Abagna HB, Akyea-Mensah K, Lo AC, Kusi KA, Gyan BA. Characterization of anti-EBA175RIII-V in asymptomatic adults and children living in communities in the Greater Accra region of Ghana with varying malaria transmission intensities. BMC Immunology. 2018;**19**(1):1-9

[67] Chowdhury P, Ray S, Chakraborty A, Sen S, Dasgupta AK, Sengupta S. Non-synonymous amino acid alterations in PfEBA-175 modulate the merozoite ligand's ability to interact with host's Glycophorin a receptor. Infection, Genetics and Evolution. 2020;**85**:104418

[68] Gaur D, Chitnis CE, Chauhan VS. Molecular basis of erythrocyte invasion by plasmodium merozoites. Advances in Malaria Research. 2016:33-86. https://doi.org/10.1002/9781118493816.ch3

[69] Chen E, Paing MM, Salinas N, Sim BK, Tolia NH. Structural and functional basis for inhibition of erythrocyte invasion by antibodies that target plasmodium falciparum EBA-175. PLoS Pathogens. 2013;**9**(5):e1003390

[70] Yang PK, Liang XY, Lin M, Chen JT, Huang HY, Lin LY, et al. Population genetic analysis of the plasmodium falciparum erythrocyte binding antigen-175 (EBA-175) gene in Equatorial Guinea. Malaria Journal. 2021;**20**(1):1-6

[71] Malpede BM. Molecular Mechanisms of Plasmodium Red Blood Cell Invasion. Louis: Washington University in St; 2015

[72] Dobaño C, Quelhas D, Quintó L, Puyol L, Serra-Casas E, Mayor A, et al. Age-dependent IgG subclass responses

to plasmodium falciparum EBA-175 are differentially associated with incidence of malaria in Mozambican children. Clinical and A Vaccine Immunology. 2012;**19**(2):157-166

[73] Abagna HB, Acquah FK, Okonu R, Aryee NA, Theisen M, Amoah LE. Assessment of the quality and quantity of naturally induced antibody responses to EBA175RIII–V in Ghanaian children living in two communities with varying malaria transmission patterns. Malaria Journal. 2018;**17**(1):1-1

[74] Broni FK, Acquah FK, Obiri-Yeboah D, Obboh EK, Sarpong E, Amoah LE. Profiling the quality and quantity of naturally induced antibody responses against Pfs230 and Pfs48/45 among non-febrile children living in southern Ghana: A longitudinal study. Frontiers in cellular and infection. Microbiology. 2021;**1169**

[75] Kumari P, Sinha S, Gahtori R, Yadav CP, Pradhan MM, Rahi M, et al. Prevalence of asymptomatic malaria parasitemia in Odisha, India: A challenge to malaria elimination. The American Journal of Tropical Medicine and Hygiene. 2020;**103**(4):1510

[76] van Eijk AM, Sutton PL, Ramanathapuram L, Sullivan SA, Kanagaraj D, Priya G, et al. The burden of submicroscopic and asymptomatic malaria in India revealed from epidemiology studies at three varied transmission sites in India. Scientific Reports. 2019;**9**(1):1-1

[77] Lin JT, Saunders DL, Meshnick SR. The role of submicroscopic parasitemia in malaria transmission: What is the evidence? Trends in Parasitology. 2014;**30**(4):183-190

[78] Shekalaghe S, Drakeley C, Gosling R, Ndaro A, Van Meegeren M, Enevold A, et al. Primaquine clears submicroscopic plasmodium falciparum gametocytes that persist after treatment with sulphadoxine-pyrimethamine and artesunate. PLoS One. 2007;**2**(10):e1023

[79] Ayanful-Torgby R, Sarpong E, Abagna HB, Donu D, Obboh E, Mensah BA, et al. Persistent plasmodium falciparum infections enhance transmission-reducing immunity development. Scientific Reports. 2021;**11**(1):1-3

[80] Healer J, McGuinness D, Carter R, Riley E. Transmission-blocking immunity to plasmodium falciparum in malaria-immune individuals is associated with antibodies to the gamete surface protein Pfs230. Parasitology. 1999;**119**(5):425-433

[81] Acquah FK, Adjah J, Williamson KC, Amoah LE. Transmission-blocking vaccines: Old friends and new prospects. Infection and Immunity. 2019;**87**(6):e00775-e00718

[82] Stone WJ, Campo JJ, Ouédraogo AL, Meerstein-Kessel L, Morlais I, Da D, et al. Unravelling the immune signature of plasmodium falciparum transmission-reducing immunity. Nature Communications. 2018;**9**(1):1-4

[83] Jones S, Grignard L, Nebie I, Chilongola J, Dodoo D, Sauerwein R, et al. Naturally acquired antibody responses to recombinant Pfs230 and Pfs48/45 transmission blocking vaccine candidates. Journal of Infection. 2015;**71**(1):117-127

[84] Muthui MK, Kamau A, Bousema T, Blagborough AM, Bejon P, Kapulu MC. Immune responses to gametocyte antigens in a malaria endemic population—The African falciparum context: A systematic review and

meta-analysis. Frontiers in Immunology. 2019;**2480**

[85] Duffy PE. Transmission-blocking vaccines: Harnessing herd immunity for malaria elimination. Expert Review of Vaccines. 2021;**20**(2):185-198

[86] Coelho CH, Tang WK, Burkhardt M, Galson JD, Muratova O, Salinas ND, et al. A human monoclonal antibody blocks malaria transmission and defines a highly conserved neutralizing epitope on gametes. Nature Communications. 2021;**12**(1):1-2

[87] Ouédraogo AL, Eckhoff PA, Luty AJ, Roeffen W, Sauerwein RW, Bousema T, et al. Modeling the impact of plasmodium falciparum sexual stage immunity on the composition and dynamics of the human infectious reservoir for malaria in natural settings. PLoS Pathogens. 2018;**14**(5):e1007034

[88] Struik SS, Riley EM. Does malaria suffer from lack of memory? Immunological Reviews. 2004;**201**(1):268-290

[89] Bousema T, Roeffen W, Meijerink H, Mwerinde H, Mwakalinga S, van Gemert GJ, et al. The dynamics of naturally acquired immune responses to plasmodium falciparum sexual stage antigens Pfs230 & Pfs48/45 in a low endemic area in Tanzania. PLoS One. 2010;**5**(11):e14114

[90] Lamptey H, Ofori MF, Kusi KA, Adu B, Owusu-Yeboa E, Kyei-Baafour E, et al. The prevalence of submicroscopic plasmodium falciparum gametocyte carriage and multiplicity of infection in children, pregnant women and adults in a low malaria transmission area in southern Ghana. Malaria Journal. 2018;**17**(1):1-2

[91] Liehl P, Meireles P, Albuquerque IS, Pinkevych M, Baptista F, Mota MM, et al. Innate immunity induced by plasmodium liver infection inhibits malaria reinfections. Infection and Immunity. 2015;**83**(3):1172-1180

[92] Spence PJ, Jarra W, Lévy P, Reid AJ, Chappell L, Brugat T, et al. Vector transmission regulates immune control of plasmodium virulence. Nature. 2013;**498**(7453):228-231

[93] Bousema T, Okell L, Felger I, Drakeley C. Asymptomatic malaria infections: Detectability, transmissibility and public health relevance. Nature Reviews Microbiology. 2014;**12**(12):833-840

[94] Okell LC, Drakeley CJ, Ghani AC, Bousema T, Sutherland CJ. Reduction of transmission from malaria patients by artemisinin combination therapies: A pooled analysis of six randomized trials. Malaria Journal. 2008;7(1):1-3

[95] Phattanawiboon B, Jariyapan N, Mano C, Roytrakul S, Paemanee A, Sor-Suwan S, et al. Salivary gland proteome during adult development and after blood feeding of female Anopheles dissidens mosquitoes (Diptera: Culicidae). PLoS One. 2016;**11**(9):e0163810

[96] Wang J, Zhang Y, Zhao YO, Li MW, Zhang L, Dragovic S, et al. Anopheles gambiae circumsporozoite protein–binding protein facilitates plasmodium infection of mosquito salivary glands. The Journal of Infectious Diseases. 2013;**208**(7):1161-1169

[97] Zhao J, Bhanot P, Hu J, Wang Q. A comprehensive analysis of plasmodium circumsporozoite protein binding to hepatocytes. PLoS One. 2016;**11**(8):e0161607

[98] Dundas K, Shears MJ, Sinnis P, Wright GJ. Important extracellular interactions between plasmodium sporozoites and host

cells required for infection. Trends in Parasitology. 2019;**35**(2):129-139

[99] Coppi A, Natarajan R, Pradel G, Bennett BL, James ER, Roggero MA, et al. The malaria circumsporozoite protein has two functional domains, each with distinct roles as sporozoites journey from mosquito to mammalian host. Journal of Experimental Medicine. 2011;**208**(2):341-356

[100] Schleicher TR, Yang J, Freudzon M, Rembisz A, Craft S, Hamilton M, et al. A mosquito salivary gland protein partially inhibits plasmodium sporozoite cell traversal and transmission. Nature Communications. 2018;**9**(1):1-2

[101] Chuang YM, Agunbiade TA, Tang XD, Freudzon M, Almeras L, Fikrig E. The effects of a mosquito salivary protein on sporozoite traversal of host cells. The Journal of Infectious Diseases. 2021;**224**(3):544-553

[102] Beristain-Ruiz DM. Pathogen Screening from Soft and Hard Ticks Isolated from Different Species in Chihuahua. Producto de investigación ICB: Mexico; 2018

Chapter 5

Estimation of Malaria Mortality in Developing Countries

Sepiribo Lucky Braide

Abstract

This chapter considered monitoring human health condition as vital variable for well-being of man/society required input data for effective daily planning. Researchers have contributed to prediction of incidence/recovery rate for malaria mortality. Modified state-estimation model based (matrix-formulation, weighted sum of squares of errors) was applied. The instrument (sphygmomanometer, etc.) is manipulated for study under investigation to examined existing state of system. Four (4) measurements data were analyzed from different geographical locations for patients with malaria endemic cases. Physician measurement data are implemented into modified state-estimation equations to estimate degree of error (s) to classify as bad measurement. Results shows bad data estimation attributed to poor instrument calibration, aging, and poor physician measurement. These reveal discrepancies between actual (true-measurement) and patient-physical measurements. Four vital measurements include blood pressure (Bp), blood sugar level (BSL), body temperature (BT), and Plasmodium ViVax with relied validation test following chi-square distribution for 2-degree freedom with 99% significance level suspected as error measurement. Model-matrix coded in MATLAB gives state-estimation results ($\boldsymbol{x_1 = 8.5225}$ ***and*** $\boldsymbol{x_2 = 13.235}$), indicating strong variation between actual and physical measurements for some patients having low pulse rate under the measurement of blood pressure (Bp). Essentially, physicians' measurements must be revalidated for accuracy before drugs prescription/administration to avoid under- or over-dose since patients' body chemistry varies significantly for different persons.

Keywords: measurement, matrix formulations, malaria, mortality, state-estimates, distribution

1. Introduction

1.1 Improved state estimation model techniques and governing equations

The analysis and investigation of basic human body diagnosis uses the vital statistics variables of physical measurement because it deals with scientific application to the life history of communities and nation. That is historical development which is a function of human society can be numerically be expressed qualitatively or quantitatively. The purpose of this study is to find out the changing composition of communities or nations with reference to sex, age, education, economic and civic status which is considered under study [1].

Evidently the state estimation model considered the numerical records of marriage, births, sickness and deaths by which the health and growth of community may be studied. The vital statistics variable provides the results of the biometry which deals with data and the laws of human mortality, morbidity and demography [2].

This technical contents considered the data or the laws which explain the phenomenon of birth, deaths, health and longevity, composition and concentration etc.

This study can also be extended to solve information particularly on fertility, mortality, maternity, urban density which is indispensable for planning and evaluation of the schemes of health, family planning and other vital amenities for purpose of efficient planning, evaluation and analysis of various economic and social policies [3].

Importantly, data collected on life expectancy at various age levels is helpful in actual calculations of risk on life policies, this means that life table called the biometer of public health and longivity helps in fixing the life insurance premium rates at various age level.

The modified state estimation model described the estimation strategy using different mathematical matrics operations to estimates the physical measurements carried out by a physician/medical doctors, on the view to determine the estimated physical measurements for malaria mortality in a developing countries, the question is how true? is the physical measurement taken by the medical doctor for purpose of placing drug dispensation and administration evidently, research studies has provided with results the measurement equations characterizing the meter readings with the view to the addition of error terms to the system model for purpose of validating physical measurement by medical practitioners [4].

Several measurement instruments and devices are used in the measurements of vital statistics variable (state-variables) of the human life expectancy. We have the sphygmomanotreter (device that measures blood pressure) thermometer (device that measures temperature), (blood sugar level), (plasmodium viviax: parasite for malaria) etc. [5].

The physical measurements data are collected from patients in the health/clinic and hospital which are not always true to some extend, the acquired data from the measurements device/instruments contains inaccuracies which is unavoidable since physical measurements cannot be entirely free from random errors or noise. These errors can be quantified in a statistical sense and the estimated values of the quantities being measured are then either accepted as reasonable or not, if certain measurement of accuracy are exceeded because of noise the true values of physical quantities are never known and we have to consider how to calculate the best possible estimates of the unknown quantities [6].

Incidentally, the techniques of least square is often used to best fit measurement data relating to two or more quantities. However, modified equations are developed and formulated to characterize measurements of the physical data collected or acquired from patients for purpose of analysis with the integration of errors terms in the system model. The best estimates are choosen which minimizes the weighted sum of squares of the measurement errors [7].

2. Background of study

State estimation techniques is the process of determining a set of values for a set of unknown systems (Engineering systems, human being systems, medical systems, biological systems, machine/instruments system etc). State variables are based on certain criterion making use of physical measurements made which are not precise due to inherent error associated with controllers/transducers and sometimes creates redundancy of measurement that does not require assessment of the true-value of the systems state variables [8]. Statistical methods are also used to estimate the true value of the system state variables with the minimum number of variables required to analyze the system in all aspects. The measurements taken by a medical practitioner are required to meet the basic records for a given circumstances intended to address particularly to the engineering systems, medical system, biological systems and related systems in order to provide good quality of reliable physical measurements for system variables [9]. Evidently, the necessary conditions for vital statistics variables analysis for administering drugs dispension to patients ensure and declared measurements records conformity to calculation of the measuring instruments, precision and tolerance for purpose of standard practice for world health organization (WHO) [10].

Importantly, if the measurement instruments introduces errors while undertaking details information variables statistics about patients status, this may results into wrong presentation of recorded data required for prescription/dispensing of drugs this will eventually results into gradual breakdown of human body system, immunity, antibodies vital tissues and sensitive organs like liver, kidney etc. in a colossal decay condition that may leads to early mortality for associated emergence of infected and transmitted diseases [11].

Essentially for purpose of good working condition of human lives, standard practice for healthy living, is strongly monitored in order to regularly checked for recalibration of measuring instruments, for purpose of high precision, tolerance and accuracy [12].

3. Materials and method

3.1 Model formulation of modified state estimation equations

The measurement set used by medical practioners consists of thermometer reading (z_1), sphygmomanometer (z_2), Blood-sugar level (z_3) and plasmodiums vivax parasite transmission measurement (z_4) etc. Where z_1, z_2, z_3 *and* z_4, are mathematical measurement parameter sowing to the physical measurements/quantities respectively.

Similarly, the symbol x represents physical quantities being estimated.

Then the measurement equations that is characterizing the meter readings/measured terms are found by adding error terms (e) to the system model as:

$$Z = Hx + e \tag{1}$$

Z : Measurement variables.
H : rectangular matrice operations.
x : State variables (the physical quantities being estimated).
e : errors term.
hx : True values of system model.

The numerical coefficient are determined by the human body circulatory components and the error terms e_1, e_2, e_3 *and* e_4 which represents errors in measurement z_1, z_2, z_3 *and* z_4 and respectively.

If the errors terms e_1, e_2, e_3, e_4 are zero, then it is an ideal condition which mean that the meter reading of the physical measurement taken by the vital statistics variable of the patients are exact and true measurements (z), which gives exact values of χ_1 *and* χ_2 *of* $\hat{\chi}_1$ *and* $\hat{\chi}_2$ which could be determined.

From the relationship of eq. (1) it can be obtained as:

$$Z_1 = h_{11}x_1 + h_{12}x_2 + e_1 = Z_{1,true} + e_1 \tag{2}$$

$$Z_2 = h_{21}x_1 + h_{22}x_2 + e_2 = Z_{2,true} + e_2 \tag{3}$$

$$Z_3 = h_{31}x_1 + h_{32}x_2 + e_3 = Z_{3,true} + e_3 \tag{4}$$

$$Z_4 = h_{41}x_1 + h_{42}x_2 + e_4 = Z_{4,true} + e_4 \tag{5}$$

Where; Z_{jtrue}: True value of the measured quantity Z_j.

Reformulating eq. (2)–(5) into vector form to obtained as;

$$\begin{bmatrix} e_1 \\ e_2 \\ e_3 \\ e_4 \end{bmatrix} = \begin{bmatrix} z_1 \\ z_2 \\ z_3 \\ z_4 \end{bmatrix} - \begin{bmatrix} z_{1true} \\ z_{2true} \\ z_{3true} \\ z_{4true} \end{bmatrix} = \begin{bmatrix} z_1 \\ z_2 \\ z_3 \\ z_4 \end{bmatrix} - \begin{bmatrix} h_{11} & h_{12} \\ h_{21} & h_{22} \\ h_{31} & h_{32} \\ h_{41} & h_{42} \end{bmatrix} \begin{bmatrix} x_1 \\ x_2 \end{bmatrix} \tag{6}$$

In compact form representation given as:

$$e = z - z_{true} = z - Hx \tag{7}$$

Which represents the error term between the actual measurement (z). and the true (but unknown) values $z_{true} \triangleq Hx$ of the measurement quantities. The true values of x_1 *and* x_2 cannot be determined but we can calculate the estimates $\hat{\chi}_1$ *and* $\hat{\chi}_2$

Substituting these estimates ($\hat{\chi}_1$ *and* $\hat{\chi}_2$) into eq. (6) gives the estimated values of the errors in the form as:

$$\begin{bmatrix} \hat{e}_1 \\ \hat{e}_2 \\ \hat{e}_3 \\ \hat{e}_4 \end{bmatrix} = \begin{bmatrix} z_1 \\ z_2 \\ z_3 \\ z_4 \end{bmatrix} - \begin{bmatrix} h_{11} & h_{12} \\ h_{21} & h_{22} \\ h_{31} & h_{32} \\ h_{41} & h_{42} \end{bmatrix} \begin{bmatrix} \hat{x}_1 \\ \hat{x}_2 \end{bmatrix} \tag{8}$$

The quantitie are estimates of the corresponding quantities.

The vector, $\hat{e}$ which represents the differences between the actual measurement (z) and their estimated values $\hat{z}_{true} \triangleq Hx$, thus in compact form is given as:

$$\hat{e} = z - \hat{z} = z - H\hat{x} = e - H(\hat{x} - x) \tag{9}$$

The criterion for calculating the estimates ($\hat{\chi}_1$ *and* $\hat{\chi}_2$) can be determined as:

$$\hat{e} = [\hat{e}_1 \hat{e}_2 \hat{e}_3 \hat{e}_4]^T \tag{10}$$

and

$$\hat{z} = [\hat{z}_1 \hat{z}_2 \hat{z}_3 \hat{z}_4]^T \tag{11}$$

Eq. (10) and (11) have to be computed for purpose of estimation analysis.

The techniques can be used to describe algebraic sum of errors to minimize positive and negative operations which may not be acceptable.

However, it is preferable to minimize the direct sum of squares of errors.

To ensure that measurement from meters or data collected of known greater accuracy are considered more favorably than less accurate measurements instrument/ device, that is in each term the sum of squares is multipled by an appropriate weighting factor (w) to give the objective function as:

$$f = \sum_{j-1}^{4} w_j e_j^2 = w_1 e_1^2 + w_2 e_2^2 + w_3 e_3^2 + w_4 e_4^2 \tag{12}$$

We select the best estimates of the state variables as those values $\hat{\chi}_1$ *and* $\hat{\chi}_2$ which cause the objectives functions (f) to take on its minimum value.

In accordance to the application of necessary conditions for minimizing function (f), the estimates $\hat{\chi}_1$ *and* $\hat{\chi}_2$ are those values of χ_1 *and* χ_2 which satisfy the equations as;

$$\frac{\partial f}{\partial x_1}\bigg| = 2\left[w_1 e_1 \frac{\partial e_1}{\partial x_1} + w_2 e_2 \frac{\partial e_2}{\partial x_2} + w_3 e_3 \frac{\partial e_3}{\partial x_3} + w_4 e_4 \frac{\partial e_4}{\partial x_4}\right]\bigg| = 0 \tag{13}$$

Similarly,

$$\frac{\partial f}{\partial x_2}\bigg| = 2\left[w_1 e_1 \frac{\partial e_1}{\partial x_1} + w_2 e_2 \frac{\partial e_2}{\partial x_2} + w_3 e_3 \frac{\partial e_3}{\partial x_3} + w_4 e_4 \frac{\partial e_4}{\partial x_4}\right]\bigg| = 0 \tag{14}$$

That is, the notation: $|_{\hat{x}} = 0$ which, indicates that the equations have to be evaluated from the state estimates $\hat{x} = [\hat{x}_1 \hat{x}_2]^T$ since the true values for the states variable are not known.

The unknown actual error (e_j) are then replaced by estimated errors $\hat{e}_j$ which can be calculated once the true estimate $\hat{x}_i$ are known.

Eq. (14) and (15) can be represented in vector form as:

$$\begin{bmatrix} \frac{\partial e_1}{\partial x_1} & \frac{\partial e_2}{\partial x_1} & \frac{\partial e_3}{\partial x_1} & \frac{\partial e_4}{\partial x_1} \\ \frac{\partial e_1}{\partial x_2} & \frac{\partial e_2}{\partial x_2} & \frac{\partial e_3}{\partial x_2} & \frac{\partial e_4}{\partial x_2} \end{bmatrix}_{\hat{x}} \begin{bmatrix} w_1 & x & x & x \\ x & w_2 & x & x \\ x & x & w_3 & x \\ x & x & x & w_4 \end{bmatrix} \begin{bmatrix} e_1 \\ e_2 \\ e_3 \\ e_4 \end{bmatrix} = \begin{bmatrix} 0 \\ 0 \end{bmatrix} \tag{15}$$

Where w is the diagonal matrix of weighting factor which have special significance to the accuracy of measurement.

The partial derivatives for substitution in eq. 15 are found from eqs. (2) through (5) to be constant given by the elements (H) given as:

$$\begin{bmatrix} h_{11} & h_{21} & h_{31} & h_{41} \\ h_{12} & h_{22} & h_{32} & h_{42} \end{bmatrix} \begin{bmatrix} w_1 & x & x & x \\ x & w_2 & x & x \\ x & x & w_3 & x \\ x & x & x & w_4 \end{bmatrix} \begin{bmatrix} \hat{e}_1 \\ \hat{e}_2 \\ \hat{e}_3 \\ \hat{e}_4 \end{bmatrix} = \begin{bmatrix} 0 \\ 0 \end{bmatrix} \tag{16}$$

Using the operation of the compact notation process of eq. (9) can be applied to also represent eq. (17) as:

$$H^T W\hat{e} = H^T W(z - H\hat{x}) = 0 \tag{17}$$

Multiplying through this eq. (17) and solving for the estimates $(\hat{x})$ as:

$$\hat{x} = \begin{bmatrix} \hat{x}_1 \\ \hat{x}_2 \end{bmatrix} = \underbrace{\left(H^T WH\right)}_{G}^{-1} = H^T WZ = G^{-1}H^T WZ \tag{18}$$

Where $\hat{x}_1$ *and* $\hat{x}_2$ are the weighted least square estimates of the state variables, It is the rectangular matrix component

The symmetrical matrix (called the gain-matrix, G) must be inverted as a single entity to give as:

$$G^{-1} = \left(H^T WH\right)^{-1} \tag{19}$$

Which is also symmetrical in the mathematical operations.

Essentially, the weighted least-squares procedure are required to estimates $\hat{x}_i$ how close to the true value x_i of the state variables,

The expression for the difference $(x_i - \hat{x}_i)$ is found my substituting for;

$$Z = Hx + e \text{ to obtain as} \tag{20}$$

$$\hat{x} = G^{-1}H^T W(Hx + e) = G^{-1}\underbrace{\left(H^T WH\right)}_{G}x = G^{-1}H^T We \tag{21}$$

It is an important consideration to check the useful operation of the dimensions of each term in the matrix product of eq. (21) which is an important idea for developing properties of the weighted least-square estimations. In this analysis we have the matrix operation: $G^{-1}H^T W$ which as an overall operation of row × column dimensions of 2 × 4, which means that any one or more of the four errors (e_1, e_2, e_3, e_4) an influence the difference between each state estimates.

The weighted least squares calculations spread the effects of the errors in any one measurements to some or all other estimates the characteristics is the basis for detecting bad data measurement.

In a similar manner we can compare the calculated values of $\hat{z} = H\hat{x}$ of the measured quantities with their actual measurements (z) by substituting for $\hat{x} = x$ from eq. (21) into eq. (7) to obtain as:

$$\hat{e} = z - \hat{z} = e - HG^{-1}H^T W_e = \left[I - HG^{-1}H^T W\right]_e \tag{22}$$

Where; I: unit or identity matrix.

4. Statistical analysis, errors and estimates

In reality we know absolutely true state of a physical operating system. Great care is taken to ensure accuracy. Unavoidable random noise enters into the measurements process to distort more or less the physical results. Repeated measurements of the same quantity under careful controlled conditions reveals certain statistical properties from which the true value can be estimated [13].

If the measured values are plotted as a function of their relative frequency of occurrence, a histogram is obtained to which a continues curve can be fitted as the number of measurement increases theoretically to any number [14].

The continuous curve commonly encountered is a ball-shaped function $p(z)$. This is the Gaussian or normal probability density function gives as:

$$p(z) = \frac{1}{5\sqrt{2\pi}} \varepsilon^{-\frac{1}{2}\left(\frac{z-\mu}{\delta}\right)^2} \tag{23}$$

The probability that z-takes on values between the point a and b in **Figure 1** is the shaded area given as;

$$pr = (a < z < b) = \int_a^b p(z)dz = \frac{1}{\sigma\sqrt{2\pi}} \int_a^b \varepsilon^{-\frac{1}{2}} = \frac{1}{\sigma\sqrt{2\pi}} \tag{24}$$

The total area under the curve p(z) between 0 and equals to 1. The value of z is certain with probability equal to 1 or 100% [15].

The Gaussian distribution plays a very important role in the measurement statistic because the probability function density cannot be directly integrated. For transfer from z to y using change of variable formula given as (**Tables 1–3**) (**Figure 2**):

$$y = \frac{z-\mu}{\delta} \tag{25}$$

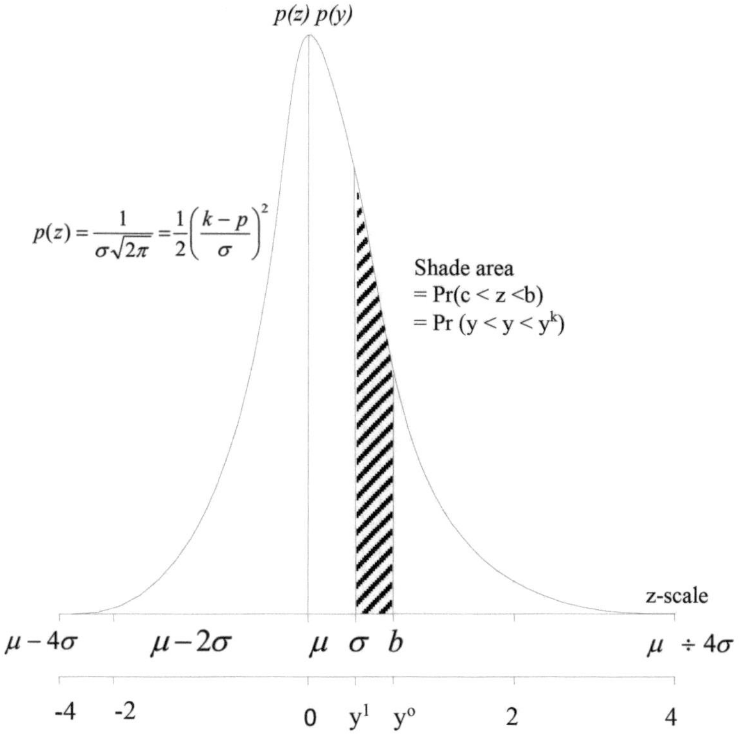

Figure 1.
Gaussian normal distribution.

K	0.05	0.025	0.01	0.005
1	3.84	5.02	6.64	7.88
2	3.99	7.38	9.21	10.60
3	7.82	9.35	11.35	12.84
4	9.49	11.14	13.28	14.86
5	11.07	12.83	15.09	16.75
6	12.59	14.45	16.81	18.55
7	14.07	16.01	18.48	20.28
8	15.51	17.54	20.09	21.96
9	16.92	19.02	21.67	23.59
10	18.31	20.48	23.21	25.19
11	19.68	21.92	24.73	26.76
12	21.03	23.34	26.22	28.30
13	22.36	24.74	27.69	29.82
14	23.69	26.12	29.14	31.32
15	25.00	27.49	30.58	32.80
16	26.30	28.85	32.00	34.27
17	27.59	30.19	33.41	33.72
18	28.87	31.53	34.81	37.16
19	30.14	32.86	36.19	38.58
20	31.41	34.17	37.57	40.00

Table 1.
Normal chi-square distribution table (values of area α to the right of $\chi_k^2 = \chi_{k,\alpha}^2$.

A	Pr(a)	a	Pr(a)
.05	0.01994	.08	0.28814
.10	0.03983	.85	0.30234
.15	0.05962	.90	0.31594
.20	0.07926	.95	0.32894
.25	0.09871	1.00	0.34134
.30	0.11791	1.05	0.35314
.35	0.13683	1.10	0.36433
.40	0.15542	1.15	0.37493
.45	0.17364	1.20	0.38493
.50	0.19146	1.25	0.39435
.55	0.20884	1.30	0.40320
.60	0.23575	1.35	0.41149
.65	0.24215	1.40	0.41924
.70	0.25804	1.45	0.42647

A	Pr(a)	a	Pr(a)
.75	0.27337	1.50	0.43319
1.55	0.43943	2.30	0..48928
1.60	0.44520	2.35	0.49061
1.65	0.45053	2.40	0.49180
1.70	0.45543	2.45	0.49286
1.75	0.45994	2.55	0.49379
1.80	0.46407	2.60	0.49461
1.85	0.46784	2.65	0.49534
1.90	0.47128	2.70	0.49597
1.95	0.47441	2.75	0.49653
2.00	0.47726	2.80	0.49702
2.05	0.47982	2.85	0.49744
2.10	0.48214	2.90	0.49781
2.15	0.48422	2.95	0.49813
2.20	0.48610	3.00	0.49841
2.25	0.48778		0.49865

Table 2.
Gaussian distribution for chi-square distribution.

Location/geographical region	Clinical suspected census	Laboratory confirmed cases	Positive predictive accuracy
Buguma city/south	161	28	17%
Ido town/south	223	64	30%
Abalama/south East	181	26	15%
Elelelema town/south east	32	6	20%
okpo town/south	13	3	24%
Sama/south east	45	13	30%
Kala-Ekwe town/south	4	2	5%
Efoko/south	33	1	3%
Tombia town/south east	8	0	0%

Table 3.
Data collected from geographical location about laboratory confirmed cases.

5. Results and discussion

The data collected from different geographical location for patients by a physician on malaria epidemic cases were estimated using the developed modified state estimation model for malaria mortality. The measurement statistics are $z:\left(z_1 = 1.5 = \frac{120}{80} mmHg\right)$,

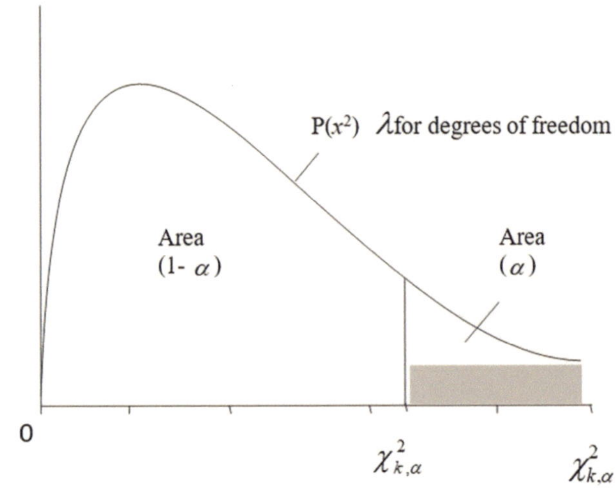

Figure 2.
Gaussian distribution skewed to the right.

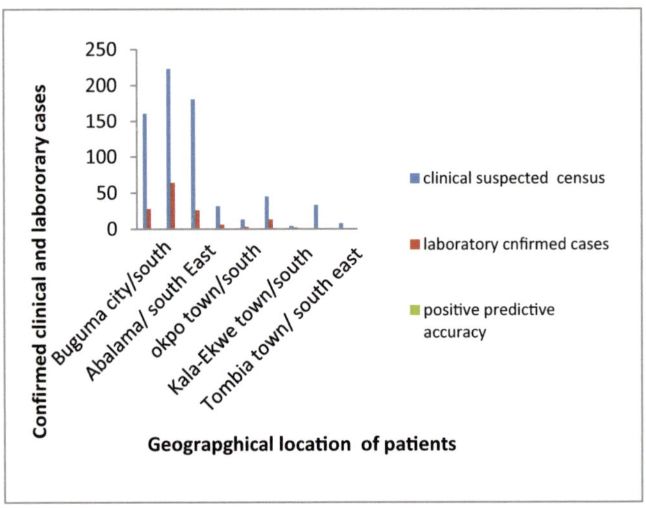

Figure 3.
A bar chart showing clinical/laboratory confirmed cases.

$\left(z_2 = 1.5 = \frac{120}{80}mmHg\right)$, $\left(z_3 = 1.8 = \frac{140}{80}mmHg\right)$, $\left(z_4 = 1.9 = \frac{150}{80}mmHg\right)$ while the estimated measurement the model $\hat{z}$: $(\hat{z}_1 = 1.4759)$,$(\hat{z}_2 = 1.4759)$, and $(\hat{z}_4 = 1.87295)$. The state estimates of the body blood pressure were determined as x_1,x_2 : 8.5225 *and* 13.235 for the respective patients under study, which indicate low-pulse rate or heart rate that required attention, which is also agree with the validated results of the coded matrix laboratory (matlab results) (**Figure 3**).

5.1 Expected values of measurements

We assume that the noise terms e_1, e_2, e_3, *and* e_4 are independent Gaussian random variables with zero means and the respective variances σ_1^2, σ_2^2, σ_3^2 *and* σ_4^2 of the physical

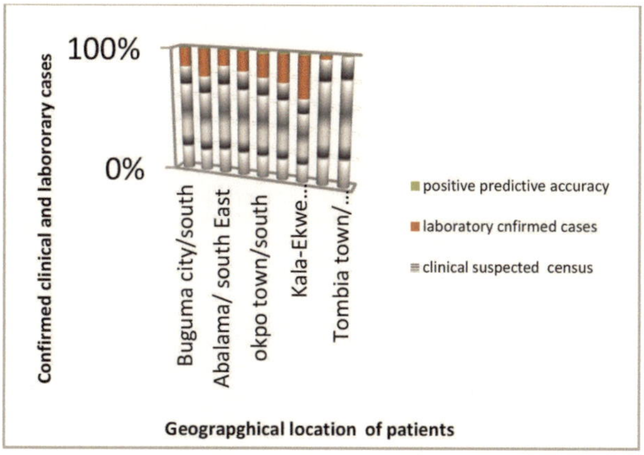

Figure 4.
A chart showing positive prediction for clinical/laboratory cases.

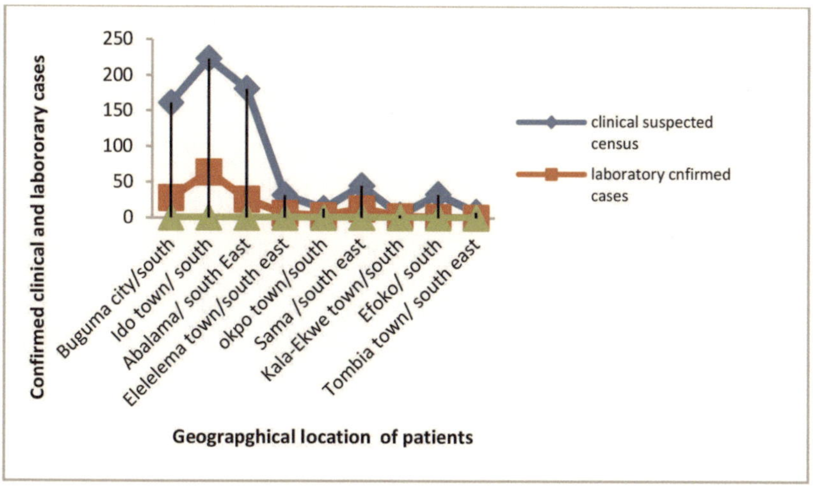

Figure 5.
A line chart showing distribution of clinical/laboratory cases.

measurement are considered (**Figure 4**). Two variables are termed independent when $E(e_ie_j) = 0\, for\ i \neq j$. The zero mean assumption implies that the error in each measurement has equal probability of taking on a positive and negative values of a given magnitudes (**Figure 5**).

The analysis of the vector (e) and its transpose $e^T = [e_1e_2e_3e_4]$ can be represented as (**Figure 6**):

$$e^T = \begin{bmatrix} e_1 \\ e_2 \\ e_3 \\ e_4 \end{bmatrix} [e_1e_2e_3e_4] = \begin{bmatrix} e_1^2 & e_1e_2 & e_1e_3 & e_1e_4 \\ e_2e_1 & e_2^2 & e_2e_3 & e_2e_4 \\ e_3e_1 & e_3e_2 & e_3^2 & e_3e_4 \\ e_4e_1 & e_4e_2 & e_4e_3 & e_4^2 \end{bmatrix} \tag{26}$$

Analysis consideration:

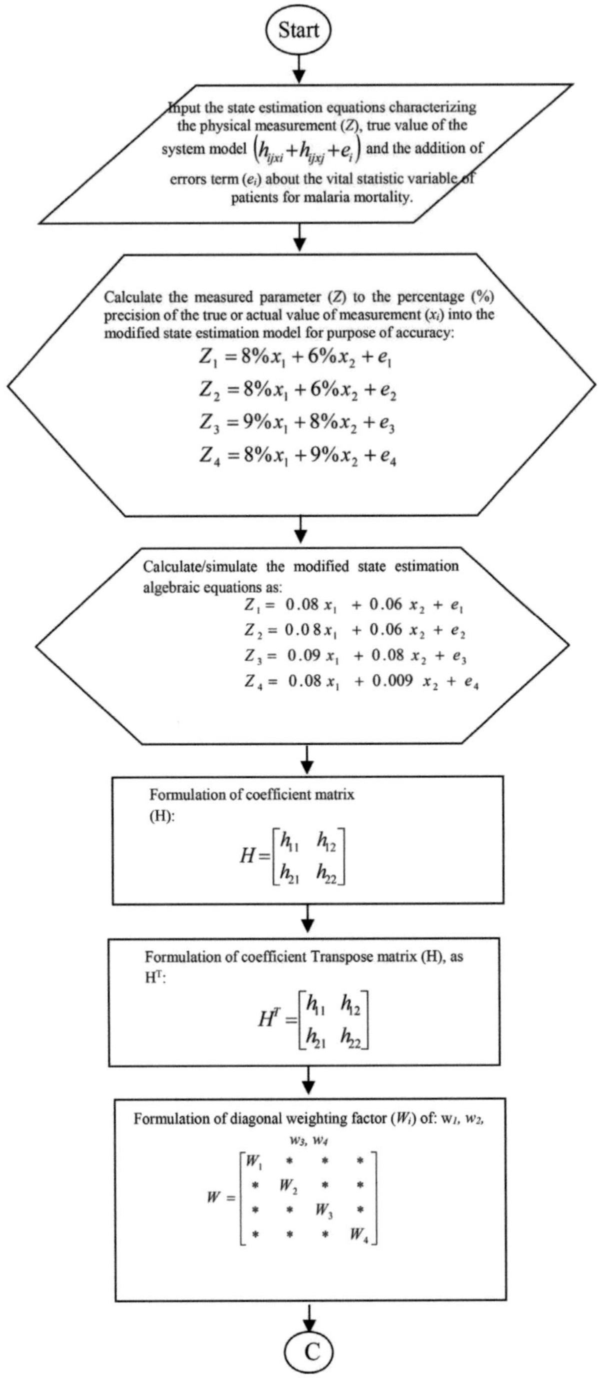
Start
Input the state estimation equations characterizing the physical measurement (Z), true value of the system model $\left(h_{ijxi}+h_{ijxj}+e_i\right)$ and the addition of errors term (e_i) about the vital statistic variable of patients for malaria mortality.
Calculate the measured parameter (Z) to the percentage (%) precision of the true or actual value of measurement (x_i) into the modified state estimation model for purpose of accuracy:
$Z_1 = 8\%x_1 + 6\%x_2 + e_1$
$Z_2 = 8\%x_1 + 6\%x_2 + e_2$
$Z_3 = 9\%x_1 + 8\%x_2 + e_3$
$Z_4 = 8\%x_1 + 9\%x_2 + e_4$
Calculate/simulate the modified state estimation algebraic equations as:
$Z_1 = 0.08\,x_1 + 0.06\,x_2 + e_1$
$Z_2 = 0.08\,x_1 + 0.06\,x_2 + e_2$
$Z_3 = 0.09\,x_1 + 0.08\,x_2 + e_3$
$Z_4 = 0.08\,x_1 + 0.009\,x_2 + e_4$
Formulation of coefficient matrix (H):
$H = \begin{bmatrix} h_{11} & h_{12} \\ h_{21} & h_{22} \end{bmatrix}$
Formulation of coefficient Transpose matrix (H), as H^T:
$H^T = \begin{bmatrix} h_{11} & h_{12} \\ h_{21} & h_{22} \end{bmatrix}$
Formulation of diagonal weighting factor (W_i) of: w_1, w_2, w_3, w_4
$W = \begin{bmatrix} W_1 & * & * & * \\ * & W_2 & * & * \\ * & * & W_3 & * \\ * & * & * & W_4 \end{bmatrix}$
C

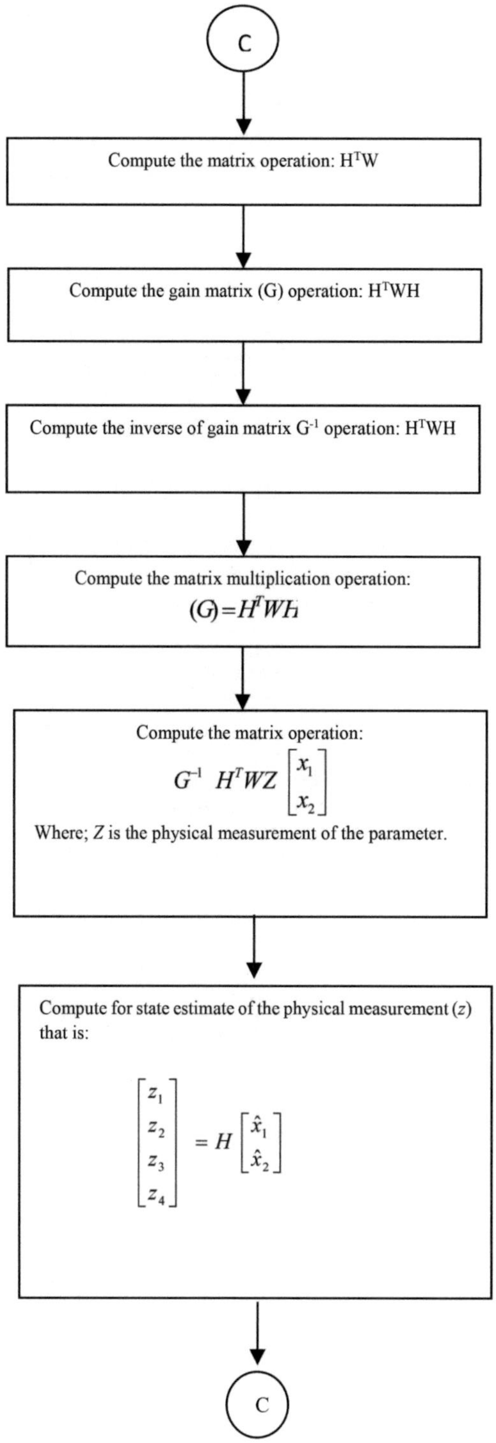
C
Compute the matrix operation: H^TW
Compute the gain matrix (G) operation: H^TWH
Compute the inverse of gain matrix G^{-1} operation: H^TWH
Compute the matrix multiplication operation:
$(G)=H^TWH$
Compute the matrix operation:
$G^{-1}\ H^TWZ\begin{bmatrix}x_1\\x_2\end{bmatrix}$
Where; Z is the physical measurement of the parameter.
Compute for state estimate of the physical measurement (z) that is:
$\begin{bmatrix}z_1\\z_2\\z_3\\z_4\end{bmatrix}=H\begin{bmatrix}\hat{x}_1\\\hat{x}_2\end{bmatrix}$
C

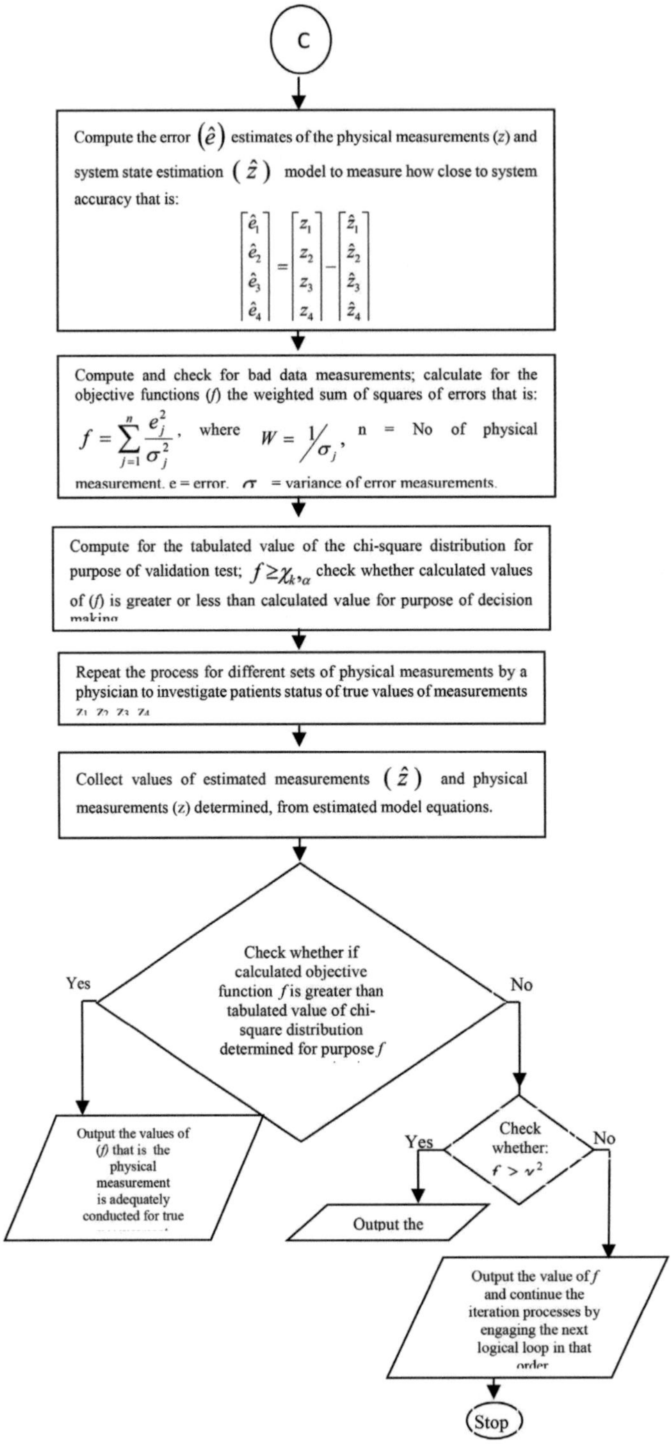

Figure 6.
Algorithms (flow-chart for modified state estimation model for malaria mortality showing different measurement system plan.

- The expected value of ee^T are found by calculating expected value of each entry in the matrix operations.
- The expected value of all the off diagonal events are zero because errors are assumed to be independent, the expected values of the diagonal events are non zero and correspond to the variance: $E\left[e_j^2\right]$ for i from 1 to 4.
- The resultant diagonal matrix are usually assigned the (R) given as:

$$E\left[ee^T\right] = R = \begin{bmatrix} E\left[e_1^2\right] & . & . & . \\ . & E\left[e_2^2\right] & . & . \\ . & . & E\left[e_3^2\right] & . \\ . & . & . & E\left[e_4^2\right] \end{bmatrix} \quad (27)$$

$$= \begin{bmatrix} \sigma_1^2 & . & . & . \\ . & \sigma_2^2 & . & . \\ . & . & \sigma_3^2 & . \\ . & . & . & \sigma_4^2 \end{bmatrix} \quad (28)$$

Evidently, the statistical properties of the weighted least-square estimation provides solution to the measurement (z), which is the sum of the Gaussian random variables (e_1) and the constant term $(h_{11}x_1 + h_{12}x_2)$ which represents the true values Z_{1true} of Z_1. The addition of the constant term to shift the curve of e_1 of the right by the amount of the true value.

Weighting Factor $(\boldsymbol{w})$

The analysis of formulating the objective function (f), the preferential weighting (w_i) is given to be more accurate measurement by choosing the weight (w_i) as the reciprocal of the corresponding to the variance $\left(\delta_j^2\right)$. This means that an errors of smaller variance have greater weight (w), hence we can specify the weighting matrix, (w) as:

$$W = R^{-1} = \begin{bmatrix} 1/\delta_1^2 & . & . & . \\ . & 1/\delta_2^2 & . & . \\ . & . & 1/\delta_3^2 & . \\ . & . & . & 1/\delta_4^2 \end{bmatrix} \quad (29)$$

The, gain matrix becomes

$$(G) = H^T R^{-1} H \quad (30)$$

The weighted sum of square of error as the objective function (f), determination.

The critical value of the statistics f can be determined using the tabulated values of $\chi_{k,\alpha}^2$ for a quantifiable level of significance, k : degree of freedom $(N_m - N_s)$. That is the calculated value can be compared to the tabulated value to measure accuracy which is given as:

$$p_r\left(f \le \chi_{k,\alpha}^2\right) = (1 - \alpha) \quad (31)$$

The weighted sum of squares equation of errors with weight (w_i) choosen equals to the reciprocal of corresponding error δ_j^2 variance which is given as:

$$f = \sum_{j=1}^{N} \frac{e_j^2}{\sigma_j^2} = \frac{(z_1 - h_1(x_1,\ x_2))^2}{\delta_1^2} + \frac{(z_2 - h_2(x_1,\ x_2))^2}{\delta_2^2} + \frac{(z_3 - h_3(x_1,\ x_2))^2}{\delta_3^2} + \frac{(z_4 - h_4(x_1,\ x_2))^2}{\delta_1^2} \tag{32}$$

Where: h_1, h_2, h_3 and h_4 are function that expresses the measured quantities in terms of the state variable while e_1, e_2, e_3 *and* e_4 are Gaussian random variables terms. The true value of χ_1 *amd* χ_2 and not known and have to be estimated from measurement: Z_1, Z_2, Z_3 *and* Z respectively.

Chi-square test statistics (*f*), as a sum of squares of error terms for purpose of validation

The analysis of physical measurement, the chi-square distribution test and validation are required to the check the presence of bad data. Then eliminate any bad data detected and recalculate subsequent resultant state estimation from the determined results.

The objective function (*f*) for chi-square distribution can be presented as:

$$\hat{f} = \sum_{j-1}^{N} \frac{\hat{e}_j^2}{\sigma_j^2} = w_1\hat{e}_1^2 + w_2\hat{e}_2^2 + w_3\hat{e}_3^2 + w_4\hat{e}_4^2 \tag{33}$$

where;

$$w = {}^{1}\!/_{\sigma^2}$$

σ: variance of measurement error

α: quantifiable level of significance for accuracy

$f \leq \chi^2_{\alpha,k}$: for a quantifiable level of significant (α) for a given degree of freedom (k). If f is greater than $\chi^2_{\alpha,k}$ then there is at least suspected bad data measurements in the analysis which required attention.

This means that the suspected measurement instrument (z) must be recalculated and subjected to test statistics and required re-measurement of the vital statistics variables of the system.

This could be traceable to human error, instrument error due to poor calibration, aging of the instrument and temperature/humidity etc.

If $f \leq \chi^2_{\alpha,k}$ is satisfied it is adequate for purpose of physical measurement accuracy, while comparing calculated and tabulated values for validation.

Standardized error estimates

The standardized error estimations can be determined using diagonal elements as:

$$\begin{aligned} \frac{\hat{\mathrm{e}}_1}{\sqrt{\mathrm{R}'_{11}}} &= \mathrm{Sde}_1 \\ \frac{\hat{e}_2}{\sqrt{R'_{22}}} &= Sde_2 \\ \frac{\hat{\mathrm{e}}_3}{\sqrt{\mathrm{R}'_{33}}} &= \mathrm{Sde}_3 \\ \frac{\hat{\mathrm{e}}_4}{\sqrt{\mathrm{R}'_{44}}} &= \mathrm{Sde}_4 \end{aligned} \tag{34}$$

Analysis of measurement for malaria mortality Using modified state estimation model

The measurement equations characterizing the physical status of patient using sphygmomanometer for blood pressure considered the true/actual value of the system model and the addition of error term in the system model were developed. The question is how true is the physical measurement carried out by the physician? Which can be represented as:

$$Z = h_{ij}x_i + \ell_i \tag{35}$$

Z: Measurement of the vital statistics variable of the patients.

h_{ij}: Account for the precision of the measurements to the accuracy of the instruments (how close to the true value).

x_i: Unknown state variable that need to be determined and accounts for the pulse/health rate for blood pressure measurement.

ℓ_i Error term introduced in the measurement which can be expressed mathematically as:

$$Z = h_{11}x_1 + h_{12}x_2 + e_1 \tag{36}$$

Eq. (36), provided the vital statistics variable measurement which is the weighted sum of squared of errors for the Gaussian distribution. Since the physical measurements of the patients is considered as a function of their relative frequency of occurrence, a histogram may be represented which is a continuous curve in relation to the number of occurrence.

Clinical Diagnosis Measurement, geographical location and distribution.

Data were collected from reputable hospitals and clinics from different location for malaria mortality using blood pressure measurements as one of the key associated parameter for the incidence of malaria parasite transmission variable (**Tables 4–6**).

S/N	Location/Geographic region	Clinical suspected census (%)	Laboratory confirmed	Positive predictive accuracy
1	Buguma city/South	161(23)	281 (0)	17% (10–24)
2	Ido town/South	223(32)	64(45)	30% (24–35)
3	Abalama/South East	181(26)	26(18)	15% (10–20)
4	Elelema town/south-Cast	32(5)	6(4)	20% (8–36)
5	Okpo town/south	13(2)	3(2)	24%(6–54)
6	Same south-east	45(6)	13 (9)	30%(16–44)
7	Kala Ekwe town/south	4(0.6)	2(1)	5%(7–93)
8	Efoko/South	33(5)	1(0.7)	3%(0.1–16)
9	Tombia/South	8(1)	0	0%(0–37)
	Total	700	143	

Table 4.
Distribution of suspected and confirmed cases of malaria parasites (plasmodium) according to the province in a developing countries.

S/N	Vital statistics variables for measuring transmitted cases of malaria parasite (plasmodium) etc	Blood (BP) Pressure Measurement	Accepted standard for blood pressure measurement.
1	Measurement 1; patients - A: Abuja City in Nigeria	$\frac{120}{80}mmHg = 1.5$	Ok (normal)
2	Measurement 2; patients –B Buguma City in Nigeria	$\frac{120}{80}mmHg = 1.5$	Ok (normal)
3	Measurement 3; Patients –C Lagos City in Nigeria	$\frac{140}{80}mmHg = 1.8$	Required attension
4	Measurement 4: Patients – D Port Harcourt City in Nigeria	$\frac{150}{80}mmHg = 1.9$	Required attension

Table 5.
Blood pressure measurement (Sphygmomano-meter) for purpose of incidence of malaria parasite transmission.

S/N	Measurements instrument Sphygmomanometer (BP)	Precision to the accuracy of measurements instruments
1	Measurements 1, Blood pressures for pulse rate estimation –Abuja City in Nigeria	8% & 6% to the true values of the system model measured
2	Measurement 2, blood pressure for pulse rate estimation – Buguma City in Nigeria	8% & 6% to the true values of the systems model measured
3	Measurements 3, blood pressure for pulse rate, estimation –Lagos city in Nigeria	9% & 6% to the true values of the systems model measured
4	Measurement 4, blood pressure for pulse rate estimation – Port Harcourt City in Nigeria.	8% & 9% to the true values of the system model measured

Table 6.
Sphygmomanometer measurement and precision for true (actual value of measurement) for associated malaria parasite transmission.

Measurements Matrix, (Z) equation given as:

$$[Z] = \begin{bmatrix} Z_1 \\ Z_2 \\ Z_3 \\ Z_4 \end{bmatrix} = \begin{bmatrix} \frac{120}{80}mmHg = 1.5 \\ \frac{120}{80}mmHg = 1.5 \\ \frac{140}{80}mmHg = 1.8 \\ \frac{150}{80}mmHg = 1.9 \end{bmatrix} \tag{37}$$

Measurements error (e) given as:

$$[e] = \begin{bmatrix} e_1 \\ e_2 \\ e_3 \\ e_4 \end{bmatrix} = \text{To be determined} \tag{38}$$

True value of system model term given as:

$$\left[h_{ij}x_{ij}\right] = h_{11}x_1 + h_{12}x_2 + e_1 \tag{39}$$

Measurement instruments precisions to the accuracy of true/actual value give as:

$$Z_1 = 8\%x_1 + 6\%x_2 + e_1 \tag{40}$$

$$Z_2 = 8\%x_1 + 6\%x_2 + e_2 \tag{41}$$

$$Z_3 = 9\%x_1 + 8\%x_2 + e_3 \tag{42}$$

$$Z_4 = 8\%x_1 + 9\%x_2 + e_4 \tag{43}$$

Eqs. (40), (41), (42), (43) can be represented as:

$$Z_1 = 0.08x_1 + 0.06x_2 + e_1 \tag{44}$$

$$Z_2 = 0.08x_1 + 0.06x_2 + e_2 \tag{45}$$

$$Z_3 = 0.09x_1 + 0.08x_2 + e_3 \tag{46}$$

$$Z_4 = 0.08x_1 + 0.09x_2 + e_4 \tag{47}$$

Where; x_1 *and* x_2 and are the state variable that is unknown that needed to be determined

Case 1: Formulations of the Coefficient matrix (H) which can be represented as:

$$H = \begin{bmatrix} 0.08 & 0.06 \\ 0.08 & 0.06 \\ 0.09 & 0.08 \\ 0.08 & 0.09 \end{bmatrix} \tag{48}$$

Case 2: Weighting factor for measuring instrument (w_i) which can be presented in diagonal matrix form as:

$$w_i = \begin{bmatrix} 100 & . & . & . \\ . & 100 & . & . \\ . & . & 50 & . \\ . & . & . & 50 \end{bmatrix} \tag{49}$$

Where

$$w_i = w_1, w_2, w_3, w_4$$

The weighing factor (w) for the measurement instrument w_1, w_2, w_3, w_4 are 100, 100, 50, 50

Case 3: Determine nation of transpose of coefficient matrix (H) given as:

$$H^T = \begin{bmatrix} 0.08 & 0.08 & 0.09 & 0.08 \\ 0.06 & 0.06 & 0.08 & 0.09 \end{bmatrix} \tag{50}$$

Case 4: Compute the matrix operation $H^T W$ as:

$$H^T W = \begin{bmatrix} 0.08 & 0.08 & 0.09 & 0.08 \\ 0.06 & 0.06 & 0.08 & 0.09 \end{bmatrix} \begin{bmatrix} 100 & . & . & . \\ . & 100 & . & . \\ . & . & 50 & . \\ . & . & . & 50 \end{bmatrix} \tag{51}$$

$$= \begin{bmatrix} 8 & 8 & 4.5 & 4 \\ 6 & 6 & 4 & 4.5 \end{bmatrix} \tag{52}$$

Case 5: Determination of gain matrix (G) given as:

$$\mathrm{G} = \mathrm{H^T W H}$$

Thus

$$G = \begin{bmatrix} 8 & 8 & 4 & 4 \\ 6 & 6 & 4 & 4.5 \end{bmatrix} \begin{bmatrix} 0.08 & 0.06 \\ 0.08 & 0.06 \\ 0.09 & 0.08 \\ 0.08 & 0.09 \end{bmatrix} \tag{53}$$

This implies;

$$G = H^T W H = \begin{bmatrix} 2.005 & 1.68 \\ 1.68 & 1.445 \end{bmatrix} \tag{54}$$

Case 6: Determination of Inverse of gain matrix (G) given as:

$$G^{-1} = \frac{I}{|G|} = \begin{bmatrix} 2.005 & 1.68 \\ 1.68 & 1.445 \end{bmatrix} \tag{55}$$

$$|\mathrm{G}| = 0.074825$$

$$G^{-1} = \frac{I}{0.074825} = \begin{bmatrix} 1.445 & -1.68 \\ -1.68 & 2.005 \end{bmatrix} \tag{56}$$

or

$$G^{-1} = \begin{bmatrix} 19.3 & -22.45 \\ -22.45 & 26.9 \end{bmatrix} \tag{57}$$

Case 7: Determination of multiplication of inverse operation of gain matrix (G^{-1}) and $H^T W$ given as:

$$G^{-1} H^T W = \begin{bmatrix} 19.3 & -22.45 \\ -22.45 & 26.8 \end{bmatrix} \begin{bmatrix} 8 & 8 & 4.5 & 4 \\ 6 & 6 & 4 & 4.5 \end{bmatrix} \tag{58}$$

This implies

$$G^{-1} H^T W = \begin{bmatrix} 19.7 & 19.7 & -2.95 & -23.825 \\ -18.8 & -18.8 & 6.175 & 30.8 \end{bmatrix} \tag{59}$$

Case 8: Determination of matrix operation $\left(G^{-1}H^TWZ\right)$ given as:

$$G^{-1}H^TWZ = \begin{bmatrix} 19.7 & 19.7 & -2.95 & -23.825 \\ -18.8 & -18.8 & 6.175 & 30.8 \end{bmatrix} \begin{bmatrix} 1.5 \\ 1.5 \\ 1.8 \\ 1.9 \end{bmatrix} \tag{60}$$

Where; $G^{-1}H^TWZ$ is represented as the matrix operations determination of the state variables estimate $\hat{x}_1$ *and* $\hat{x}_2$ given as:

$$\begin{bmatrix} \hat{x}_1 \\ \hat{x}_2 \end{bmatrix} = G^{-1}H^TWZ = \begin{bmatrix} 8.5225 \\ 13.235 \end{bmatrix} \tag{61}$$

Case 9: Determination of the matrix operation Hx as a function of the estimate of the physical measurements $(Z_1Z_2Z_3Z_4)$ given as:

$$\hat{Z} = H\hat{X} \tag{62}$$

$$Similarly, \begin{bmatrix} \hat{Z}_1 \\ \hat{Z}_2 \\ \hat{Z}_3 \\ \hat{Z}_4 \end{bmatrix} = H \begin{bmatrix} X_1 \\ X_2 \end{bmatrix} \tag{63}$$

Where;

$$H = \begin{bmatrix} 0.08 & 0.06 \\ 0.08 & 0.06 \\ 0.09 & 0.08 \\ 0.08 & 0.09 \end{bmatrix}, \hat{x} = \begin{bmatrix} X_1 \\ X_2 \end{bmatrix} = \begin{bmatrix} 8.5225 \\ 13.235 \end{bmatrix} \tag{64}$$

Thus; the estimates of the measurement $\left(\hat{Z}\right)$ becomes as:

$$\begin{bmatrix} \hat{Z}_1 \\ \hat{Z}_2 \\ \hat{Z}_3 \\ \hat{Z}_4 \end{bmatrix} = \begin{bmatrix} 0.08 & 0.06 \\ 0.08 & 0.06 \\ 0.09 & 0.08 \\ 0.08 & 0.09 \end{bmatrix} \begin{bmatrix} 8.5225 \\ 13.235 \end{bmatrix} \tag{65}$$

This implies as:

$$\begin{bmatrix} \hat{Z}_1 \\ \hat{Z}_2 \\ \hat{Z}_3 \\ \hat{Z}_4 \end{bmatrix} = \begin{bmatrix} 1.4759 \\ 1.4759 \\ 1.825825 \\ 1.87295 \end{bmatrix} \tag{66}$$

Case 10: Determination of number of physical measurement (N_m) and states variable (N_s) on the view to determine redundancy (K) for a quantifiable level of significance.

$N_m = Z_1, Z_2, Z_3$ *and* $Z_4 = 4$ (four physical measurements)
$N_s = x_1 \& x_2 = 2$ (blood pressure for pulse/heart rate)

$$\text{Redundancy}(K) = N_m - N_s = 4 - 2 = 2 \tag{67}$$

Case 11: Determination of errors estimates$(\hat{e})$ of the physical measurements and estimated measurements$(\hat{z})$ are presented as:

$$\hat{e} = [Physical\ measurement\ (Z)] - [estimated\ measurement\ (\hat{z})] \tag{68}$$

That is;

$$\begin{bmatrix} \hat{e}_1 \\ \hat{e}_2 \\ \hat{e}_3 \\ \hat{e}_4 \end{bmatrix} = \begin{bmatrix} Z_1 \\ Z_2 \\ Z_3 \\ Z_4 \end{bmatrix} - \begin{bmatrix} \hat{Z}_1 \\ \hat{Z}_2 \\ \hat{Z}_3 \\ \hat{Z}_4 \end{bmatrix} \tag{69}$$

Where

$$\begin{bmatrix} Z_1 \\ Z_2 \\ Z_3 \\ Z_4 \end{bmatrix} = \begin{bmatrix} 1.5 = 120/80mmHg \\ 1.5 = 120/80mmHg \\ 1.8 = 140/80mmHg \\ 1.9 = 180/80mmHg \end{bmatrix}; \begin{bmatrix} \hat{Z}_1 \\ \hat{Z}_2 \\ \hat{Z}_3 \\ \hat{Z}_4 \end{bmatrix} = \begin{bmatrix} 1.4759 \\ 1.4759 \\ 1.825825 \\ 1.87295 \end{bmatrix} \tag{70}$$

Thus,

$$\begin{bmatrix} \hat{e}_1 \\ \hat{e}_2 \\ \hat{e}_3 \\ \hat{e}_4 \end{bmatrix} = \begin{bmatrix} 0.0241 \\ 0.0241 \\ -0.025525 \\ 0.02705 \end{bmatrix} \tag{71}$$

Case 12: Determination of sum of Squared of Errors (e) Measurement

If calculated weighted sums of squares of errors calculated $(f_{calculated})$ is greater than chi-square distribution it can be deduced that there is suspected error (or bad data in the measurement sets).

Similarly,

If calculated objective function $(f_{calculated})$ is less than chi-square distribution value, it is concluded or declared a violations which does not satisfy the measurements criteria for decision making for purpose of diagnosing human body conditions.

6. Results and discussion

Case 13. Estimate of measurements error (e)

The objectives function (f) of the weighted sum of squares of errors can be presented as:

$$\mathrm{f} = \sum_{j=1}^{n} \frac{e_j^2}{\sigma_j^2} = 100(e_1)^2 + 100(e_2)^2 + 50(e_3)^2 + 50(e_4)^2$$

$$\text{where} : e_1 = 0.0241, e_2 = 0.0241, e_3 = -0.025525, e_4 = 0.02705$$

$$f = \sum_{j=1}^{n} \frac{e_j^2}{\sigma_j^2} = 100(0.0241)^2 + 100(0.0241)^2 + 50(-0.025525)^2 + 50(0.02705)^2$$

$$= 100(0.00058081) + 100(0.00058081) + 50(0.000651525625) + 50(0.0007317025)$$

$$= 0.058081 + 0.058081 + 0.03257628125 + 0.036585125$$

$$= 0.185323125$$

Similarly,

The chi-square distribution from tabulated results given as: $\left(\chi^2_{k,\alpha} = 9.21\right)$

$$f_{\text{calculated}} \leq \chi^2_{k,\alpha}$$

where;

$$K = N_m - N_s = 4 - 2 = 2$$

For, α = 1% quantifiable level of significant = 0.01($\alpha = 0.01$)
(Significance level, $\alpha = 0.01$)

The probability of $((1 - \alpha) = (1 - 0.01)) = 99\%$ declared confidence level for a degree of freedom, $K = N_m - N_s = 2$

From the tabulated result obtained for a given degree of freedom and a quantifiable level of significance of $\alpha = 0.01$, for $k = 2$ given as 9.21 which means that the calculated value of $(f_{calculated})$ is greater than the critical value of the chi-square distribution value. Thus, the chi-square of f provides a test statistics for validating the error measurements of bad data or probably suspected adverse health condition that required attensions for purpose of ensuring good status healthy conditions.

```
%MATTIX LABORATORY
%PROGRAM: MATLAB FOR MALARIA MORTALITY
%AUTHUR: BRAIDE, SEPIRIBO LUCKY
%TECHNICAL PAPER PORESENTAION
%First iteration calculation using a flat start values (,k,t which
%represent the static variables x1 and x2);
k = 1;
t = 1;
% measurement instrument represented as z: z1 z2 z3 z4
z1 = 1.5;
z2 = 1.5;
z3 = 1.8;
z4 = 1.9;
z = [1.5; 1.5; 1.8; 1.9];
% estimated measurement represented as zk1 zk2 zk3 zk4
zk1 = 1.4759;
zk2 = 1.4759;
zk3 = 1.825825;
zk4 = 1.87295;
% measurement error represented as e1 e2 e3 e4
e1 = z1-zk1;
e2 = z2-zk2;
```

```
e3 = z3-zk3;
e4 = z4-zk4;
% Jacobianmatrix represented as H
H = [0.08 0.06;0.08 0.06;0.09 0.08;0.08 0.09];
%Transpose of jacobian matrix T represented as H
T = H'
% Diagonal matrix of the weighting factor as W
W = [100,0,0,0; 0,100,0,0;0,0,50,0;0,0,0,50];

% MUutiply Transpose of jacobian matrix H' and weighting factor W as
D=H'*W

% Multiply the matrix operation D and jacobian matrix H to obtain gain matrix
represented as
G = D*H
% The inverse of gain matrix G represented as F
F = inv.(G)
% multiply the matrix operation F and matrix D be represented as
M = F*D

% multiply matrix M and Z representation as N = M*Z state variable [xi x2]

% Determination of matrix operation of state estimation [x1 x2] = N
for z = [1.5; 1.5; 1.8; 1.9];
v = M*z
end
T =
0.0800 0.0800 0.0900 0.0800
0.0600 0.0600 0.0800 0.0900
D =
8.0000 8.0000 4.5000 4.0000
6.0000 6.0000 4.0000 4.5000
G =
2.0050 1.6800
1.6800 1.4450
F =
19.3117–22.4524
−22.4524 26.7959
M =
19.7795 19.7795–2.9068-23.7888
−18.8440-18.8440 6.1477 30.7718
v =
8.9075
13.0003
```

7. Recommendation

Considering the fact that health is wealth the relationship between the two is frequently misconstrued. That is there is strong need for healthy living to create wealth for man and society.

Measurement of malaria endemictiy is basically on vector or parasites measurement especially for infected cases on transmission of plasmodium parasite etc. which may seriously leads to some vital sign and symptom: Temperature rise beyond normal level, headache, blood pressure become abnormal, blood-sugar concentration level may also be affected medically etc.

Evidently, the mapping of malaria transmission have demonstrated a wider geographical distribution of the parasite (plasmodium, etc). The number of clinical report cases due to malaria infection resulted into early mortality which is becoming an increase on daily basis across the world. Particularly in south America, where *P. Vivax* is currently the most predominant malaria species. Although control measures and programs have had a significant impact on malaria associated cases. Consequently the centers for disease control and prevention (CDC) Saving lives, protecting people in various states of America have considered regular, rapid and accurate diagnosis of malaria which is an integral part to the appropriate treatment of affected individuals. It is also requested that the CDC: Health care providers should always obtain a travel history form patients, especially person who traveled in a malaria epidemic area, must be evaluated for check using appropriate tests (for malaria) for purpose of healthy free environment. This technical paper having carried out thorough extensive investigation especially to this robust medically affected case of earthly malaria mortality for man which may also be associated to bad measurement for vital statistics variables about a patients. The detail history of patients measured must be checked for accurate, precision, tolerance, error etc. to the true value declared by standard world health organization (like WHO etc). Therefore physical measurements taken by medical practioner from patient must:

i. Regularly check for instrument calibration measurement for effectiveness before drug prescription/administration.

ii. Consider and satisfy many associated variables measurement to the particular emergence of incidence of malaria species before placing drugs administration and dispensing to avoid over-does or under-dose problems which may leads to early malaria mortality.

iii. Considering adequate treatments procedures for malaria cases which may depends on disease severity, species of malaria parasites infections on the view to determine the organism that is resistant to certain anti-malarial drugs in order to provide adequate alternative provisions.

iv. Check for vaccine effectiveness to affected cases of malaria patients particularly to age, sex, community (habitant or group of people) and other associated multivariable's parameter like vaccination histories etc. to avoid gradual destruction of sensitive organs like liver and kidney etc.

v. Check for bad data measurement: the status of human body state which may be affected by surrounding circumstances, aging of measuring instrument, human error, temperature/humidity, sensitivity of measurement etc.

vi. This work can also be extended to include the estimation of malaria mortality the estimation of malaria mortality and recovery rates of plasmodium falciparium parasitaemic, using the model equations:

The transition rates: h *and* r can be estimated from transition frequencies: α *and* β with

$$\hat{h} = \frac{\alpha}{t(\alpha + \beta)} \ln \frac{1}{1 - (\alpha - \beta)}$$

$$\hat{r} = \frac{\beta}{t(\alpha - \beta)} \ln \frac{1}{1 - (\alpha + \beta)}$$

Where;
t : time interval for estimation
h : incidence rate
r : recovery rate

8. Conclusion

The analysis of modified state estimation model is developed for estimated measurement of malaria mortality in a case of a developing countries. This model help to identify detect and flag measurement error which is classified as bad data measurement; whose result may be received on drug prescription and administration for early malaria mortality rate especially when measurement instruments are not regularly calibrated for efficiency. This technical paper for purpose of analysis and scope considered the associated vital statistic variables like blood-pressure (BP) using sphygmomanometer as a key driver for this analysis. The techniques establishes a mathematical modified state estimation model that characterizes the physical measurement of the patient to the acceptable value of $\left(BP = \frac{120}{80} mmHg\right)$ in order to satisfy the operating normal conditions.

The true value of the system model equations and error term addition are considered for purpose of estimating measurements made by physician instrument. Data were collected from four (4) geographical area in a developing countries for purpose of validation of the modified estimation model. The techniques allow for an algebraic summation operation of measurement for the weighted sum provided the declared standard measurement of blood pressure of $\left(\frac{120mm}{80} Hg \text{ is not violated}\right)$.

The analysis technical paper identified bad data measurement which required urgent attention for check: The surrounding circumstance of the patients, human error, calibration error etc. for the purpose of determining the state of the body system configuration.

The paper also validated this work research via the objective function (f) as the calculated value versus chi-square distribution (tabular form) for 99% level of significance with 2 degree of freedom in quantitative measures.

This paper also establishes a string conformity, uniquencie and synergy between measured ad estimated measurements which eventually validated with objective function calculated (f) and chi-square distribution and between matrix operations and matrix laboratory code programs for a test statistics.

Author details

Sepiribo Lucky Braide
Department of Electrical Engineering, Rivers State University, Port Harcourt, Rivers State, Nigeria

*Address all correspondence to: braidesepiribo@yahoo.com; sepiribo.braide@ust.edu.ng

References

[1] World Health Organization. Global Malaria Programme: World Malaria report. 2011. Available from: http://www.who.int/malaria/World malaria/WMR2011noprofiles lowres.pdf

[2] Braide SL, Idoniboyeobu DC. Determinants of estimated measurement for malaria mortality using modified state estimation model in a case of a developing country. In: Proceedings of the World Congress on Engineering and Computer Science. San Francisco, USA; WCECS; 22-24 Oct 2019. ISBN: 978-988-14048-79, ISSN: 2078-0966 (Online)

[3] Guerra CA, Snow RW, Hay SI. Mapping the global extent of malaria In 2005. Trends Parasltology. 2006;**22**: 353-358

[4] Marques AC. Human migration and the spread of malaria in Brazil. Parasitology Today. 1987;**3**:166-170

[5] Alves FP, Durlacher RR, Menezes MJ, Kriger H, Silva LHP, et al. High prevalence of asymptomatic *plasmodium* wax and *plat* infections in native amazonian populations. The American Journal of Tropical Medicine and Hygiene. 2002;**66**:641-648

[6] Qliveira-Ferr Bira J, Lacerda MVO, Brasil P, Ladislau JLB, Tauil PL, et al. Malaria in Brazil: an overview. Malaria Journal. 2010;**9**:115

[7] Coura JR, Suarez-Mutis M, Ladeia-Andrade S. A new challenge for malaria control in Brazil: Asymptomatic *plasmodium* infection. Memorias do Instituto Oswaldo Cruz. 2006;**101**:229-237

[8] Braide SL, Idoniboyeobu DC. Gas turbine blade reliability of generator availability for electric power supply using optimal estimation of Weilbull probability distribution. Internal Journal of Scientific & Engineering Research. 2022;**13**(3):340-357

[9] Price RN, Tjitra E, Gunrra CA, Young S, Whlto NJ, et al. Vivax malaria; neglected and not benign. The American Journal of Trc Hygiene. 2007;**77**:79-87

[10] Guerra CA, Howes RE, Patll AP, Gething PW, Van Boeckel TP, et al. The international limits and population at risk of *Plasmadi* transmission in 2009. PLoS Neglected Tropical Diseases. 2010;**4**:e774

[11] Braide SL, Idoniboyeobu DC. Development of error estimation model (ESM) for radial distribution system. International Journal of Academic Research. Sept 2011;**3**(5):439-452

[12] Mueller I, Gallnski MR, Baird JK, Carlton JM, Kochar DK, et al. Key gaps in the knowledge of *plasmodium vivax,* a neglected h parasite. The Lancet Infectious Diseases. 2009;**9**:555-566

[13] Ladeia-Andrade S, Ferreira MU, De Carvalho ME, Curado I, Coura JR. Age-dependent acquisition of protective immunity to man populations of the Amazon Basin of Brazil. The American Journal of Tropical Medicine and Hygiene. 2009;**80**:452-459

[14] Silva-Nunes M, Moreno M, Conn JE, Gamboa D, Abeles S, et al. Amazonian malaria: Asymptomatic human reservoirs, diagno environmentally driven changes in mosquito vector populations, and tho mandate for sustainable control strategies. Acta Tropica. 2012;**121**(3):281-291

[15] Brasil P, Costa AP, Pedro RS, Bressan CS, Silva S, et al. Unexpectedly long incubation period of *plasmodium vivax* malaria, in chamoprophylaxis, in patients diagnosed outside the transmission area in Brazil. Malaria Journal. 2011;**10**:122

Section 4

Malaria Prevention

Chapter 6

Bio-Efficacy of Insecticide-Treated Bednets (ITNs) Distributed through the Healthcare Facilities in a Boundary Community in Nigeria

Ezihe K. Ebuka, Emmanuel Obi, Nwangwu C. Udoka, Ukonze B. Chikaodili, Nwankwo N. Edith, Udezue Nkemakonam, Egbuche M. Chukwudi and Okeke C. Peter

Abstract

This study was conducted to evaluate the susceptibility and efficacy of three insecticidal treated bednets; Olyset®, PermaNet2.0® and MAGNet® collected from the different health facilities, against *Anopheles* mosquitoes under laboratory conditions. PermaNet3.0 was used as a positive control. Larval collections were carried out and reared at the insectary of National Arbovirus and Vector Research Centre, Enugu State. *Anopheles Kisumu* mosquitoes were used as the standard control in the cone bioassay test. The bioassay showed that the wild *An. gambiae* s.l. and *An. gambiae* Kisumu strains were susceptible (100% mortality) to the PermaNet3.0® used as positive control while the wild-caught *Anopheles* were resistant to the mono-treated ITNs. The mortality effect of the net brands showed that the brands have a statistically significant effect on the mosquito mortality after 24 hours F (2, 18) = 14.32, $p < .001$), while the sides of the net did not have a statistically significant effect on the mosquito mortality (F (3, 18) = 1.67, $p = .209$). This study also suggests the need to develop and adopt routine monitoring of the ITNs at the health facilities, as it will inform the replacement of ineffective nets. However, a mass campaign of PBO nets is necessary for the state to achieve and maintain the universal coverage of ITNs.

Keywords: bednet, efficacy, bioassay, malaria, Nigeria

1. Introduction

Noticeable progress has been made in the fight against malaria and most of this progress can be attributed to the scale-up of malaria control interventions. The interventions include insecticidal treated nets (ITN), indoor residual spraying

(IRS), chemo-prevention for pregnant women and children and treatment with artemesinin-based combination therapy [1]. Insecticide-treated nets (ITNs) are a widely used tool that has been proven to be effective in the prevention and control of malaria in malaria endemic countries [2].

ITNs are mosquito nets treated with insecticides that do not require any re-impregnation. They are designed to retain their efficacy against mosquito vectors for a minimum of 3 years or 20 standard washes under laboratory conditions [3, 4]. However, it has been recommended that ITNs should be made available to all individuals at risk in endemic areas, regardless of age, universal access [5, 6], which is defined as the availability of one mosquito net for every two individuals [7]. Of the 663 million cases that were avoided owing to malaria control interventions between 2001 and 2015 in sub-Saharan Africa, it is estimated that 69% were circumvented with the use of ITNs, 21% with artemisinin-based combination therapy, and 10% with IRS [8].

Between 2008 and 2016, more than 1 billion ITNs have been distributed in Africa through mass campaigns and replacement programmes; and the scale-up has contributed immensely to the drop in malaria incidence by 68% [9, 10]. WHO recommends that countries maintain universal coverage through a combination of health facility distribution and continuous distribution through community-based channels [3].

Monitoring the insecticide performance of the ITNs distributed through a mass campaign is a priority for the Integrated Vector Management (IVM) sub-committee of the National Malaria Elimination Programme (NMEP), as studies have confirmed insecticide survival time rate of 3–4 years in Nigeria [11], 2.5 years in Tanzania [12], 3.1–3.3 years in Zanzibar [13] and 2.5–3 years in Zambia [14].

The study aims to determine the insecticidal effectiveness of the net sides and brands (PermaNet 2.0®, Olyset® net and MAGNet®) distributed through the primary healthcare facilities in the boundary community with known high pyrethroid resistance status using the WHO cone bioassay. The study also intends to compare the efficacy of the mono-treated nets (PermaNet 2.0®, Olyset® net and MAGNet®) with a PBO net (PermaNet3.0®).

2. Methodology

A cross sectional study on the efficacy of different sides and brands of ITNs (PermaNet2.0®, Olyset® and MAGNet) collected from the Primary Health Care (PHC) Centres were assayed. The PHCs includes Amechi-Idodo Health Centre, Ohani (6.44326'N, 7.71239′E) and Eziama Health Centre (6.41989'N, 7.71880′E) in Amechi-Idodo, Nkanu East of Enugu state, Nigeria. Two nets of each of the 3 net brands were collected from the health facility for the assessment.

Mosquito larvae were collected from the four communities (Eziobodo, Obinagu, Eziama and Ohani) in Amechi Idodo. A geo-referenced map of the collection points was created to show that these villages are contiguous as well as borders Ebonyi State, Nigeria as seen in **Figure 1**.

3. Collection of *Anopheles* mosquito larvae

The test requires a 2–5-day old female adult mosquito so the larval population of *Anopheles* mosquitoes were collected from the four communities. The larvae were

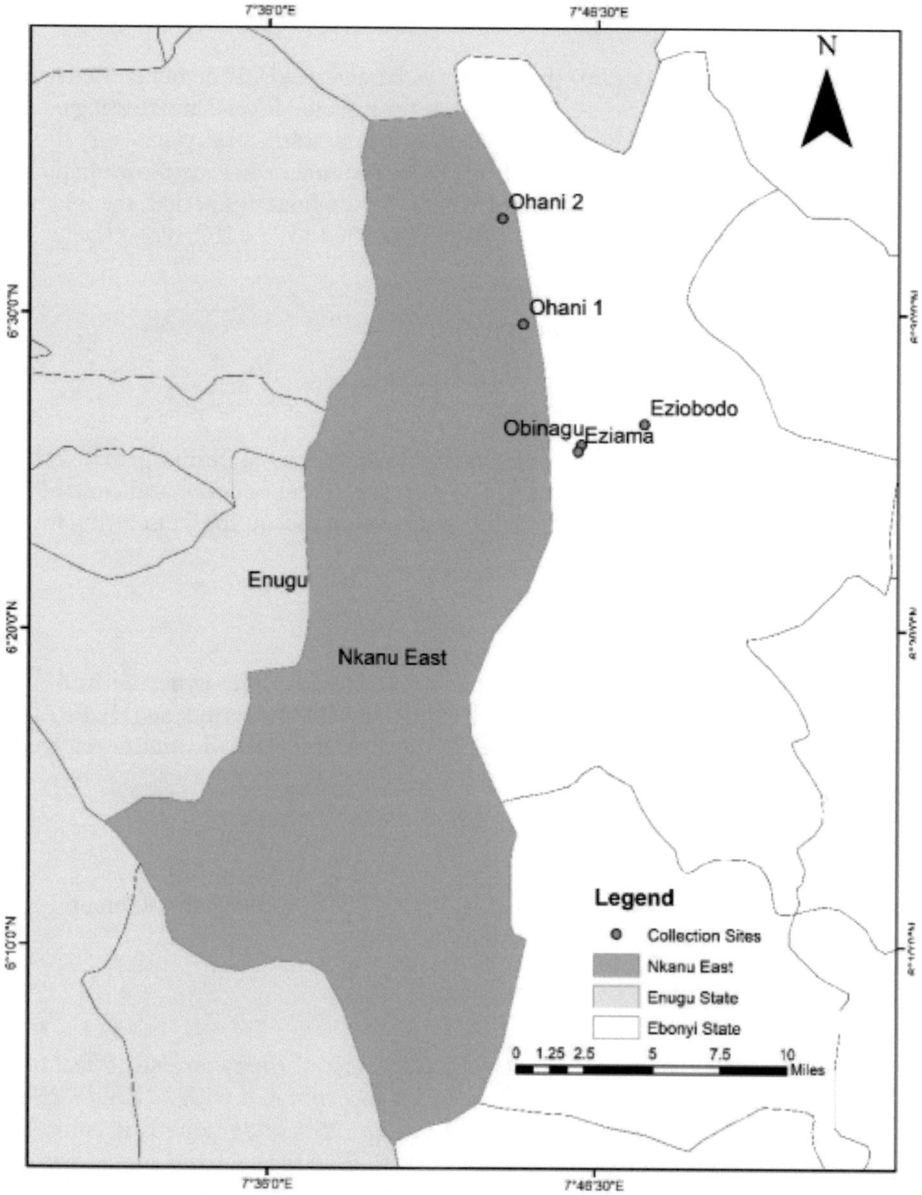

Figure 1.
Map of larval collection sites in Amaechi-Idodo, Nkanu east L.G.a.

collected according to the method of Service (1993). The larvae collected from sunlit, open pools were carefully transferred in a slightly covered container to the insectary of National Arbovirus and Research Centre Enugu (NAVRC) where they were reared to adult.

The field-collected larvae were reared to the adult stage with part of the water from the breeding habitat according to Chukwuekezie et al. [15]. Care was taken to remove all the predators from the collections.

4. *Anopheles gambiae* Kisumu colony used as standard

A. gambiae s.s. (Kisumu strain) that has been characterized and demonstrated to be susceptible to insecticides was used for the bioassay. Insecticide resistance testing using the WHO test procedure [16] on the *An. gambiae* Kisumu strain takes place every three months to ascertain that the susceptibility of the mosquitoes to insecticides is maintained. The strain is colonized at the insectary of NAVRC, Throughout this period, the relative humidity and temperature were maintained at 80 ± 10% and 25 ± 2°C, respectively.

5. Test insecticide treated nets (ITNs)

5.1 Olyset net

Olyset® net is a pre-qualified net by WHO with 2% w/w of permethrin insecticide incorporated into the fibers of the nets. The net uses hybrid polymer and controlled insecticide release technology to repel, kill and prevent mosquitos from biting for up to five years.

5.2 MAGNet®

MAGNet® net is also a pre-qualified net by WHO with alpha-cypermethrin insecticide incorporated with the 150-denier high density Polyethylene (HDPE) filament which diffuses to the surface of the net slowly and this small amount released is enough to kill a mosquito.

5.3 PermaNet®

PermaNet 2.0® is a pre-qualified net by WHO. It is a knitted poly filament polyester fiber which are infused with deltamethrin.

5.4 PermaNet3.0®

PermaNet3.0® was used as positive control because of the synergistic effect of the PBO. It is made mainly of polyethylene fabric incorporated with 2.1 g/kg ± 25% of deltamethrin alone (on the upper sides) and 4 g/kg ± 25% of deltamethrin combined with 25 g/kg of a synergist piperonyl butoxide (PBO) on the roof and coated with 2.8 g/kg ± 25% of deltamethrin on the lower sides, also called borders. The lower sides are reinforced with polyester fabric [17].

5.5 Cone test

The WHO cone bioassay was carried out at the Entomology Laboratory of the National Arbovirus and Vectors Research Centre, Enugu. The cone test was used to assess the insecticidal effectiveness of the three WHO pre-qualified ITNs. The test was conducted following the WHO protocol. Four sub-samples (replicates namely the sides A, side B, Side C and the Roof) measuring 25 cm × 25 cm were cut from each of the three nets as indicated in **Figure 2**. The same net sides as seen in **Figure 2** were cut from an untreated bednet without insecticide and was evaluated alongside the assay. Each net was fastened to the cone and five non-blood-feed, 2–5-day-old

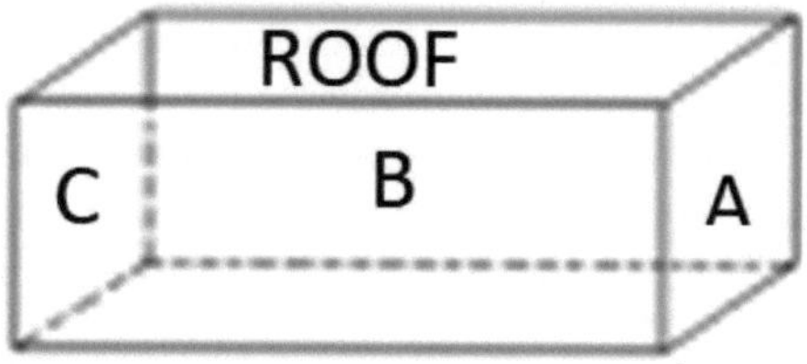

Figure 2.
Net sides and the roof of the net brands cut out for cone bioassay.

female *Anopheles* mosquitoes were exposed to each piece of netting for 3 minutes according to the protocol of WHO [3]. The mosquitoes were then removed from the cones and transferred to resting tubes with access to 10% sugar solution. The number of knockdown (KD) was recorded every 10 minutes for up to 60 minutes after exposure and effective mortality was assessed 24 hours after exposure.

6. Data analysis

According to the WHOPES, the two main outcomes proposed in its guidelines to assess the bio-efficacy of LLIN on mosquitoes exposed for three minutes are: (i) mortality after 24 hours≥80%, and (ii) a KD rate after 60 minutes ≥95%. Although the standard protocol recommends using the two outcomes, i.e., mortality of 80% or KD ≥ 95% [3, 18].

The result were subjected to descriptive statistics such as mean and standard deviation (SD) to determine the average number of mosquitoes that died after 24 hours and those that were knocked down at 30 minutes and 60 minutes post-exposure to the different brands and different sides of nets. The Global Validation of Linear Model Assumption (GVLMA) was used to assess the data for conformity to linear model assumptions. Inferential statistics the analysis of variance (ANOVA) were used to compare the means of mosquito knockdown and mortality across the different groups of net brands (Olyset®, PermaNet2.0®, and MAGNet®), sides of the net (A, B, C, and roof), and mosquito status (wild or Kisumu). The interaction effect, simple main effect or main effect of the different groups on the mortality or knockdown of the mosquitoes were assessed, accordingly. BeforeThe Tukey's post hoc test was used for pairwise comparison of the means in groups that had statistically significant differences. Statistical significance was determined at 5% probability level ($p < 0.05$). However, for the simple main effect, statistical significance was determined at a probability level of 0.01 to avoid Type 1 error. The statistical analysis was performed in R version 4.1.1 [19], using the packages; dplyr [20], gvlma [21], ggplot2 (Hadley [22]), and emmeans [23].

7. Results

7.1 Effect of net brands on the mortality of wild *An. gambiae* s.l. for different sides of the net

Mortality observed with the positive control (PermaNet3.0®) for all the nets tested was 100% irrespective of the net side. On the other hand, the treatment recorded the least mortality in MAGNet® for all the sides to which the mosquitoes were exposed. A two-way ANOVA was performed to analyze the effect of net brands and net side on the mortality of wild *An. gambiae* s.l. The result as shown in **Figure 3** revealed that there was not a statistically significant interaction between the effects of net brands and the net side (F (6, 12) = .92, p = .513). The main effect analysis showed that the net brands have a statistically significant effect on the mosquito mortality after 24 hours (F (2, 18) = 14.32, p < .001), while the sides of the net did not have a statistically significant effect on the mosquito mortality (F (3, 18) = 1.67, p = .209). Tukey's test for multiple comparisons revealed that the mean mortality was significantly different between Olyset® and MAGNet® (p = .003) and between PermaNet2.0® and MAGNet® (p < .001). There was no statistically significant difference in mean mortality between Olyset® and PermaNet2.0® (p = .495).

7.2 Comparison of the effect of nets brands on the mortality of wild and susceptible *An. gambiae* s.l.

Least percentage mortality with the wild mosquitoes was observed in MAGNet®, irrespective of the net side to which the mosquitoes were exposed to. A similar observation was recorded in the susceptible mosquitoes except for mosquitoes exposed to Side B, where the least percentage mortality was observed in Olyset®. It was shown in **Figure 4** that irrespective of the side of the net the mosquitoes were exposed to, the susceptible *An. gambiae* s.l. recorded higher mortality than the wild mosquitoes in all the nets tested. A two-way ANOVA was performed to analyze the effect of net brands and mosquito status on mortality. The result revealed that there was not a statistically significant interaction between the effects of net brands and mosquito status (F (2, 42) = 2.54, p = .091). The main effect analysis showed that the net brands and the mosquito status both have a statistically significant effect on the mosquito mortality after 24 hours (F (2, 44) = 16.60, p < .001 and F (1, 44) = 44.08, p < .001,

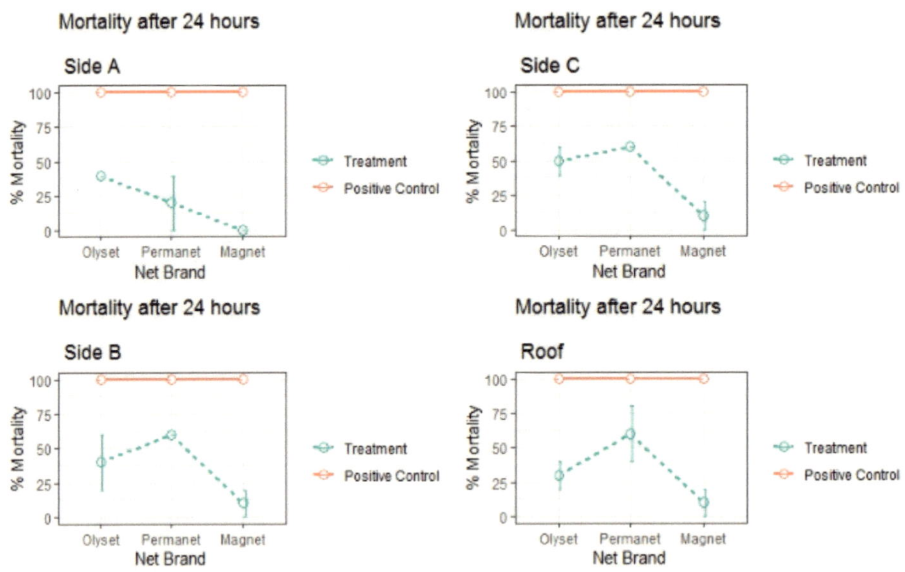

Figure 3.
Effect of net brands on the mortality of wild An. gambiae *s.l. for different sides of the net.*

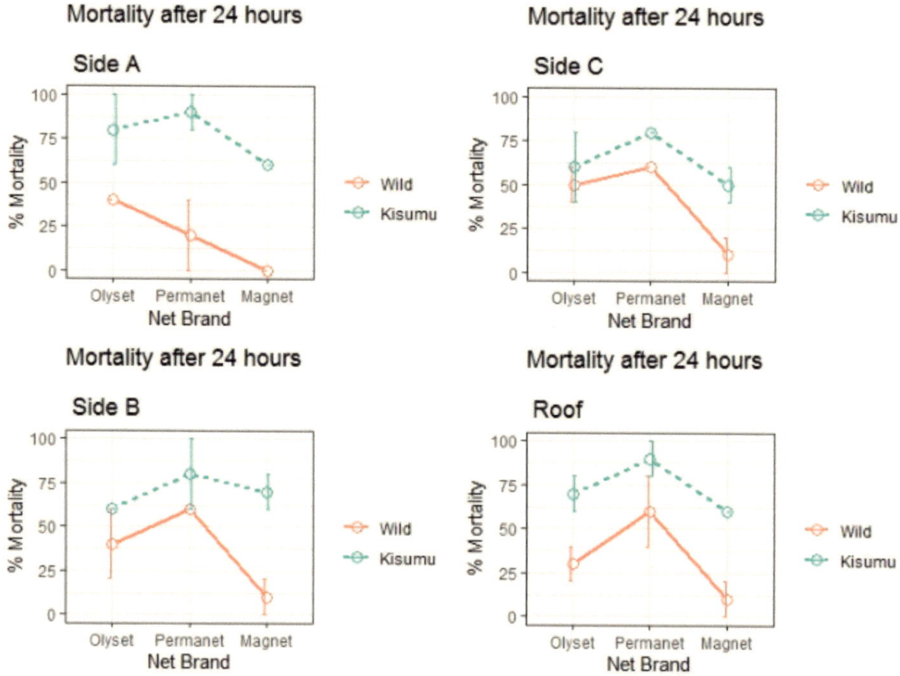

Figure 4.
Comparison of the effect of nets brands on the mortality of wild and susceptible An. gambiae *s.l.*

respectively). Tukey's test for multiple comparisons revealed that the mean mortality was significantly different between PermaNet® and MAGNet® (p = .001). There was no statistically significant difference in mean mortality between Olyset® and PermaNet® (p = .260) or between Olyset® and MAGNet® (p = .083).

7.3 Knockdown effect (30 minutes post-exposure) of net brands on wild *An. gambiae* s.l. exposed to the different sides of the net

The treatment recorded the highest knockdown (30 minutes) in mosquitoes exposed to Side C of both the PermaNet2.0® and MAGNet® nets as shown in **Figure 5**.

The result of a two-way ANOVA performed to analyze the effect of net brands and the side of nets on knockdown after 30 minutes revealed that there was not a statistically significant interaction between the effects of net brands and the side of the net (F (6, 12) = 1.13, p = .404). The main effect analysis showed that both the net brands and the side of the net do not have a statistically significant effect on the knockdown after 30 minutes (F (2, 18) = 1.08, p = .361 and F (3, 18) = .96, p = .433, respectively).

7.4 Knockdown effect (60 minutes post-exposure) of net brands on wild *An. gambiae* s.l. exposed to the different sides of the net

In both PermaNet 2.0® and MAGNet®, the treatment recorded the highest knockdown (60 minutes) in mosquitoes exposed to Side B of the nets, while the least was observed on Side A as seen in **Figure 6**.

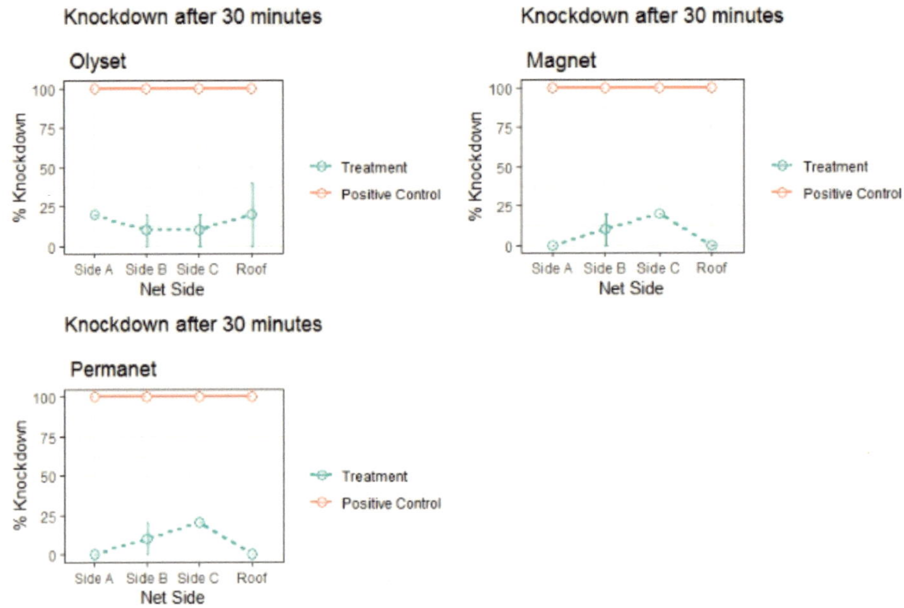

Figure 5.
Knockdown effect (30 minutes post-exposure) of net brands on wild An. gambiae *s.l. exposed to the different sides of the net.*

The result of a two-way ANOVA performed to analyze the effect of net brands and the side of nets on knockdown after 60 minutes revealed that there was not a statistically significant interaction between the effects of net brands and the side of the net (F (6, 12) = 1.49, p = .263). The main effect analysis showed that the net brands did not have a statistically significant effect on knockdown after 60 minutes of exposure (F (2, 18) = .13, p = .877). The net side, on the other hand, has a statistically significant effect on knockdown after 60 minutes (F (3, 18) = 4.46, p = .017). Tukey's test for multiple comparisons revealed that the mean knockdown (60 minutes) was significantly different between sides A and B (p = .006) only.

7.5 Comparison of the knockdown (after 30 minutes) effect of nets side on wild and susceptible *An. gambiae s.l*

Susceptible mosquitoes recorded a higher mean percentage knockdown (after 30 minutes) in all the nets tested. The result of a two-way ANOVA performed to analyze the effect of the side of nets and mosquito status on knockdown after 30 minutes revealed that there was a statistically significant interaction between the effects of the side of the net and the mosquito status (F (3, 40) = 10.35, p < .001). At an alpha level of .012, the mosquito status effect within the Side A group was statistically significant (p = .001). On Side A of the nets, the mean knockdowns after 30 minutes was 0 for the wild mosquito and 3 for the Kisumu as seen in **Figure 7**.

7.6 Comparison of the knockdown (after 60 minutes) effect of nets side on wild and susceptible *An. gambiae* s.l.

The result of a two-way ANOVA performed to analyze the effect of the side of nets and mosquito status on knockdown after 60 minutes revealed that there was a

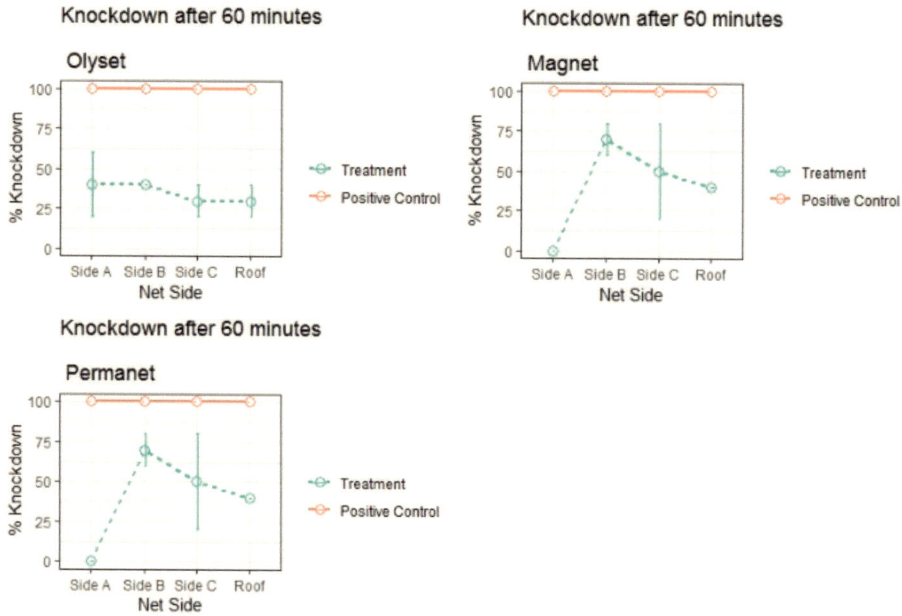

Figure 6.
Knockdown effect (60 minutes post-exposure) of net brands on wild An. gambiae *s.l. exposed to the different sides of the net.*

statistically significant interaction between the effects of the side of the net and the mosquito status (F (3, 40) = 4.5, p = .008). At an alpha level of .012, the mosquito status effect within the Side A group was statistically significant (p = .001). On Side A of the nets, the mean knockdowns after 60 minutes was 1 for the wild mosquito and 4 for the Kisumu. It was shown in **Figure 8** that the susceptible mosquitoes recorded a higher mean percentage knockdown (after 60 minutes) in all the nets tested.

8. Discussion

This study is one of the first conducted in the South-east of Nigeria to compare the response of local malaria vectors in a boundary community known to have pyrethroid-resistant malaria vectors to ITNs available in the health facilities. Pyrethroid insecticides used to treat nets have an excito-repellent effect that adds a chemical barrier to the physical barrier. The insecticide kills mosquito that encounters the ITNs, thus reducing the vector population [24]. Variations in the mortality of malaria vectors to different types of ITNs used for the study were generally low, especially with nets treated with pyrethroids only. Several studies have shown a decrease in the bio-efficacy of ITNs against local pyrethroid-resistant vectors [25, 26]. The highest mortality of 62.5% attained in the study with PermaNet2.0® is still below the 80% mortality and 90% KD60 approved by the WHOPES. The mortality recorded using PermaNet2.0® treated with deltamethrin was found to be significant compared to other net brands (Olyset® and MAGNet®). Irrespective of the sides of the net tested, higher mortality was recorded especially between Olyset® and PermaNet2.0® when the susceptible mosquitoes were exposed to the nets as compared to the mortality in

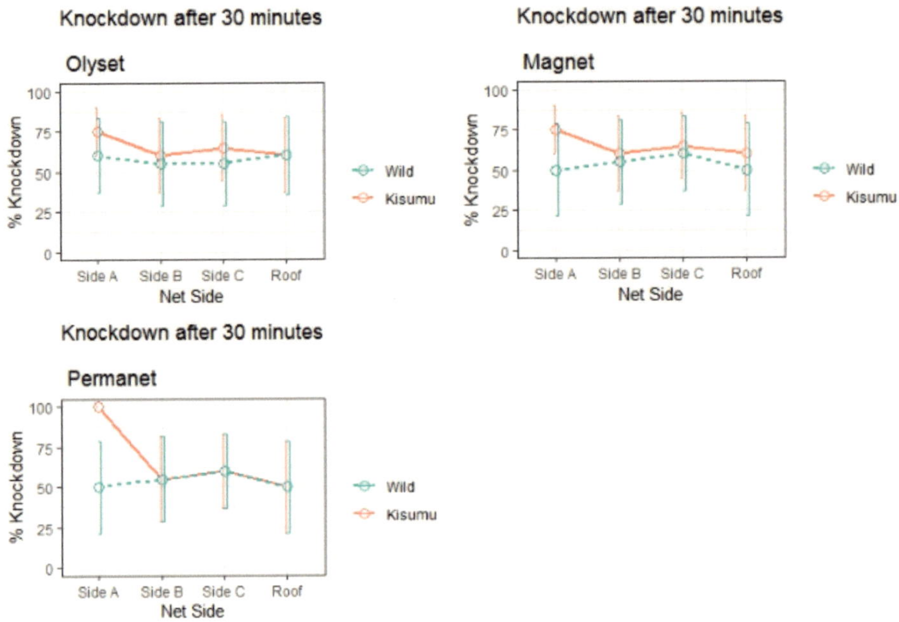

Figure 7.
Comparison of the knockdown (after 30 minutes) effect of nets side on wild and susceptible An. gambiae s.l.

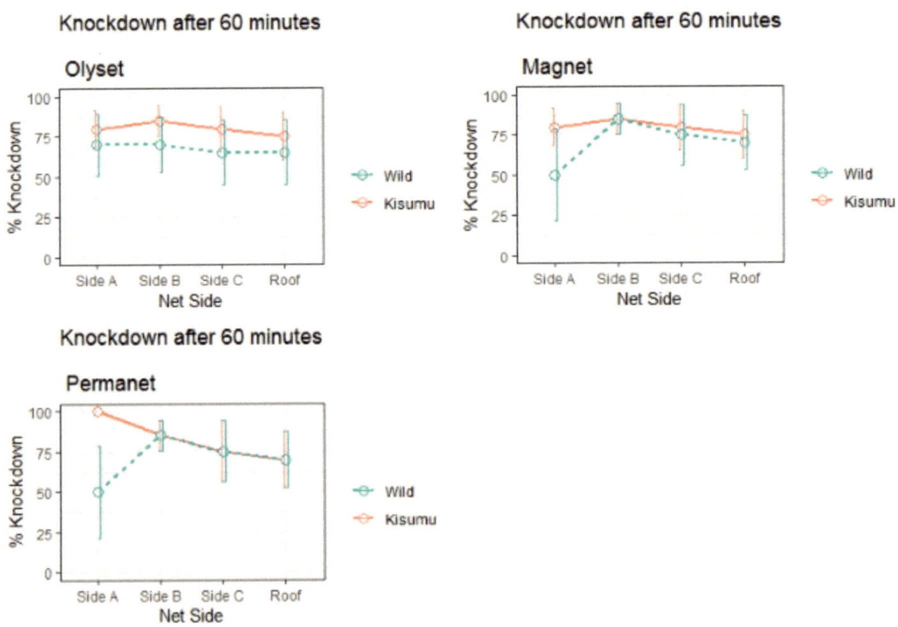

Figure 8.
Comparison of the knockdown (after 60 minutes) effect of nets side on wild and susceptible An. gambiae *s.l.*

the wild mosquitoes. The findings observed in the study showed that mortality was brand-dependent and not side-dependent. However, the efficacy of ITN treated with alpha-cypermethrin (MAGNet®) was generally lower than that of the other ITNs irrespective of the sides tested. *Anopheles* mosquitoes in Amechi-idodo was shown to be resistant to the pyrethroids in the PMI entomological surveillance studies [27], especially for the three insecticides used in impregnating the three brands of nets. According to the findings by PMI [27] in Amechi-Idodo, using WHO susceptibility bioassay showed that *Anopheles gambiae* complex in the study site had a mortality of 19% for Permethrin, 68% for alpha-cypermethrin and 84% for deltamethrin which are the insecticides used in impregnating Olyset®, MAGNet® and PermaNet2.0® respectively. The comparison of ITNs bio-efficacy performed in this study provides the necessary information for the selection of appropriate ITNs for mass distribution. The reduced efficacy of pyrethroid-only ITNs could be attributed to the selection pressures exerted using the same class of insecticide for pest control in agriculture which describes Amechi-Idodo as agrarian and as seen in the studies of [28, 29]. A similar finding was observed in southwestern Ethiopia by Yewhalaw et al. [25] and in Uganda [30] where the researchers recorded a reduced efficacy of mono-treated ITNs against wild-resistant *An. gambiae* s.l. in comparison with the response of the same mosquito population to PermaNet3.0® treated with deltamethrin + PBO. The new-generation ITN with pyrethroids and PBO (PermaNet3.0®) in the study showed higher efficacy than mono-treated ITNs (PermaNet2.0®, MAGNet® and Olyset®). However, the strong resistance of local vectors to pyrethroids especially deltamethrin suggests that the combination of deltamethrin + PBO will be the most appropriate strategy against local vectors in the study area for now. According to the findings of PMI [31], synergist test with PBO showed a complete restoration to pyrethroid susceptibility (54–98% for permethrin and 90–100% for deltamethrin) of *A. gambiae* s.l collected from Ohaukwu, an adjourning local government in Ebonyi state and this was observed in the study that the use of PBO net significantly showed an increased in the mortality of mosquitoes.

The results of this study, therefore constitute important evidence that can guide decision making in the selection and distribution of high-efficacy ITNs in the eastern region of Nigeria, as evidence has shown in the studies of [15, 32] that *A. gambiae* s.l is resistant to all pyrethroids. The use of ITNs that showed high bio-efficacy against the local vector populations should be encouraged to significantly reduce the transmission of malaria indoors. Indoor biting in the study area has shown to occur mainly from 10 pm to 6 am [27] and the infectivity rate in the neighboriong state is as high as 6.6%, highlighting the importance of ITNs [31] thereby a need for an efficient ITNs.

Despite the importance of our findings, there are some limitations. An epidemiological survey concerning the protection offered by the ITNs would have been ascertained to see the real efficacy of the nets in the study area. The evaluation of the efficacy of the ITNs would have been better if tunnel tests were conducted on nets, as none of the nets met the criteria of 80% mortality with resistant mosquito strains. Also, chemical analysis of the ITNs prior to the start of the study would have improved the quality of the results and also the effect of temperature and relative humidity on the stored ITNs and for how long will also help in answering the question of the low efficacy obtained.

This study recommends the need to develop and adopt routine monitoring of the ITNs at the health facilities, as it will inform the replacement of ineffective nets. However, a mass campaign of PBO nets is necessary for the state to achieve and maintain the universal coverage of ITNs as the Antenatal care and Expanded programme on immunization channels are no longer sufficient for the continuous distribution of ITNs.

Author details

Ezihe K. Ebuka[1*], Emmanuel Obi[2], Nwangwu C. Udoka[3], Ukonze B. Chikaodili[4], Nwankwo N. Edith[5], Udezue Nkemakonam[5], Egbuche M. Chukwudi[5] and Okeke C. Peter[6]

1 Malaria Consortium, Abuja, Nigeria

2 PMI VectorWorks Project, Tropical Health LLP, Abuja, Nigeria

3 National Arbovirus and Vectors Research Centre, Federal Ministry of Health Enugu, United States

4 School of Biological Science, Universiti Sains, Malaysia

5 Department of Parasitology and Entomology, Nnamdi Azikiwe University, Awka, Nigeria

6 Opec Research Consult, Awka, Anambra State, Nigeria

*Address all correspondence to: eziheebuka@yahoo.com

References

[1] Kesteman T, Randrianarivelojosia M, Rogier C. The protective effectiveness of control interventions for malaria prevention: A systematic review of the literature. F1000Research. 2017;**6**:1932

[2] Njumkeng C, Apinjoh TO, Anchang-Kimbi JK, et al. Coverage and usage of insecticide treated nets (ITNs) within households: Associated factors and effect on the prevalance of malaria parasitemia in the Mount Cameroon area. BMC Public Health. 2019;**19**:1216

[3] WHO. Vector Control Technical Expert Group Report to MPAC September 2013: Estimating Functional Survival of Long-Lasting Insecticidal Nets from Field Data. Geneva: World Health Organization; 2013

[4] World Health Organization. Guidelines for Monitoring the Durability of Long-Lasting Insecticidal Mosquito Nets under Operational Conditions. Geneva: World Health Organization; 2011

[5] Mboma ZM, Festo C, Lorenz LM, Massue DJ, Kisinza WN, Bradley J, et al. The consequences of declining population access to insecticide-treated nets (ITNs) on net use patterns and physical degradation of nets after 22 months of ownership. Malaria Journal. 2021;**20**:171

[6] Olapeju B, Choiriyyah I, Lynch M, et al. Age and gender trends in insecticide-treated net use in sub-Saharan Africa: A multi-country analysis. Malaria Journal. 2018;**17**:423

[7] Koenker H, Arnold F, Ba F, Cisse M, Diouf L, Eckert E, et al. Assessing whether universal coverage with insecticide-treated nets has been achieved: Is the right indicator being used? Malaria Journal. 2018;**17**:355

[8] Sousa JO, de Albuquerque BC, Coura JR, Suárez-Mutis MC. Use and retention of long-lasting insecticidal nets (LLINs) in a malaria risk area in the Brazilian Amazon: A 5-year follow-up intervention. Malaria Journal. 2019;**18**(1):100

[9] Bhatt S, Weiss D, Cameron E, et al. The effect of malaria control on *plasmodium falciparum* in Africa between 2000 and 2015. Nature. 2015;**526**:207-211

[10] Milliner J. Net Mapping Project. 2016. Available from: http: //alliance formalariaprevention.com/working-groups/net-mapping-project/

[11] Obi E, Okoh F, Blaufuss S, Olapeju B, Akilah J, Okoko OO, et al. Monitoring the physical and insecticidal durability of the long-lasting insecticidal net DawaPlus® 2.0 in three states in Nigeria. Malaria Journal. 2020;**19**:124

[12] Lorenz LM, Bradley J, Yukich J, Massue DJ, Mboma ZM, Pigeon O, et al. Comparative functional survival and equivalent annual cost of three long-lasting insecticidal net (LLIN) products in Tanzania: A randomised trial with 3-year follow-up. PLoSMed. 2020;**17**:e1003248. DOI: 10.1371/journal.pmed.1003248

[13] Haji KA, Khatib BO, Obi E, Dimoso K, Koenker H, Babalola S, et al. Monitoring the durability of the long-lasting insecticidal nets Olyset® and PermaNet®2.0 in similar use environments in Zanzibar. Malaria Journal. 2020;**19**:187

[14] Tan KR, Coleman J, Smith B, Hamainza B, Katebe-Sakala C,

Kean C, et al. A longitudinal study of the durability of long-lasting insecticidal nets in Zambia. Malaria Journal. 2016;**15**:106. DOI: 10.1186/s12936-016-1154-4

[15] Chukwuekezie O, Nwosu E, Nwangwu U, et al. Resistance status of *Anopheles gambiae* (*s.l.*) to four commonly used insecticides for malaria vector control in south-East Nigeria. Parasites Vectors. 2020;**13**:152

[16] WHO. World Malaria Report 2016. Geneva: World Health Organization; 2016

[17] Tungu P, Magesa S, Maxwell C, et al. Evaluation of PermaNet 3.0 a deltamethrin-PBO combination net against *Anopheles gambiae* and pyrethroid resistant *Culex quinquefasciatus* mosquitoes: An experimental hut trial in Tanzania. Malaria Journal. 2010;**9**:21

[18] Boyer S, Pothin E, Randriamaherijaona S, et al. Testing bio-efficacy of insecticide-treated nets with fewer mosquitoes for enhanced malaria control. Scientific Reports. 2018;**8**:16769

[19] R Core Team. R: A Language and Environment for Statistical Computing. Vienna, Austria: R Foundation for Statistical Computing; 2021

[20] Wickham H, François R, Henry L, Müller K. Dplyr: A grammar of data manipulation. 2021. R package version 1.0.7. Available from: https://CRAN.R-project.org/package=dplyr

[21] Pena EA, Slate EH. Gvlma: Global validation of linear. 2019. Models Assumptions. R package version 1.0.0.3. Available from: https://CRAN.R-project.org/package=gvlma

[22] Hadley Wickham. Ggplot 2: Elegant graphics for data analysis. New York: Springer-Verlag; 2016

[23] Lenth RV. Emmeans: Estimated Marginal Means, aka Least-Squares Means. 2021. R package version 1.7.0. Available from: https://CRAN.R-project.org/package=emmeans

[24] Choi L, Pryce J, Garner P. Indoor residual spraying for preventing malaria in communities using insecticide-treated nets. The Cochrane Database of Systematic Reviews. 2019;**5**(5):CD012688

[25] Yewhalaw D, Asale A, Tushune K, Getachew Y, Duchateau L, Speybroeck N. Bio-efficacy of selected long-lasting insecticidal nets against Pyrethroid resistant *anopheles arabiensis* from South-Western Ethiopia. Parasites & Vectors. 2012;**5**:159

[26] Zainab G, Zainab T. Post-intervention assessment of long-lasting insecticide nets (LLINs) distributed in the Kano metropolis, Kano state, Nigeria. Advances in Entomology. 2013;**1**:38-41

[27] AIRS. Nigeria Final Entomology Report. November 2014–December 2015, Africa Indoor Residual Spraying Project. Abt Associates Inc.; 2015. pp. 1-73

[28] Gnanguenon V, Agossa FR, Badirou K, Govoetchan R, Anagonou R, Oke-Agbo F, et al. Malaria vectors resistance to insecticides in Benin: Current trends and mechanisms involved. Parasite and Vectors. 2015;**8**:223

[29] Ranson H, Abdallah H, Badolo A, et al. Insecticide resistance in *Anopheles gambiae:* Data from the first year of a multi-country study highlight the extent of the problem. Malaria Journal. 2009;**8**:299

[30] Okia M, Ndyomugyenyi R, Kirunda J, et al. Bioefficacy of long-lasting insecticidal nets against pyrethroid-resistant populations of *Anopheles gambiae s.s.* from different

malaria transmission zones in Uganda. Parasites Vectors. 2013;**6**:130

[31] AIRS. Nigeria Final Entomology Report. January–December 2017, Africa Indoor Residual Spraying Project (IRS 2). Rockvill, Maryland, USA: Abt Associates Inc.; 2017. pp. 1-50

[32] Nwankwo EN, Okorie PN, Acha CT, Okonkwo OE, Nwangwu UC, Ezihe EK. Insecticide resistance in *Anopheles gambiae s.l.* mosquitoes in Awka, Anambra state, Southeast Nigeria. Journal of Mosquito Research. 2017;7:32-37

Chapter 7

Interventions and Practical Approaches to Reduce the Burden of Malaria on School-Aged Children

Andrew Macnab

Abstract

Robust evidence indicates school-aged children are particularly vulnerable to malaria and need special measures to protect them. Calls are widespread for better diagnostic approaches and innovative programs that benefit children, because current levels of malaria-related morbidity and mortality are so high. Problematically, most national malaria control programs do not specifically target school-aged children; although the literature describes options for child-focused strategies, there is no consensus on the optimal intervention; and where a strategy is advocated, it is almost always one identified through systematic review. While understandably the scientific "gold standard," such reviews exclude many potentially useful and valid approaches, because reports describing them do not meet the inclusion criteria of being randomized controlled trials. Such trials are inevitably limited in number due to cost and complexity, and many excluded reports describe locally developed innovation based on World Health Organization diagnostic and therapeutic guidelines with the potential to benefit children. This chapter frames how practical interventions such as these can be put in place by school communities, and in parallel, how approaches advocated by the WHO and Lancet Commission to promote health literacy and access to essential health services can create ways to reduce the burden of malaria on school-aged children.

Keywords: artemisinin combination therapy, cognitive impairment, intermittent protective treatment, health promotion, rapid diagnostic testing, seasonal malaria chemoprophylaxis, school-based prophylaxis, task shifting, teachers, WHO health promoting school (HPS) model

1. Introduction

Malaria exemplifies how health inequity negatively impacts children's lives and their ability to benefit from education. While global investment in recent years to fight malaria has led to millions of malaria deaths being averted, and this progress has certainly benefited young children [1], bold decisions are still needed to control the disease [2], and especially to meet the longstanding calls for specific interventions to reduce the burden of disease in school-age children [3–6]. Overall, policies to address the high prevalence of malaria infection in this age group are lacking, and school-age children continue to attract little attention as a group in need of special measures to protect them [4, 7].

Although leading authors have recommended that malaria should be included as a key component of school health programs, the clear ideas and defined approaches required to effectively improve malaria control among school-age children remain unforthcoming [5]. Even a recent Lancet commentary largely echoed prior (unheeded) calls for interventions specifically targeting this age group by reporting more trials which had failed to define a universally applicable intervention, and offering the potential cost of programs and lack of policy support as continuing barriers to progress [3]. However, effective school-based approaches do exist that can positively impact morbidity. Importantly they include elements that are simple and broadly applicable, and will improve health and wellbeing and in doing so increase the capacity of children to learn [1, 7, 8]. Many also have the ability to benefit the broader community beyond the school in the context of malaria.

In a prior review (2020), Macnab described the global impact of malaria on school children, and outlined the principal school-based strategies tried as a way to reduce the adverse effects of infection on the health of children, their ability to attend school and on their long-term academic potential [7]. Such strategies continue to include seasonal chemoprophylaxis, intermittent protective treatment and antimalarial therapy linked to mass drug administration for neglected tropical diseases. This review also emphasized the global need for children to be educated about malaria at school so that they understand how it is caused, how it can be prevented, and the importance of early diagnosis and prompt treatment. This is a fundamental need in addition to being a necessary component that must be provided in parallel with any preventive or therapeutic strategy if it is to be fully effective.

Expanded and innovative strategies are needed to regain momentum over malaria control, including new and better diagnostic approaches to address malaria in children because of the current levels of morbidity and mortality [9]. The WHO estimates widespread deployment of insecticide-treated bed nets, vector control programs, rapid diagnostic testing, new treatments and prophylactic strategies have averted 7·6 million deaths since 2000. But recently stated global targets to reduce case incidence and mortality rates by at least 90% by 2030 are now at risk, and emphasize again that a disproportionate disease burden falls on children [10].

Schools are important in the fight against malaria on several levels. Simple and inexpensive additions to the curriculum can increase children's knowledge and improve their health, and where teachers are engaged and taught the necessary skills schools can provide their pupils with timely diagnosis and treatment. School-based programs that educate children broadly on the causation and prevention of malaria and what care is required, reduce child morbidity. But health promotion in schools is also known to benefit the broader community, as where children receive appropriate guidance they can act as agents for change both within and beyond the school and spread the knowledge they acquire to their families and beyond [3, 11, 12]. This willingness and ability to share learned concepts and practices also indicates that children educated in this way acquire higher levels of health literacy [13].

As early as 2005 Afenyadu et al. proposed improving access to treatment for children with malaria by engaging teachers in care [14]. But the first endorsement of this approach came from the International Pediatric Association (IPA) following a

2-year trial in rural Uganda of a community participatory intervention model where teachers were taught to screen all sick children using rapid point-of-care diagnostic testing (RDT) and treat those testing positive promptly [15]. The IPA identified this model as applicable worldwide in areas where malaria is endemic, because it significantly reduced morbidity from malaria in school-aged children, and the diagnostic and treatment components were based on the approaches recommended by the World Health organization (WHO) [16].

School-based health care delivery has the potential to benefit more than 1 billion children worldwide [17]. The WHO 'Health Promoting School' (HPS) model is one potential way to initiate school health programs [18]. The model is based on simple concepts and is flexible. The aim is to generate life-long learning through additions to the curriculum that enable children to acquire both relevant health 'knowledge' and practical 'skills' with the overarching objective of positively influencing social determinants of health [19]. Many schools initiate basic health promotion programs independently, others require varying levels of teacher training, resource provision and ongoing support [20]. The WHO now endorses school programs as a way to address specific health challenges worldwide.

Effective engagement of schools in health promotion and care delivery is most readily achieved where policies to do so are in place and practical support is provided [17, 21]. Currently there are calls to improve the overall health of children as a way to promote their learning and enable them to achieve their full potential [7]. This has come about because of the growing recognition that good health at school improves educational outcomes, which in turn builds human capital: "the sum of a population's health, skills knowledge and experience that is central to a country's economic growth" [3]. Importantly, addressing malaria in school-age children is now an element in this goal to build human capital.

There is growing evidence of 'what works and why' in the context of health promotion in school settings. Gaps remain in our understanding of the optimal intervention and programing needed in the context of malaria, and ongoing efforts to conduct research to identify effective programs is essential, and ideally followed by the conduct of randomized controlled trials [7]. Cohee has described school health as "the key to unlocking the potential of the world's children," and that "schools offer a uniquely sustainable platform for health delivery in low resource settings, while at the same time influencing community change through their education role" [3].

Importantly, the literature describes several approaches employed successfully to address malaria in school-aged children, and while many have significant limitations in terms of being broadly applicable, these too may still be the right approach in defined circumstances. New strategies are also being proposed; many are innovative modifications of prior approaches, some are specific refinements to address challenges like emerging drug resistance, and of course the new recommendation for the first malaria vaccine to be rolled out on a large scale now has to be factored into national programs to fight malaria [22, 23]. The aim must be to find broadly applicable, socially acceptable, cost effective, interventions to reduce mortality and morbidity in school children. Such programs in turn will ensure that malaria does not negatively impact the ability of participating children to achieve their academic potential by minimizing the risk of short- and long-term cognitive impairment, and that the broader community becomes better informed about the challenge of malaria and ways to address it, through the 'trickle down' effect of pupils sharing knowledge and skills learned with their families [24]. Where programs successfully reduce the incidence of infection in children, the broader community also benefits through the overall local reduction in the reservoir of malaria transmission [8].

2. Therapeutic and interventional approaches

Despite being preventable, detectable and curable, malaria remains one of the main causes of mortality and significant morbidity due to infectious disease [9]. Trialed approaches to reduce morbidity in school-age children include prophylaxis, intermittent protective treatment (IPT), mass drug administration (MDA) and combination of rapid diagnosis and treatment. Preventive treatment to protect school-aged children significantly decreases P. falciparum prevalence, malaria-related anemia, and also the risk of subsequent clinical infection across transmission settings. Hence the logic of policies to make therapeutic intervention strategies broadly available to protect this age group; this approach could also provide benefit by decreasing transmission, and thereby advance the goal of malaria elimination [8].

2.1 Prophylaxis

In areas where malaria is endemic prophylaxis is generally not recommended for children due to poor adherence to prescribed regimens, limited compliance due to cost, side effects over time, and the risk of emergence and drug resistance [25].

2.2 Intermittent protective treatment (IPT)

IPT involves periodic drug administration at defined intervals of a full therapeutic dose of a single drug, or drugs in combination, to those at high risk regardless of their infection status. Trials have involved two main approaches, seasonal malaria chemoprevention and intermittent parasite clearance. An example of IPT delivery through schools is described by Fernando et al. from Sri Lanka [26]. In a randomized double-blind placebo-controlled trial school children aged 6–12 years were given weekly chloroquine or placebo for 9 months. The incidence of malaria fell in the treated group, and a significant difference in absence from school and a marked improvement in school performance was found between them and those pupils receiving a placebo. Evidence from several African countries has shown that seasonal malaria chemoprevention measures can be highly effective, with most severe malaria eradicated, and a reduction in P. falciparum prevalence, the incidence of clinical uncomplicated malaria, and malaria-related anemia [27].

Trials data generally indicate that IPT regimens benefit school-age children by reducing rates of infection, improving health, decreasing absence from school, enhancing academic achievement, and protecting cognitive ability [28, 29]. There is consensus that IPT is a safe and simple strategy that offers remarkable protection in school-aged children in high-malarial-transmission settings, and preferable to prophylaxis. Effective strategies are seen as a potentially valuable addition to school health programs [30]. Evidence from several African countries has also shown that SMC using SP-AQ is highly effective, eradicating most severe malaria, and leading to strong reduction in P. falciparum prevalence, the incidence of clinical uncomplicated malaria, and malaria anemia; two systematic reviews and meta-analyses on efficacy and safety summarize the pros and cons of specific drug regimens [31, 32].

2.3 Mass drug administration (MDA)

MDA is a WHO endorsed strategy to control 7 of a group of 13 major, disabling and 'neglected' tropical diseases (NTDs) (ascariasis, trachoma, trichuriasis, hookworm, schistosomiasis, lymphatic filariasis, and onchocerciasis) [33]. MDA has been combined with the delivery of other care entities in school-based settings. In Ghana, combining IPT for malaria with MDA to control intestinal soil-transmitted helminths benefited measures of anemia, sustained attention and recall [34]. And, in Malawi the approach was found to be well-tolerated, safe for teachers to administer, beneficial, and well-received by parents; all findings of obvious practical importance [35]. Adding malaria IPT to already established NTD control programs also increases the cost-effectiveness of both interventions, particularly where teachers are trained to be part of program delivery.

2.4 Combined rapid diagnosis and treatment

Diagnosis and treatment in combination employs the use of rapid diagnostic test kits (RDT) and treatment of those testing positive with artemisinin combination therapy (ACT). This has primarily been a clinic-based strategy, and is an approach endorsed by the WHO as the first-line of treatment in areas where malaria is endemic [7, 16]. In order to increase access to this standard of care, several countries have reported expanding the role of pharmacists by training them how to do RDTs [36]. Reports have also followed of successful 'downstream' expansion through school-based programs where appropriately trained volunteer teachers administer RDT to all children who are sick at school, and administer ACT promptly to those testing positive [15, 37].

RDTs are an inexpensive diagnostic approach, reliably estimate infection in low and high prevalence categories, and have the major advantage that they make immediate treatment feasible [38]. The sensitivity and specificity of RDTs are good enough for them to replace conventional testing for malaria. The positive impact of RDTs on malaria management has been widely demonstrated, and effective roll-out and sustained use on a national scale has been achieved through well planned implementation [39]. Basic training in their use also enables teachers and other providers without a healthcare background to use them reliably [40]. When employed for school-based diagnosis it has been shown that practical aids in the form of step-by-step usage guides can improve performance. Like any technology, refinement will likely be needed over time to keep to keep RDTs a cutting edge diagnostic entity.

ACTs are a unique class of antimalarial drugs. Developed from plant-based peroxides they kill young intraerythrocytic malaria parasites before they can develop into more harmful mature forms; this achieves a robust parasitological response which results in rapid clinical improvement [41]. More than 20 years ago the WHO recommended ACT as the first-line treatment for P. falciparum malaria in all countries with endemic disease [42]. The benefits of genuine ACTs are considerable, and include their fast action, high efficiency, minimal adverse effects, low cost, and the potential to lower the rate at which resistance emerges and spreads [43]. However, care must be taken over the choice of the preparation used, because sub-standard and counterfeit products with little or no efficacy pose severe threats to human health, and there is increasing concern over the emergence of resistance to this class of drugs [44].

Where the efficacy of ACTs is high, more could be achieved through increasing their availability. But in spite of the large body of evidence for both the efficacy and safety of ACTs this drug class is not being used as widely or as comprehensively as it should be [45]. An additional concern is that even when they are available, the way ACTs are used does not always conform to international guidelines [46]. There are of course many practical challenges to making ACTs more available globally, including cost, and finding effective ways to distribute and administer ACTs to a greater number of children, who are arguably the population who needs them most [47]. Continuing to search for innovative ways to increase ACT availability and promote their appropriate use are two essential components for improving malaria control in school-aged children. Approaches to date with promise include: a community case management approach, where a variety of trained providers are used to deliver ACTs [48], distribution through agents in drug stores, pharmacies and private medical clinics [49], and of course via teachers in school health programs [15, 37].

Importantly, the use of RDT and ACT is endorsed by the WHO, and arguably, increasing access to this combined diagnostic and treatment approach is one of the simplest and potentially most cost-effective ways to reduce malaria morbidity among school-aged children. This is especially true in countries that are already using RDT and ACT in government hospitals and clinics, as expansion of bulk purchasing and scale up of distribution offer a more economic proposition than developing new programs which will potentially require other drugs and alternative infrastructure. The use of RDT and ACT in non-traditional outlets is particularly applicable in rural areas where distance limits ready access to hospital and clinic facilities.

2.5 Multiple first line therapies

Use of multiple first-line therapies (MFT) is an emerging strategy where several ACTs are prescribed together rather than a single first-line ACT. Because antimalarial treatment currently depends so heavily on artemisinins, the evolution of resistance to ACTs in some parts of the world seriously threatens the overall effectiveness of antimalarial treatment [50]. The emergence of resistance is compounded by use of these drugs in some of the poorest countries in the world, where the dosage used is often incorrect, ineffective counterfeit products are widespread, poor quality drugs are commonly purchased due to their lower cost, and a complete course of treatment is not taken as some is held back to use with future illness [44].

The WHO has also identified that the dosage recommendations for a number of antimalarials used in children have not always been optimal. This is largely evident where schedules are derived from adult dosing regimens [46]. This too creates increased selection pressure for the emergence and spread of resistance. However, while there is growing concern that resistance to ACTs could spread rapidly, modeling predicts that using MFT rather than a single first-line ACT will reduce the number of treatment failure in the long term, and prolong the effective life of this important class of drugs [51].

3. School-based community teacher-driven intervention models

3.1 History

As early as the 1920's it was recognized that use of malaria suppressive drugs for special groups might be beneficial. Quinine was tried in Ghana (Gold Coast) in 1925 with little success. In the 1950's several school-based trials of the synthetic antimalarial pyrimethamine were conducted in sub-Saharan Africa; these showed that malaria could be successfully controlled, and treated children were found to have significantly better general health and average weight gain compared to untreated children [7].

In 1955 Colbourne reported using a combination of amodiaquine and pyrimethamine to suppress malaria in 7-year-old children in a school in Accra, Ghana. In the regimen used, children received amodiaquine at the beginning of each term to clear parasitemia followed by pyrimethamine weekly to provide suppression. A control group received comparable placebo. In treated children a 50% reduction in absenteeism resulted; the first use of this measure as a surrogate for morbidity from malaria [52].

3.2 Teacher administered RDT and ACT

This community participation teacher-driven model was first implemented in 4 low resource communities in Uganda where sick children were usually just sent home for parents to manage, and teachers had identified the burden malaria was taking on the health and academic potential of their pupils [15]. In order to ensure that the resources and will of the community were behind any program implemented, the principles of respectful engagement were followed by engaging in dialog with community leaders, teachers and parents and exploring a range of possible interventions. The plan the community chose as the best, locally achievable approach was for two volunteer teachers in the each of the schools to be trained how to use RDT kits to test for malaria in all the children falling sick at school on a daily basis, and administer ACT promptly to all those testing positive.

In order to evaluate the effect, the schools were taught to formally record their regular daily census of which pupils were present or absent at school, and how to document numeric and descriptive data on the children requiring the planned intervention. The daily census data documenting when and how long any child was absent were then recorded for a full year prior to testing and treatment beginning. During that time a local clinic ran training days to teach all required skills and safety procedures to the teachers [53], orient the schools on data collection, screening and treatment, and set up delivery of the RDT kits and ACT supplies. The same data collection on absenteeism was then continued during the following year; the consecutive 2 year timeline was to ensure no bias from seasonal variations in malarial infection. In addition, the number of children found to be sick each day, tested using RDT, found to be RDT positive for malaria, and who received ACT was documented. A brief clinical history for each child treated also noted the time line for their return to class. A single dose ACT preparation was used to ensure a full course of treatment was completed.

Results: In the pre-intervention (year 1) 953 of 1764 pupils were sent home due to presumed infectious illness. At home, parental management only approached WHO standards for accurate diagnosis and prompt treatment of malaria in 1:4 children, and the mean duration of absence from school was 6.5 school days (SD: 3.17). During school-based teacher-administered RDT/ACT (year 2) 1066 of 1774 pupils were identified as sick, 765 of these had a positive RDT and received ACT, and their duration of absence fell to 0.6 (SD: 0.64) days $p < 0.001$. Many of the children felt well enough to return to class within hours of being treated; this was presumed due their malaria being diagnosed early in its evolution, and the prompt treatment with ACT being effective.

Overall, absence from school was reduced by 60.8% during this intervention. If the same percentage of children sent home in year one had malaria as were diagnosed using RDTs in year two, this would equate to 1358 cases in 1775 children over the 2 years - a malaria incidence rate of 79% across the 4 schools. The significant decrease in the duration of absence due to malaria from 6.5 school days to <1 day was maintained in the subsequent 3 years when the schools themselves sustained this teacher-driven program. Of interest, these outcome data are directly comparable to Colbourne's initial estimate that 5–6 school days were saved per child with malaria suppression, in her landmark studies 60 years earlier [52]. Importantly, delivery of care using this model was readily implemented and sustained, teachers participated willingly, pupils reported health benefits, and their parents also saw the intervention as positive [7].

A similar approach was successfully trialed subsequently in primary schools in Malawi and was comparably effective. Absence from school was again decreased and the trained teachers were identified to be trusted providers of malaria care [37]. The authors of both studies concluded that training teachers to "test and treat" was well received, supported national health and education policies and was seen to be a worthwhile intervention by the community. Importantly, teachers were enthusiastic about taking part and sustainability was demonstrated by ongoing data from Uganda; the target schools independently continued RDT/ACT post intervention (until the school closures necessitated by the Covid-19 pandemic) and the significant reduction in malaria morbidity (reduction in absenteeism) was sustained; there is also robust evidence of greater knowledge about many aspects of malaria among the school-children and in the broader community.

RDT and ACT are widely employed, but their use by trained teachers in a school-based initiative to address the health related consequences of malaria on absenteeism had not previously been implemented. Training teachers is an approach that reflects government policy in many countries to promote RDT use by non-medical personnel [36, 49]. The intervention incorporates diagnostic and treatment entities advocated by WHO [16, 38, 42]. The model is now endorsed by the International Pediatric Association as a community-based approach applicable worldwide where morbidity from malaria is high. Integrating 'test and treat' strategies for malaria control into larger health, nutrition and education platforms that schools can offer, is a pathway that would also help in achieving the current health-related UN sustainable development goals [54].

4. School-based approaches to reduce morbidity

There are a range of practical measures not directly related to formal additions to the curriculum or the introduction of school-based therapeutic options that can be put in place by school communities to reduce the burden of malaria on their school-aged children. The most applicable ones are those that individual schools develop themselves in response to local needs that their community identifies, or which grow out of collaborative activities to achieve a defined public health or educational goal. In any given community local needs and resources will differ, so individual initiatives need to be tailored accordingly, and, for instance, accommodate differences between urban and rural settings. Ideally each initiative will be broad and multifaceted enough to leverage as many components of the malaria education/prevention/treatment equation as are required to comprehensively meet the needs of the target school community.

Centering malaria programs on children in schools is an example of the type of innovative, content specific intervention called for by the WHO Commission on

Social Determinants of Health to support health behaviors, and empower young people to take control of their lives [55]. Such 'task shifting' to school-based programs has already increased the delivery of other essential health services for children [23]. Hence, a particularly effective way to develop the measures an individual school or larger community requires, is to use the strategic approaches advocated by the WHO Commission and the Lancet Commission on the future of health in sub-Saharan Africa to improve health literacy and achieve health equity through action [55, 56].

Six of the WHO/Lancet Commission approaches relevant to enabling school communities to reduce the burden of malaria on children are:

- Community empowerment
- People-centered strategies
- Innovative education
- Novel and improved tools
- Training to respond to local needs
- Use of non-traditional avenues and outlets

4.1 Community empowerment

There are multiple health benefits to be gained through community empowerment and this approach is needed to promote health in all sections of society [57, 58]. Campaigns that inform, consult, involve, collaborate and empower for example can be used to engage stakeholders in sub-populations at particular risk from malaria. Parents need to be engaged in particular, as care for sick children obviously generally devolves to them. The central problem parents need help with is that many lack the knowledge and/or resources necessary to provide what their child needs when she/he becomes sick and may have malaria. There is evidence that the current lack of understanding about the approach required to diagnose and treat malaria means that only around 25% of children with early malarial infection receive accurate diagnosis and prompt, effective treatment within 24 hours of the onset of illness, as advocated by WHO [1, 7, 15].

The widespread practice of teachers generally sending home children found to be sick at school compounds this problem, as the end result is that appropriate diagnosis and treatment often do not occur, or at best, the required interventions are delayed [7, 59]. In many communities most febrile illnesses are treated empirically without any diagnostic procedure [44]. Also, dependence on care by traditional healers or trust in prayer often dictates the care a child receives, and there is strong reliance on non-specific medication for fever; preference for such entities contributes to morbidity [60].

Second-order ramifications of malaria morbidity are also compounded in this way. These include loss of schooling due to repeated or prolonged absence, malaise following sub-optimal treatment that prevents full attention and participation in class, and loss of cognitive ability and fine motor skills where a child is left with neurological sequalae. These all negatively impact a child's ability to learn and ultimately rob many of the ability to achieve their long term academic potential [28, 61, 62].

School communities in endemic areas are generally aware of the immediate impact malaria takes on children of school age, but often do not equate infection with impairment of academic performance over time. Parents can be empowered by learning about this association and, in turn, be guided to learn more about the many ways in which they can protect their children against malaria. For example, through the use of insecticide-treated bed nets, indoor spraying, reduction of breeding sites, and other methods for vector control [63, 64].

Communities should be encouraged to see their schools as platforms for the basic education required to inform children adequately about malaria in endemic areas, and be encouraged to lobby for 'test and treat' capacity in schools where the local mindset and/or infrastructure do not make WHO levels of diagnosis and treatment available for children.

4.2 People-centered strategies

Where low public confidence exists in health care services people-centered strategies can improve low public confidence [56]. Constructive solutions are best arrived at through listening and respectful dialog. What needs to be identified is where the real issues lie, and where distrust is based on misconceptions or misinformation. Practical training in social listening and the use of role-play helps caregivers to respond in a non-judgmental manner.

Where there is a lack of knowledge or practical skills, the best people-centered programs are ones that are flexible, so as to allow the people they are for to get as much benefit from them as their abilities or circumstances allow. If misinformation is an issue, small group discussion will be preferable for many older parents, while internet and social media-generated dissemination of appropriate facts can be used to engage younger segments of the population.

Misinformation on malaria on the internet is not as prevalent as for other health issues such as vaccination or Covid-19 containment. But, it pays to identify and recommend sites with accurate facts and good resources. But, in parallel, reinforce the obvious, that not everything that people read online is true or reliable, and if there are important facts about malaria that anyone does not understand, someone that person trusts should be asked to explain what the key facts are.

Enabling people to understand the importance of controlling malaria and the need to protect children especially is not usually that difficult to achieve. However, strategic planning and dialog are particularly important to ensure understanding over issues that people will see as divisive. An example is the consideration being given to using gene drive approaches as part of future integrated strategies to combat malaria. Gene drive is an advanced form of genetic modification where a lab-created gene is introduced into an organism that targets and removes a specific natural gene. But, importantly this new gene can also automatically replicate itself in a way that ensures virtually all resulting offspring have the lab-created gene. This is in contrast to conventional genetic engineering where only about 50% of offspring are altered. Radical steps of this type are being considered because both the malaria mosquito and the malaria parasite are becoming increasingly resistant to current control methods. Gene drive technology is only authorized for laboratory research at present, but people are already concerned over its potential to impact species other than mosquitoes when it is used in the wild.

4.3 Innovative education

School-based programs that educate children broadly on the causation and prevention of malaria, and what care is required can reduce morbidity, and, in particular, increase access to timely diagnosis and treatment. The WHO health promoting school (HPS) model in particular lends itself to education on malaria, as a core concept is teaching children knowledge and practical skills through focused additions to the curriculum [17, 18]. Elements of the HPS model can be applied in various ways to either generate an overarching health ethos in the school or focus on a locally relevant health issue like malaria [18].

Award schemes should be explored as a way to foster HPS activity; a variety of support and recognition strategies can be put in place that will encourage individual schools, and create a spirit of competition between schools that is synergistic [21]. Although not evaluated specifically in the context of malaria education, the experience in African schools following the WHO HPS model is that health promotion activities benefit from local recognition and spread from one school to another through healthy rivalry between neighboring schools [65].

Innovative education can be used to address inequitable distribution of knowledge about malaria and promote understanding about the fundamentals of causation, preventive measures and timely diagnosis and treatment. Data on the use of insecticide-treated bed nets for instance suggest focused school-based education positively impacts their use; the need has also been identified for households to learn to make nets available for use by school-aged children [66]. Health promotion messaging should be tailored to address specific need such as this, and framed so that the message resonates with the age group being targeted. Sometimes non-traditional messengers prove to be particularly effective as communicators, for example, young people are drawn to celebrities endorsing health promotion through music videos and social media are an example [67].

In 2020 the World Economic Forum, UNICEF and the World Food Program announced an innovative approach to helping children achieve their full potential. The aim is to improve their health throughout the first 8000 days of life, and thereby build on current investment focused on improving health during the first 1000 days based on developmental origins of health and disease (DOHaD) science [68]. The mechanism proposed will be the development of integrated school programs that combine strategies that improve the health of school-age children. And the goal, to thereby promote their academic potential, achieve better educational outcomes and build human capital [3].

Clearly the education and school-based management strategies required for malaria will be part of this model in future. Integrated school health packages will be based on experience gained from a variety of successful school-based health interventions, and the expectation is that such integration will lead to synergistic effects where combined aims are met through delivery in a single program. Evidence already available from trials of combined health approaches in schools indicates that benefit will also accrue from shared costs, and the stronger health returns anticipated over programs where individual interventions are delivered alone [8, 69, 70].

Schools should also encourage teachers to create and share innovative educational approaches that engage their pupils. For example, clean-up programs can be initiated where children collect discarded plastic bottles, bags and bottle caps on their way to and from school. This approach is innovative as it provides evidence-based learning on how these items offer a breeding habitat for mosquito larvae, and an introduction to larval source management; a preventive approach with the dual benefit of reducing the numbers of house-entering mosquitoes and those that bite outdoors [64, 65]. Practical learning approaches like this can be complimented by in-class question and answer sessions, and the generation of visual aids for the classroom wall by the pupils that show other effective prevention practices and key facts about malaria.

4.4 Novel and improved tools

When the use of RDTs was introduced in community pharmacies this form of testing was not a new tool, but its application in this setting was novel, as was the later expansion of RDT kit use to include teachers in school-based programs [15, 48]. RDT use in both settings resulted in a significant improvement in the reach of this diagnostic tool, as it made testing more readily available and accessible to a larger proportion of the population. In school-based programs RDTs also provided a long called for way to improve care of the school-aged child, by providing an immediate and accurate diagnosis which then allows teachers to treat sick children promptly and with confidence [38].

ACTs continue to be the WHO endorsed first-line therapy in most parts of the world. However, the novel strategy of using multiple first-line therapies rather than a single ACT is a treatment innovation that will help counter emerging resistance to ACTs, and thereby allow this class of drug to remain therapeutically useful as antimalarial drugs for longer [50, 51].

While it is well recognized that the malaria targets for the Millennium Development Goals for 2015 were achieved even though the tools used and the ways in which they were applied were often imperfect [71], it is important that the search continues for better tools for all aspects of malaria control. But in parallel, ways should be explored to expand access to the tools we have that work well, ensure that they are used optimally, and find innovative ways in which they can be modified to meet a new need or counter the very real risk of emergence of drug resistance.

In 2021, the WHO made the historic announcement that a long awaited vaccine for malaria was now recommended for the prevention of P. falciparum malaria in children living in regions with moderate to high transmission [22]. A vaccine against malaria has long been sought, but has proved elusive, in part due to the complexity of the parasite and its numerous immune evasion mechanisms [72]. The RTS,S/AS01 vaccine (RTS,S) is designed to induce antibodies against the sporozoite phase of the lifecycle; this blocks infection of the liver, where the parasite would normally mature and multiply before re-entering the bloodstream to further infect erythrocytes.

RTS,S is the first parasite vaccine to obtain regulatory approval, and there are caveats regarding its current place in malaria control, particularly related to the dosing strategy required, the period of protection provided and partial efficacy, all of which leave room for improvement [73]. Currently the vaccine requires 4 doses from 5 months of age, and for the foreseeable future, vaccinated children will also require some form of chemoprophylaxis in addition, in order to achieve optimum vaccine efficacy. Because of the target age group, programs to immunize will obviously not be school-based [74], but awareness that child vaccination is now an option should be incorporated into school-based health education. This investment will mean that the next generation of young parents will know that this form of prevention is available for their children.

Modifications in dose and schedule have contributed to improved vaccine performance, and further variations may follow [75]. But, as important and historic as vaccine use will be, WHO is calling for the introduction of this novel tool to be used to reinvigorate the fight against malaria in parallel with vaccine rollout programs [22]. This is an important opportunity to respond more effectively than in the past to the repeated calls to scale up and improve malaria control in school-age children [23].

National policies will need to be established and strategies developed to promote local programs that incorporate child vaccination. Creating and implementing the programs required will require both inspired leadership and inter-sectorial collaboration, funding, and support in order for communities to 'buy into' the concept and participate successfully. In addition to the public education and engagement needed regarding the vaccine, clear direction and recommendations are also necessary at the same time on how to deliver and sustain the components of the scaled up malaria control programs for children called for by the WHO to accompany introduction of the vaccine [23].

Meanwhile, several other malaria vaccines with different modes of action are under development. Pre-erythrocytic forms continue to be some of the most promising; pre-erythrocytic agents target antigens from the Plasmodium sporozoite and liver stages when infection is in its earliest stages following inoculation and clinically silent. Induction of antibodies and T cell responses clear sporozoites or block their invasion of hepatocytes [73]. Circumsporozoite protein is a specific target in ongoing research; this is the major antigen on the surface of sporozoites. Various approaches are being applied to develop RTS,S derivatives that improve immunogenicity; recent trials indicate that the R21/MM vaccine appears safe and very immunogenic in African children, and promises high-level efficacy [72].

Novel use of technology can also impact vector control and improve the logistics of delivering supplies needed to test and treat malaria in rural areas. The deployment of drones is an example. Use of this technology in Zanzibar has made it possible to map difficult to find water pools which enables breeding sites to be targeted before larvae turn into adult mosquitoes, and it was learned during the Covid-19 pandemic that drones can be employed effectively to deliver urgently needed supplies when vaccines required in remote areas were provided in this way.

4.5 Training personnel to respond to local needs

The majority of teachers understand the toll malaria takes on their pupil's health, but many need training to fully understand how they and their school can contribute to strategies to reduce the impact the disease can have on their pupils. For instance, not all recognize that repeated absence from class or a pupil dropping out of school altogether can be due to the cumulative effects of malaria. Also, full realization of the negative impact that severe or repeated infection can have often only comes when the beneficial effects of a school-based diagnostic and treatment program become evident through the school's improved performance in national exams.

It is well documented in the literature that the duration of malaria-related absence, frequency of absence due to repeated infection, residual malaise from sub-optimal treatment and transient neurological complications due to malaria can all compromise a child's potential to learn. In this context, it is important that teachers and parents learn about the negative neurologic effects malaria can cause, and that repeated infection can have detrimental effects that are cumulative, and lead to permanent loss of cognition and learning ability [28, 30, 62]. While the exact mechanisms underlying long-term detriment are debated, a clear relationship exists between the severity of infection and the magnitude of the adverse cognitive effect. An excellent schematic that helps in teaching how adverse effects probably come about and their importance was published in 2010 based on a series of studies examining cognitive function and school performance in children after infection with P. falciparum and P. vivax malaria [62].

Nutrition programs are the most widespread school-based initiatives to promote child health. When personnel are trained to implement them well, such programs can improve children's learning ability and academic potential as well as their physical and mental well-being. Children who are well nourished are better positioned to recover from infectious illnesses, including malaria; significantly it is the most disadvantaged children who often benefit the most from school-based nutrition programs [76]. School garden projects can provide produce for lunch programs to feed children in need. Parents can be trained to collaborate and help run school gardens. A systematic review indicates that multiple life skills are learned and educational benefits accrued by pupils who are actively involved in tending gardens and the growing, harvesting and sale of produce [77].

Teachers in many low and middle income countries have been trained successfully to administer specific health programs in schools in response to identified local needs; examples include: the provision of intermittent anti-malarial therapy in Kenya [25, 78], prophylactic chloroquine in Sri Lanka [26], and nationwide anti-helminth treatment in India, Ghana and Uganda [34, 79]. Tetanus prophylaxis and now vaccination against human papilloma virus are also widely administered by individuals trained to deliver them through schools.

Training of staff in pharmacies to use RDT kits could provide sufficient additional capacity in some communities for this to be an alternative to setting up school-based testing and treatment. Programs developed to train non-medical personnel, including teachers, have been evaluated, and the knowledge and skills such training provides enables practitioners to be both safe and effective [53]. Integrating teachers trained to test and treat for malaria into larger health, nutrition and education platforms offered through schools would likely result in cost-benefit over providing individual health interventions singly, and also deliver combined benefits that would contribute towards achieving the sustainable development goals for health [54].

4.6 Non-traditional avenues and outlets

To be effective, any intervention that employs a non-traditional outlet or approach must be context-specific and tailored to meet the needs and available resources of the community that will implement and sustain it [3, 23]. The number, variety and scale of the problems communities in low-and-middle-income countries face regarding malaria requires ingenuity and creativity across society to seek out and trial non-traditional solutions that offer potential benefit. School-based health promotion is an example, and interventions with the potential to reduce malaria morbidity in children range from the provision of basic education about malaria through to 'test and treat' programs that implement WHO malaria management criteria.

Schools are still viewed as non-traditional outlets for health delivery, in spite of the many school-based programs that have been shown to provide benefits for the communities they serve. Importantly, evidence of program efficacy includes interventions to reduce the burden of malaria on school-aged children, including ones developed as a practical response to calls from teachers and community leaders. Unfortunately, not every country has a school system where teachers' morale and motivation make teacher-driven health initiatives feasible [24, 65]. But in the majority, the small number of teachers in each school required to run a 'test and treat' program for malaria are likely to be forthcoming. Certainly, where teachers are aware of the impact malaria has and the improvements intervention can achieve, enough are likely to be willing and able to be taught how to screen children found to be sick at school, treat those testing positive promptly, and refer those children with severe or atypical disease to a conventional health outlet like a clinic or hospital.

From a practical standpoint, community participatory intervention models based in schools are also broadly applicable, and a low cost and flexible approach with considerable potential to meet the longstanding calls for interventions to reduce the burden of disease on school-age children [3, 4, 8]. In addition these models can comply fully with WHO-endorsed diagnostic and treatment principles, follow local government guidelines, and help achieve national goals for malaria control.

Importantly, integration of any avenues that can improve the delivery of health services in a community, or increase access by those needing care will impact the challenge of delay in the treatment of fever [44]. Waiting too long before seeking care for a child likely to have malaria, and failure to obtain an accurate diagnosis and prompt treatment are both major obstacles to achieving the goal of reducing malaria morbidity. Studies indicate that in sub-Saharan Africa <50% of sick, febrile children receive artemisinin combination therapy (ACT) within 24 hours [15, 45, 59, 80]. Approaches that remedy this situation would in themselves go a long way towards reducing the current burden of malaria on children.

5. Conclusion

Bold decisions are needed to control of malaria and particularly to improve the situation in school-aged children. The longstanding recognition that they are a large and especially vulnerable population has not been matched by clear strategies that can be broadly applied to reduce their burden of disease. School-based interventions to control malaria have obvious logic, as schools allow access to the relevant target population. Suitable initiatives exist that are applicable worldwide and have the potential to benefit millions of children. Education to provide a basic level of health literacy about malaria causation, prevention and management should be a universal component of the school curriculum where the disease is endemic. There is also evidence that school-based health care delivery, such as teacher-driven test and treat programs for malaria, offer a cost effective option alone, and especially if combined with other health interventions.

Acknowledgements

The delivery and evaluation of key school-based projects described was made possible through support from the Stellenbosch Institute for Advanced Study at Stellenbosch University in South Africa. Funding for the novel teacher-driven 'test and treat' program in Uganda was provided by a grant from the Hillman Medical Education Fund in Canada.

Conflict of interest

The author declares no conflict of interest.

Author details

Andrew Macnab[1,2]

1 Faculty of Medicine, University of British Columbia, Vancouver, Canada

2 Stellenbosch Institute for Advanced Study (STIAS), Wallenberg Research Centre at Stellenbosch University, Stellenbosch, South Africa

*Address all correspondence to: ajmacnab@gmail.com

References

[1] WHO. World Malaria Report 2014. Geneva: World Health Organization; 2014. Available from: http://www.who.int/entity/malaria/publications/world_malaria_report_2014/wmr-2014-no-profiles.pdf?ua=1. [Accessed: May 11, 2022]

[2] Mullen Z. Malaria: Bold decisions needed. The Lancet Global Health. 2015;**3**(12):e724

[3] Cohee LM, Nankabirwa JI, Greenwood B, et al. Time for malaria control in school-age children. The Lancet Child & Adolescent Health. 2021;**5**(8):537-538. DOI: 10.1016/S2352-4642(21)00158-9

[4] Nankabirwa J, Brooker SJ, Clarke SE, et al. Malaria in school-age children in Africa: An increasingly important challenge. Tropical Medicine & International Health. 2014;**19**(11):1294-1309

[5] Drake TL, Okello G, Njagi K, et al. Cost analysis of school-based intermittent screening and treatment of malaria in Kenya. Malaria Journal. 2011;**10**(1):1-11

[6] Bundy DA, De Silva N, Horton S, Jamison DT, editors. Disease Control Priorities, (Volume 8): Child and Adolescent Health and Development. World Bank; Washington, DC; 2017

[7] Macnab AJ. School-based initiatives to reduce malaria morbidity and mortality and promote academic achievement in children. In: Macnab AJ, Daar A, Pauw C, editors. Health in Transition – Translating Developmental Origins of Health and Disease Science to Improve Future Health in Africa. Stellenbosch, South Africa: Africa Sun Media; 2020. pp. 247-290

[8] Cohee LM, Opondo C, Clarke SE, et al. Preventive malaria treatment among school-aged children in sub-Saharan Africa: A systematic review and meta-analyses. The Lancet Global Health. 2020;**8**(12):e1499-e1511

[9] Bell D, Fleurent AE, Hegg MC, Boomgard JD, McConnico CC. Development of new malaria diagnostics: Matching performance and need. Malaria Journal. 2016;**15**(1):406

[10] Editorial. Malaria vaccine approval: A step change for global health. Lancet. 2011;**398**(10309):1381

[11] Ayi I, Nonaka D, Adjovu JK, et al. School-based participatory health education for malaria control in Ghana: Engaging children as health messengers. Malaria Journal. 2010;**9**(1):98

[12] Simovska V, Carlsson M. Health-promoting changes with children as agents: Findings from a multiple case study research. Health Education. 2012;**112**(3):292-304

[13] St Ledger L. Schools, health literacy and public health: Possibilities and challenges. Health Promotion International. 2001;**16**(2):197-205

[14] Afenyadu GY, Agyepong IA, Barnish G, Adjei S. Improving access to early treatment of malaria: A trial with primary school teachers as care providers. Tropical Medicine & International Health. 2005;**10**(10):1065-1072

[15] Macnab AJ, Mukisa R, Mutabazi S, Steed R. Malaria in Uganda: School-based rapid diagnostic testing and treatment. International Journal of Epidemiology.

2016;**45**(6):1759-1762. DOI: 10.1093/ije/dyw262

[16] WHO. WHO World Malaria Report 2015. 2015. http://www.who.int/malaria/publications/world-malaria-report-2015/wmr2015-without-profiles.pdf?ua=1. [Accessed: May 11, 2022]

[17] Macnab AJ. The Stellenbosch consensus statement on health promoting schools. Global Health Promotion. 2013;**20**(1):78-81

[18] World Health Organization. What Is a Health Promoting School? WHO. Geneva; 2013. Available from: http://who.int/school_youth_health/gshi/hps/en/index.html. 2013 [Accessed: May 15, 2022]

[19] Viner RM, Ozer EM, Denny S, et al. Adolescence and the social determinants of health. Lancet. 2012;**379**(9826):1641-1652

[20] Tang K, Nutbeam D, Aldinger C, et al. Schools for health, education and development: A call for action. Health Promotion International. 2008;**24**(1):68-77

[21] Lee A. The Healthy Settings Approach in Hong Kong. Sustainable Development for Population Health. City Hong Kong: University of Hong Kong Press; 2021

[22] WHO. 2021. Available from: https://www.who.int/news/item/06-10-2021-who-recommends-groundbreaking-malaria-vaccine-for-children-at-risk. [Accessed: May 11, 2022]

[23] Macnab AJ. Malaria: What does the RTS, S/AS01 vaccine mean for children in Africa? Journal of Community Medicine and Public Health Care. 2021;**8**:096

[24] Macnab AJ, Stewart D, Gagnon F. Health promoting schools: Initiatives in Africa. Health Education. 2014;**114**(4):246-259

[25] Temperley M, Mueller DH, Njagi JK, et al. Costs and cost-effectiveness of delivering intermittent preventive treatment through schools in western Kenya. Malaria Journal. 2008;**7**(1):1-9

[26] Fernando D, De Silva D, Carter R, et al. Randomized, double-blind, placebo-controlled, clinical trial of the impact of malaria prevention on the educational attainment of school children. The American Journal of Tropical Medicine and Hygiene. 2006;**74**(3):386-393

[27] Cairns M, Roca-Feltrer A, Garske T, et al. Estimating the potential public health impact of seasonal malaria chemoprevention in African children. Nature Communications. 2012;**3**:881

[28] Nankabirwa JI, Wandera B, Amuge P, et al. Impact of intermittent preventive treatment with dihydroartemisinin-piperaquine on malaria in Ugandan schoolchildren: A randomized, placebo-controlled trial. Clinical Infectious Diseases. 2014;**58**(10):1404-1412

[29] Thera MA, Kone AK, Tangara B, et al. School-aged children based seasonal malaria chemoprevention using artesunate-amodiaquine in Mali. Parasite Epidemiology Control. 2018;**3**(2):96-105

[30] Clarke SE. Impact of a malaria intervention package in schools on plasmodium infection, anaemia and cognitive function in schoolchildren in Mali: A pragmatic cluster-randomised trial. BMJ Global Health. 2017;**2**:e000182

[31] Wilson AL. A systematic review and meta-analysis of the efficacy and safety of intermittent preventive treatment of malaria in children (IPTc). PLoS One. 2011;**6**(2):e16976

[32] Matangila JR, Mitashi P, da Luz RA, Lutumba PT, Van Geertruyden JP. Efficacy and safety of intermittent preventive treatment for malaria in schoolchildren: A systematic review. Malaria Journal. 2015;**14**(1):450

[33] Hotez PJ, Molyneux DH, Fenwick A, et al. Control of neglected tropical diseases. NEJM. 2007;**357**(10):1018-1027

[34] Opoku EC, Olsen A, Browne E, et al. Impact of combined intermittent preventive treatment of malaria and helminths on anaemia, sustained attention, and recall in northern Ghanaian school children. Global Health Action. 2016;**9**:32197

[35] Cohee LM, Chilombe M, Ngwira A, et al. Pilot study of the addition of mass treatment for malaria to existing school-based programs to treat neglected tropical diseases. The American Journal of Tropical Medicine and Hygiene. 2018;**98**(1):95-99

[36] Visser T, Bruxvoort K, Maloney K, et al. Introducing malaria rapid diagnostic tests in private medicine retail outlets: A systematic literature review. PLoS One. 2017;**12**(3):e0173093

[37] Mphwatiwa T, Witek-McManus S, Mtali A, et al. School-based diagnosis and treatment of malaria by teachers using rapid diagnostic tests and artemisinin-based combination therapy: Experiences and perceptions of users and implementers of the Learner Treatment Kit, southern Malawi. Malaria Journal. 2017;**16**(1):318

[38] WHO. WHO Global Technical Strategy for Malaria 2016-2030. Geneva: World Health Organization; 2015 Available from: http://www.who.int/malaria/areas/global_technical_strategy/en

[39] Thiam S, Thior M, Faye B, et al. Major reduction in anti-malarial drug consumption in Senegal after nation-wide introduction of malaria rapid diagnostic tests. PLoS One. 2011;**6**(4):e18419

[40] Counihan H, Harvey SA, Sekeseke-Chinyama M, et al. Community health workers use malaria rapid diagnostic tests (RDTs) safely and accurately: Results of a longitudinal study in Zambia. The American Journal of Tropical Medicine and Hygiene. 2012;**87**(1):57-63

[41] Eastman RT, Fidock DA. Artemisinin-based combination therapies: A vital tool in efforts to eliminate malaria. Nature Reviews. Microbiology. 2009;**7**(12):864-874

[42] International Artemisinin Study Group. Artesenuate combinations for treatment of malaria: Meta-analysis. Lancet. 2004;**363**(9402):9-17

[43] Benjamin J, Moore B, Lee S, et al. Artemisinin-naphthoquine combination therapy for uncomplicated pediatric malaria: A tolerability, safety, and preliminary efficacy study. Antimicrobial Agents and Chemotherapy. 2012;**56**(5):2465-2471

[44] White NJ. Qinghaosu (artemisinin): The price of success. Science. 2008;**320**:330-334

[45] Mutabingwa TK. Artemisinin-based combination therapies (ACTs): Best hope for malaria treatment but inaccessible to the needy. Acta Tropica. 2005;**95**(3):305-315

[46] Ashley EA, Poespoprodjo JR. Treatment and prevention of malaria in children. The Lancet Child & Adolescent Health. 2020;**4**(10):775-789

[47] Whitty CJM, Chandler C, Ansah E, Leslie T, Staedke SG. Deployment of ACT antimalarials for treatment of malaria: Challenges and opportunities. Malaria Journal. 2008;**7**(1):1-7

[48] Akweongo P, Agyei-Baffour P, Sudhakar M, et al. Feasibility and acceptability of ACT for the community case management of malaria in urban settings in five African sites. Malaria Journal. 2011;**10**(1):240

[49] Mbonye AK, Magnussen P, Lai S, et al. A cluster randomized trial introducing rapid diagnostic tests in registered drug shops in Uganda: Impact on appropriate treatment of malaria. PLoS One. 2015;**10**(7):e0129545

[50] Boni MF, White NJ, Baird JK. The community as the patient in malaria-endemic areas: Preempting drug resistance with multiple first-line therapies. PLoS Medicine. 2016;**13**(3):e1001984

[51] Nguyen TD, Olliaro P, Dondorp AM, et al. Optimum population-level use of artemisinin combination therapies: A modelling study. The Lancet Global Health. 2015;**3**(12):e758-e766

[52] Colbourne MJ. The effect of malaria suppression in a group of Accra school children. Transactions of the Royal Society of Tropical Medicine & Hygiene. 1955;**49**(4):356-369

[53] Witek-McManus S, Mathanga DP, Verney A, et al. Design, implementation and evaluation of a training programme for school teachers in the use of malaria rapid diagnostic tests. BMC Public Health. 2015;**15**(1):1-3

[54] Costanza R, Daly L, Fioramonti L, Giovannini E. Modelling and measuring sustainable wellbeing in connection with the UN Sustainable Development Goals. Ecological Economics. 2016;**130**:350-355

[55] Marmot M, Friel S, Bell R, et al. Commission on social determinants of health. Closing the gap in a generation: Health equity through action on the social determinants of health. Lancet. 2008;**372**(9650):1661-1669

[56] Agyepong IA, Sewankambo N, Binagwaho A, et al. The path to longer and healthier lives for all Africans by 2030: The lancet commission on the future of health in sub-Saharan Africa. Lancet. 2017;**390**(10114):2803-2859

[57] Gilmore B, Ndejjo R, Tchetchia A, et al. Community engagement for COVID-19 prevention and control: A rapid evidence synthesis. BMJ Global Health. 2020;**5**(10):e003188

[58] Airhihenbuwa CO, Makoni S, IwelunmorJ, MunodawafaD. Sociocultural infrastructure: Communicating identity and health in Africa. Journal of Health Communication. 2014;**19**(1):1-5

[59] Rutebemberwa E, Kallander K, Tomson G, Peterson S, Pariyo G. Determinants of delay in care-seeking for febrile children in eastern Uganda. Tropical Medicine & International Health. 2009;**14**:472-479

[60] Källander K, Nsungwa-Sabiiti J, Peterson S. Symptom overlap for malaria and pneumonia—Policy implications for home management strategies. Acta Tropica. 2004;**90**(2):211-214

[61] Fernando SD, Rodrigo C, Rajapaske S. The 'hidden' burden of malaria: Cognitive impairment following infection. Malaria Journal. 2010;**9**(1):1-11

[62] Thuilliez J, Sissoko MS, Toure OB, et al. Malaria and primary education in Mali: A longitudinal study in the village

of Doneguebougou. Social Science & Medicine. 2010;**71**(2):324-334

[63] Swana EK, Makan GY, Mukeng CK, et al. Feasibility and implementation of community-based malaria case management with integrated vector control in the Democratic Republic of Congo. Malaria Journal. 2016;**15**(1):413

[64] De Silva PM, Marshall JM. Factors contributing to urban malaria transmission in sub-Saharan Africa: A systematic review. Journal of Tropical Medicine. 2012;**2012**:819563. DOI: 10.1155/2012/819563 [Article ID 819563]

[65] Macnab AJ. The World Health Organization's health promoting school model: A potential avenue for developmental origins of health and disease education in Africa. In: Macnab AJ, Daar A, Pauw C, editors. Health in Transition – Translating Developmental Origins of Health and Disease Science to Improve Future Health in Africa. Stellenbosch, South Africa: Africa Sun Media; 2020. pp. 203-232

[66] Olapeju B, Choiriyyah I, Lynch M, et al. Age and gender trends in insecticide-treated net use in sub-Saharan Africa: A multi-country analysis. Malaria Journal. 2018;**17**(1):1-2

[67] Macnab AJ, Mukisa R. Celebrity endorsed music videos: Innovation to foster youth health promotion. Health Promotion International. 2019;**34**(4):716-725

[68] Barker D. Developmental origins of adult health and disease. Journal of Epidemiology and Community Health. 2004;**58**(2):114

[69] Drake TL, Okello G, Njagi K, et al. Cost analysis of school-based intermittent screening and treatment of malaria in Kenya. Malaria Journal. 2011;**10**(1):273

[70] Laxminarayan R, Chow J, Shahid-Salles SA. Intervention cost-effectiveness: Overview of main messages. In: Breman JG, Measham AR, Alleyne G, et al., editors. Disease Control Priorities for Developing Countries. Oxford: Oxford University Press; 2006. pp. 35-86

[71] Alonso P, Noor AM. The global fight against malaria is at crossroads. Lancet. 2017;**390**(10112):2532-2534

[72] Datoo MS, Natama MH, Somé A, et al. Efficacy of a low-dose candidate malaria vaccine, R21 in adjuvant matrix-M, with seasonal administration to children in Burkina Faso: A randomised controlled trial. Lancet. 2021;**397**(10287):1809-1818

[73] Duffy PE, Patrick GJ. Malaria vaccines since 2000: Progress, priorities, products. npj Vaccines. 2020;**5**(1):1-9

[74] Greenwood B, Dicko A, Sagara I, et al. Seasonal vaccination against malaria: A potential use for an imperfect malaria vaccine. Malaria Journal. 2017;**16**(1):182

[75] Draper SJ, Sack BK, King CR, Nielsen CM, Rayner JC, Higgins MK, et al. Malaria vaccines: Recent advances and new horizons. Cell Host & Microbe. 2018;**24**(1):43-56

[76] Kristjansson B, Petticrew M, MacDonald B, et al. School feeding for improving the physical and psychosocial health of disadvantaged students. Cochrane Database of Systematic Reviews. 2007;**10**:1830-1839

[77] Royal Horticultural Society. Food Growing in Schools Taskforce Report. Royal Horticultural Society, Coventry, UK. 2012. pp. 1-66. Available from: http://www.gardenorganic.org.uk

[78] Okello G, Ndegwa SN, Halliday KE, Hanson K, Brooker SJ, Jones C. Local

perceptions of intermittent screening and treatment for malaria in school children on the south coast of Kenya. Malaria Journal. 2012;**11**(1):1-4

[79] Brooker S, Kabatereine NB, Fleming F, Devlin N. Cost and cost-effectiveness of nationwide school-based helminth control in Uganda: Intra-country variation and effects of scaling-up. Health Policy and Planning. 2008;**23**(1):24-35

[80] Simba DO, Warsame M, Kakoko D, Mrango Z. Who gets prompt access to artemisinin-based combination therapy? A prospective community-based study in children from rural Kilosa, Tanzania. PLoS One. 2010;**5**(8):e12104-e12108

Chapter 8

Prevention, Treatment and Malaria Control: A Southern America Perspective

Carol Yovana Rosero-Galindo, Gloria Isabel Jaramillo-Ramirez, Cesar Garcia-Balaguera and Franco Andres Montenegro-Coral

Abstract

Malaria is one of the diseases with the highest morbi-mortality rate worldwide, including Colombia, where it is endemic in several regions of the country. Although the incidence of this disease in the Department of Meta and the Atlantic Coast is not as high as in Nariño, the number of reported cases has held steady over time. It is still an event of great interest in public health. The struggle against malaria is part of one of the Millennium Development Goals and has generated global and national programs that have been implemented at a national and global level, whose main goal is to control and eradicate malaria. These programs have stood out for their vertical nature and for the low level of community participation. Health sector needs to include, at a micro-level, the voices of the community represented in their discourses and actions in the face of the disease, its prevention, and treatment. Therefore, a community and institutional look at these elements, in relation to the disease and the vector, should be provided, which will allow the vector and disease control programs to be improved, designing strategies to bring community and government agencies together to propose public health policies and programs.

Keywords: Colombia, community, government agencies, malaria, control programs

1. Introduction

Malaria remains a global public health problem, with nearly 3.2 billion people in 97 countries at risk of being infected and developing the disease, leading to a high social and economic burden. According to the World Health Organization, malaria cases have increased since 2015, showing a significant increase not only in morbidity but also in mortality in 2020, due in part to the COVID-19 pandemic [1]. Significant progress has been made in malaria control over the past two decades in America, but in recent years, there has been stagnation and an increase in the number of cases in countries such as Venezuela (811.5% between 2010 and 2017) and Nicaragua (1482.2% between 2010 and 2017) [2]. During 2021, 72,022 cases of malaria occurred in Colombia; 70,838 of them were non-complicated malaria, and 1184 were complicated malaria (1.64%). The annual parasite index was 8.93 cases per 1000 inhabitants, with a predominance of *Plasmodium falciparum* (49.6%) and *P. vivax* (49.4%). Mixed infections accounted for only 0.9%. During that year, major outbreaks occurred in 13 municipalities of the country, and the most affected departments where Choco, Nariño, Cordoba, Amazonas, Antioquia, Meta, and Caqueta. 57.8% of the cases occurred in men, and 738 cases were reported in pregnant women [3].

Malaria is a multicausal disease, and therefore, new approaches to control it are comprehensive and include individual, community, and institutional participation to strengthen the capacity of local response to achieve a sustainability of actions with an emphasis on promoting good health and preventing malaria [4]. However, despite existing policies, plans, and programs, malaria remains a serious public health problem in the country. Since the dawn of the twentieth century and during the time of public hygiene, malaria and anemia produced by uncinaria have been considered one of the priorities for control [5]. Between 1956 and 1993, a vertical control program was carried out in Colombia headed by the Ministry of Health's Direct Campaigns Directorate and the Malaria Eradication Service (SEM by its Spanish acronym), a program that ran parallel to the National Health System [6]. During the nineties, profound reforms to the health system were carried out through Law 100 of 1993, which led to the dismantling of the programs headed by the state, transforming the fight against malaria into a control program with several actors involved [7].

Nevertheless, malaria is a disease that is closely related to the level of poverty in a community. It slows economic growth and perpetuates the vicious cycle of poverty. Rural areas are the most vulnerable since buildings and living facilities are deficient and generally have little or no protection against mosquitoes [8].

In Colombia, rural areas reveal concerning levels of health indicators; high levels of malnutrition; low levels of schooling of the population; higher illiteracy rates; and low coverage of basic public utilities, including potable water, sewerage, and electricity. This problem is largely due to the geography, the great distances and topographic difficulties of the terrain that make it difficult to enter certain areas, and also public order issues due to the presence of armed conflict participants and very low or lack of presence of health service providers [9]. These socio-economic factors play an important role in malaria transmission and in other human activities that foster movement of populations, such as migration and wars, leading to the spread of both the parasite and the vector [10].

According to the programs derived from the health system reform, malaria control activities are divided into collective actions (headed by the state) and individual actions (headed by health insurers and health services providers). The following activities are carried out as part of the collective activities included in Collective Interventions Plan (PIC by its Spanish acronym) headed by local authorities, vector control, intra- and peri-domiciliary fumigation, handing out bed nets (mosquito nets), and the supervision of the event by the municipality [11] (National Health Institute, 2014). However, programs are designed without the participation of the communities involved, ignoring local knowledge and socio-political and cultural dynamics surrounding their main health problems, in this case malaria. This leads to imposing out-of-context control measures that reduce the coverage and impact of interventions [12].

Communities forge discourses and knowledge about health and illness that are reflected in attitudes and individual actions that can contribute to the success or failure of the program. Community participation in health programs requires measurable changes in behaviors that allow for active personal involvement in decision-making regarding the health of their own families. Health personnel also have their own views of community affairs from their knowledge, hierarchies, and practices. These discourse and activities draw paths of malaria prevention, treatment, and control, often parallel to and with no contact between them. This is the reason why the community perspective needs to be incorporated into institutional programs.

In light of the aforementioned, the health sector needs to include, at a micro-level, the voices of the community represented in their discourses and actions in the face of the disease, its prevention, and treatment. It is important to note that the studies carried out so far in Colombia have focused on areas with high endemic rates. Nonetheless, it is important to keep an eye on community and governmental dynamics in areas where the number of cases is not high but has remained constant throughout the years and where outbreaks eventually occur.

2. Epidemiological depiction of malaria in the world and in Colombia

Malaria, a disease transmitted by mosquitoes of the genus *Anopheles* and produced by parasites of the genus *Plasmodium*, remains a global public health problem, with nearly 3.2 billion people in 97 countries at risk of being infected and developing the disease, leading to a high social and economic burden [13]. Between 2000 and 2020, an estimated 1.7 billion cases and 10.6 million deaths worldwide were estimated, falling from 896,000 in 2000 to 558,000 in 2015. However, there was an increase (627,000) partly due to the COVID-19 pandemic [1].

By 2020, there were 18 endemic countries in the Americas, accounting for 0.3% of the total malaria cases in the world. Brazil, Colombia, and Venezuela accounted for 77% of the cases in the region. In the past 20 years, significant advances have been made in decreasing the incidence in endemic countries, from 14.1 to 4.6 cases per 1000 inhabitants at risk and a 58% reduction in overall cases. Mortality also decreased from 0.8 to 0.3 deaths per 100,000 inhabitants at risk. Despite this, countries such as Venezuela have significantly increased the number of infections, from 35,500 in the year 2000 to more than 467,000 in 2019, affecting the statistics in the region. Other countries such as Bolivia, Haiti, Honduras, Nicaragua, and Panama showed substantial increases in 2020 in comparison to 2019 [1].

In Colombia, malaria is present in more than 80% of the national territory, with five macro-foci of variable and active transmission: the Pacific Region (departments of Choco, Nariño, and Cauca and the district of Buenaventura in Valle del Cauca), the Amazone-Orinoquia Region (departments of Amazonas, Vichada, Guainia, and Guaviare), Magdalena Medio (Antioquia, Bolivar, and Cordoba), and a recent focus on the border with Venezuela (department of Norte de Santander) [14]. Thanks to its extensive and diverse social and environmental conditions that have led to the transmission and endemicity of this disease in the country [15], malaria still represents a serious public health issue.

During the year 2015, 56,705 malaria cases were reported in the system in Colombia. 55,866 were cases of non-complicated malaria, and 839 were cases of complicated malaria. 18 deaths from this disease were reported. Choco, Nariño, and Antioquia headed the list of reports, accumulating more than 75% of total cases in the country [16]. By 2016, the increase in cases was evident, with 84,742 reports, of which 83,227 were non-complicated malaria and 1515 were complicated malaria. Additionally, 26 confirmed deaths and 10 deaths classified as compatible cases were reported [17]. During 2017, the decline in cases was evident, with a total of 55,117 reports across the country. The departments of Choco, Nariño, Antioquia, Cordoba, Guainia, Amazonas, Cauca, and Vichada registered 90.7% of cases of non-complicated malaria [18]. For the year 2018, there was a 14.6% increase compared to the previous year, with a total of

63,143 reported cases of malaria in the country. 54% of the cases came from the Pacific region, with the department of Choco (27.7%) being the largest reporter of cases, followed by the department of Nariño, with 21.8% [19]. For the year 2019, there was a situation of sustained malaria outbreak throughout the year, with a total of 80,415 cases reported in the system, of which 79,120 (98.3%) were classified as non-complicated malaria and 1295 (1.6%) were classified as complicated malaria [20]. Similar numbers were observed during 2020, with a total of 80,236 malaria reports in the public health monitoring system. Despite the health emergency caused by COVID-19 and the mandatory preventive isolation that occurred in the country from epidemiological week 12 to week 32, the country was hit by a malaria outbreak situation from epidemiological week 18 to week 23 and then from week 30 to week 53. Historically, Choco, Nariño, and Antioquia remain the departments with the highest incidence of the disease [14]. The year 2021 showed a decrease of 11.4% with respect to the previous year, with a total of 70,838 cases reported. 14 municipalities reported outbreak situations. During this year, 1291 cases of coinfection between malaria and COVID-19 were reported [14].

3. Community-based knowledge and actions regarding malaria

From a cultural perspective, the health system is made up of hierarchies or levels: the popular, the folkloric, and the professional level. An approximation among the three represents pluralism in the healthcare of a particular social group [21].

The so-called third sector, or professionals, has a technical language that separates it from their patients—their own body of knowledge. It emphasizes on the disease and is often based on technology. This perspective applies both to health care and to the generation of policies, plans, and programs that are vertically established, ignoring the conception of local medicine, which is part of a larger system of beliefs, behaviors, and attitudes.

It is important to emphasize that part of the verticality with which most health programs are established originates from this hierarchical sectoring specific to the area's staff. Knowledge and training, different from those of the community, create a gap that separates them. The community that "does not know" can be diagnosed and treated because its cultural baggage is not recognized as it is another type. In addition, this alleged "superiority" leads to a paternalistic treatment, a position generally adopted in relation to vulnerable communities.

These views of what the community is, from a professional perspective, draw disease prevention, treatment, and control paths, which are often parallel and have no contact between them. Thus, the community perspective needs to be incorporated into institutional programs. Programs are designed with no participation from the communities involved, ignoring local knowledge and the socio-political and cultural dynamics around their main health problems, in this case malaria. This leads to imposing out-of-context control measures that reduce the coverage and impact of interventions [12].

4. Malaria control programs in America

Because malaria transmission is highly heterogeneous, control programs in the Americas have to adapt to these different environments [22]. Reactive strategies are the most feasible ones and are endorsed by the World Health Organization [23]. Reactive case detection (RACD) tests and treats all household members related with a positive malaria case detected in a health facility; sometimes the neighbors are also treated [24]. Other strategies try to test the whole community that has at least one diagnosed case; this strategy is called mass screen and treat (MSAT). Or they test the whole population even if there is not a confirmed case of malaria, called mass test and treat (MTAT) [25]. The best strategy depends on the resources and their objectives, and these activities have to be attached to an effective vector control program and a strong health system [26].

5. Malaria control programs in Colombia

Since the dawn of the twentieth century and during the time of public hygiene, malaria as well as anemia produced by uncinaria have been considered disease control priorities, because they affected those areas where the production of coffee and oil began to be fundamental to the economy of the country [4].

The public health programs that marked the beginning of the twentieth century were designed from the perspective of the control and power that dominated the context of the new century. Europe was uniting at the expense of great wars, and the eyes of the great powers turned to Latin America's resources for the reconstruction of their economies. International health agencies were born in response to the need to control the prevailing tropical diseases in which North American companies began to reap benefits from the newly discovered products, channeling the expansion of the exchange in the Americas under civilizing, modernizing, and hygenizing slogans [27].

Between 1956 and 1983, a vertical control program was carried out in the country headed by the Ministry of Health's Direct Campaigns Directorate and the Malaria Eradication Service (SEM by its Spanish acronym), a program that ran parallel to the National Health System [5], and it stood out for its warmongering conception of the disease with a marked use of military terminology [28].

This period was marked by the implementation of the strategy of the Pan-American Health Organization (now known as PAHO), which in the face of communicable diseases such as yellow fever and malaria focused its activities on eradicating the vector and, consequently, the disease, introducing the use of residual-acting insecticides (DDT: dichloro-diphenyl-trichloroethane), which were initially used as pediculicide against a typhus epidemic in Naples between 1943 and 1944. The objective of the campaign was to achieve the eradication of malaria throughout the national territory, and it was carried out in four phases: preparatory, attack, consolidation, and maintenance phases [27].

During the 1980s and 1990s, there were profound reforms to the health system. Between 1983 and 1990 and in line with the State decentralization reforms, the program went from being run by the nation to the being run by the departments [29]. Between 1991 and 1994 and specifically after Law 100 of 1993, the programs run by the State ended, transforming the fight against malaria into a control program with several stakeholders dividing malaria control activities into collective actions (headed by the State) and individual actions (headed by health insurers) [7].

From the market perspective of the health system in force since 1993 and with the corresponding loss of control on the part of the state, malaria management programs have deteriorated due to the fragmentation of actions, leading to the loss of information due to the lack of robust data-gathering and analysis systems, the dismantling of the diagnostic capability installed, and the deterioration of the indicators of disease control [6]. During 2010–2015, the "Malaria Project" was carried out, with the general purpose of reducing malaria morbidity and mortality in the departments, with the highest concentration of cases in Colombia. The objectives were aimed at designing and implementing communication and social mobilization plans to increase protective factors [30]. However, none of the departments involved in our study were within the Malaria Project action plans.

6. Malaria control, prevention, treatment, and access issues in rural communities

Diseases such as malaria mainly affect populations under poor socio-economic conditions, living in precarious housing, with limited access to basic public utilities such as potable water and basic sanitation; under deteriorated environmental conditions; and with barriers to access health services. Other human activities that foster population movements, such as migration and wars, lead to the spread of both the parasite and the vector. Generally, these vulnerable populations live in rural or peri-urban areas [16]. High prevalence of this disease diminishes economic growth and perpetuates the vicious cycle of poverty. Rural areas are the most vulnerable since buildings and poor housing facilities have very little or no protection against mosquitoes [8, 10]. In Panamá, malaria cases have progressively increased in prevalence in the past 20 years. Factors such as a weak control program have affected the indigenous settlements in a major proportion [31].

In Colombia, housing conditions and basic needs are very variable; in the Olaya Herrera municipality (Pacific region), only 33.6% of the population has aqueduct, 8.2% has sewerage, and 65% has garbage collection [32]. In Vista Hermosa (a hilly landscape and alluvial plains area of the eastern plains), electrical services coverage is only 89%, and the garbage collection service reaches 85%. A similar percentage of coverage is found in the aqueduct and sewerage services, reported only by 78% of the inhabitants. Similar conditions are evident in San Jose del Guaviare (transition area between the Orinoquia and Amazon regions), where the water supply service reaches only 60% of these communities and the sewerage service reaches 53.4%. Likewise, garbage collection reaches 87.4%. Overall, these conditions have led to a significant deterioration of environmental conditions, and the population's low awareness of these issues adds to these issues. In many areas of the municipalities, garbage can be seen on the streets and water source contamination is very evident.

Child mortality from malaria could be reduced by up to 20% if people were to sleep under insecticide-treated (mosquito) bed nets. Fast access to effective treatment can further reduce deaths. Intermittent preventive malaria treatment during pregnancy can significantly reduce the proportion of low-birth-weight babies and maternal anemia [8].

In Colombia, the provision of health services in dispersed rural areas is hampered due to the geographical isolation of many communities; distances and topographic difficulties of the terrain make entering these areas difficult. Public order issues due to the presence of participants of the armed conflict do not allow the approach and adequate provision of health services. In remote rural areas of the country, quality of life indicators lag behind. There are reports of high fertility; high infant and maternal mortality rates; low life expectancy; high levels of malnutrition; low levels of schooling; high illiteracy rates; and low levels of basic sanitation services coverage for potable water, sewerage, and electricity in the population. On the other hand, ethnic groups with different cultures, knowledge, and activities related to health issues, with a greater emphasis on the ancestral medicine of their communities, predominate in these areas, which poses a challenge to their healthcare [9].

7. Knowledge, attitudes, practices, and intervention related to malaria in Colombia

Since it is one of the most malaria endemic areas, several studies have been carried out in the Pacific to implement and evaluate strategies to improve the quality of life there, starting with the reduction of malaria cases in communities. Educational strategies can improve prevention practices in communities, and this is reflected in the decrease in the incidence of malaria cases in the areas under intervention [33]. In addition, the inclusion of educational strategies integrated in national control program activities leads to a decrease in institutional costs and a reduction in cases [34].

In the municipality of Bahia Solano, it was discovered that more than 70% of the people surveyed know that malaria is transmitted by a mosquito bite. However, about 55% do not go to a health center for treatment but take herbal infusions or baths prepared with plants [35]. In the municipality of Olaya Herrera, 61% of the people surveyed claimed to have contracted malaria, and 75.37% considered the disease a problem for them and their families [32].

In the eastern plains, in the municipality of Vista Hermosa, 43% of respondents reported having had malaria at some point in their lives, and 90% still consider this disease a problem for themselves and their families. In terms of knowledge about the disease, 63% recognized that a mosquito is the vector of malaria, although they did not specifically identify which mosquito it is. In the municipality of San Jose de Guaviare, 59% of respondents said that they had malaria at some point in their lives, and 16.5% do not consider malaria a health problem for themselves and their families. 76% knew that the disease is transmitted by any mosquito bite, and only 6% knew that the Anopheles mosquito was specifically the vector of this pathology.

Despite growing community awareness of the way in which the disease is transmitted, they have no confidence in care centers. 38.7% of respondents said that they did not receive good care from health officials when they were suffering from malaria, while 90.98% of those who had malaria went to health centers and followed the treatments prescribed by doctors. 43% claimed that the office of the secretary of health makes no effort to reduce malaria in the municipality, and 51% said that there is no malaria awareness education [32]. In Vista Hermosa, most of the disease control actions are individual, among which are the drainage of lagoons and ponds at 32% and the use of bed nets (mosquito nets) at 74%. None of the respondents reported using household awnings to prevent mosquito entry, only 9% said they sprayed their homes with insecticides, and 10% used repellents.

It is possible that disconnection between communities and government agencies may be influencing malaria control programs so that they are not very ineffective.

Author details

Carol Yovana Rosero-Galindo[1*], Gloria Isabel Jaramillo-Ramirez[2], Cesar Garcia-Balaguera[2] and Franco Andres Montenegro-Coral[1]

1 Medicine Faculty, Cooperativa de Colombia University, Pasto-Nariño, Colombia

2 Medicine Faculty, Cooperativa de Colombia University, Villavicencio-Meta, Colombia

*Address all correspondence to: carol.roserog@campusucc.edu.co

References

[1] Word Health Organization. State of Inequiality HIV, Tuberculosis and Malaria. Geneva, Switzerland: Word Health Organization; 2021

[2] Sanchez A, Camaño L, Ruano AL, Rodriguez E. Hacia un mundo libre de malaria: utopía o realidad. Boletín de Malariología y Salud Ambiental. 2021;**LX1**(3):373-382

[3] Instituto Nacional de Salud. Informe de Evento - Malaria - Periodo epidemiológico XIII Colombia, 2021. Bogotá: INS; 2021

[4] Ministerio de la Protección Social. Plan Nacional de Salud Publica. Gestión para la vigilancia entomológica y control de la transmisión de malaria. Colombia: Ministerio de la Protección Social; 2010

[5] Quevedo E. Café y gusanos, Mosquitos y petroleo. In: Quevedo E, editor. Café y gusanos, Mosquitos y petroleo. Bogotá: Universidad Nacional; 2004. p. 420

[6] Jiménez M. Reformas sanitarias e impacto del control de malaria en dos áreas endémicas de Colombia, 1982-2004. Colombia Médica. 2007;**2007**:113-131

[7] Valero MV. Malaria in Colombia: Retrospective Glance during the Past 40 Years. Revista de salud pública. 2006;**141**:149

[8] UNICEF. Salud. 2015. Retrieved from El Paludismo: http://www.unicef.org/spanish/health/index_malaria.html

[9] Murillo OL. Desafios de la prestación de servicios de salud en zonas rurales de Colombia. "Experiencia del proyecto malaria fondo mundial". Universidad Nacional de Colombia. Bogotá: Universidad Nacional de Colombia; 2012. 0vector/05599416.2012.pdf

[10] Vargas Herrera J. Prevención y control de la malaria y otras enfermedades transmitidas por vectores en el Perú. Revista Peruana de Epidemiología. 2003;**11**(1):1-19

[11] Instituto Nacional de Salud. Protocolo para la vigilancia en salud pública de la malaria. Bogotá: INS; 2014

[12] Fernández J. Los dominios culturales de la malaria: una aproximación a los saberes no institucionales. 2014. DOI: 10.7705/biomedica.v34i2.1629

[13] World Health Organization. World Malaria Report 2014. Geneva, Switzerland: WHO; 2014

[14] Instituto Nacional de Salud. Informe de evento malaria, Colombia, 2020. Bogotá: INS; 2020a

[15] Organización Panamericana de la Salud. Informe de la situación del paludismo en las Américas, 2008. Washington. 2010. Retrieved from: http://www2.paho.org/hq/dmdocuments/2011/PAHO_SPA_Malaria_LR.pdf

[16] Instituto Nacional de Salud - Organización Panamericana de la Salud. Protocolo para la vigilancia en salud pública de malaria. 24. Colombia. 2015

[17] Instituto Nacional de Salud. Informe final de evento malaria, 2016, Colombia. Bogotá: INS; 2016

[18] Instituto Nacional de Salud. Informe final de evento malaria, 2017, Colombia. Bogotá: INS; 2017

[19] Instituto Nacional de Salud. Informe final de evento malaria, 2018, Colombia. Bogotá: INS; 2018

[20] Instituto Nacional de Salud. Informe final de evento malaria, 2019, Colombia. Bogotá: INS; 2019

[21] Helman C. Culture, Health and Illness. Londres: Oxford University press; 2007

[22] Stresman GH, Mwesigwa J, Achan J, Giorgi E, Worwui A, Jawara M, et al. Do hotspots fuel malaria transmission: a village-scale spatio-temporal analysis of a 2-year cohort study in The Gambia. BMC Medicine. 2018;**16**(1):160

[23] Word Health Organization. Malaria Surveillance, Monitoring & Evaluation: A Reference Manual. Geneva, Switzerland: Word Health Organization; 2018

[24] Yukich J, Bennett A, Yukich R, Stuck L, Hamainza B, Silumbe K, et al. Estimation of malaria parasite reservoir coverage using reactive case detection and active community fever screening from census data with rapid diagnostic tests in southern Zambia: a re-sampling approach. Malaria Journal. 2017;**16**:1

[25] Sturrock HJ, Hsiang MS, Cohen JM, Smith DL, Greenhouse B, Bousema T, et al. Targeting asymptomatic malaria infections: Active surveillance in control and elimination. PLoS Medicine. 2013;**10**(6):e1001467

[26] Stresman G, Whittaker C, Slater H, Bousema T, Cook J. Quantifying Plasmodium falciparum infections clustering within households to inform household-based intervention strategies for malaria control programs: An observational study and metaanalysis from 41 malaria-endemic countries. PLoS Medicine. 2020;**17**(10):e1003370

[27] Organización Panamericana de la Salud. La Organización Panamericana de la Salud y el estado colombiano 1902-2002. Bogotá: OPS; 2002

[28] Franco Agudelo S. El paludismo en América Latina. Guadalajara: Editorial Universidad de Guadalajara; 1990

[29] Blair S. Retos para la eliminación de la malaria en Colombia: un problema de saber o de poder. 2011. Available from redalyc: http://www.redalyc.org/pdf/843/84323434013.pdf. [Accessed: 15 Feb 2015]

[30] Fondo Mundial Malaria. Uso de la inteligencia epidemiológica con participación social, para fortalecer la gestión del programa, mejorar el acceso al diagnóstico y tratamiento y ejecutar intervenciones eficaces para la prevención y control de la malaria, Colombia 2010-2015. Bogotá: Instituto Nacional de Salud, Universidad de Antioquia, FONADE, Ministerio de Protección Social; 2012

[31] Hurtado L, Cumbrera A, Rigg C, et al. Long-term transmission patterns and public health policies leading to malaria elimination in Panamá. Malaria Journal. 2020;**19**:265

[32] Rosero CY, Jaramillo GI, Montenegro FA, Garcia C, Coral A. Community perception of malaria in a vulnerable municipality in the Colombian Pacific. Malaria Journal. 2020;**19**(1):343

[33] Alvarado BE, Gomez E, Serra M, Carvajal R, Carrasquilla G. Evaluación de una estrategia educativa en malaria aplicada en localidades rurales del Pacífico colombiano. Biomédica. 2006;**26**:342-352

[34] Girón S, Mateus J, Castellar C. Análisis de costo efectividad de dos inervenciones para el control de la malaria en el area urbana de Buenaventura, Colombia. Biomédica. 2006;**26**:379-386

[35] Guzman V, Correa AM, Fonseca J, Blair S. Seguridad alimentaria y nutricional en un espacio de riesgo para la malaria. Archivos Latinoamericanos de Nutrición. 2003;**53**(3):1-12

Section 5

Malaria Treatment

Chapter 9

Current Antimalarial Treatments: Focus on *Artemisia annua* Dry Leaf

Richa Goel

Abstract

Since a lot of drugs that were used for the treatment of malaria has shown resistance to the *Plasmodium* species. Even the ACT (Artemisia combination therapy) is not effective in certain cases. There is a need to look for some alternatives, which are effective in the clinical treatment of malaria and affordable for the general population. A therapy called *Artemisia annua* dry leaf antimalarial therapy (ALT) has been shown to be effective against artemisinin-resistant malarial infections and its treatment is resilient to resistance development in animal model systems. This proves to be an effective alternative to presently available antimalarials. This review defines the characteristics of different species of malaria-causing parasites, their vectors, endemicity, and features of the disease development, followed by properties of currently used (approved) antimalarials. The choices and methodologies of administration of antimalarials to adult, child, pregnant, and lactating women patients with acute and complicated malaria are described, followed by strategies to combat drug-resistant malaria, especially artemisinin resistance. A special emphasis on the origin, empirical basis, evidence on clinical efficacy, and cost aspects of ALT is given, along with the focus on the possibilities of repurposing ALT as a treatment for a variety of autoimmune, metabolic, and cancerous diseases.

Keywords: malaria, *Artemisia annua* dry leaf antimalarial therapy, currently used antimalarial drugs, drug-resistant malaria, *Artemisia*, artemisinin

1. Introduction

Malaria, which results from the transmission of the malarial parasite infection to humans by the bites of infected mosquitoes, is the deadliest infectious disease in tropical and subtropical climates. In recent years (such as 2015 and 2016), 3.5 billion people in 97 countries were at risk of getting infected with the malarial parasite(s). Actually, each of these years, several hundred million humans got malaria-infected and about half a million patients, preponderantly young children, elderly, and pregnant women, succumbed to the disease. In 2016, about 90% of malaria in southeast-cum-south Asia region was contributed by India [1].

In the last about ten years, since the introduction of artemisinin combination therapy (ACT) as the treatment of malaria and regulation of parasite transmission, at least ten countries have become largely malaria-free. During this period, due to

IntechOpen

success in the control of the disease-causing parasite by chemotherapeutic treatments, such as ACT, prophylaxis, and control of mosquito attacks by use of pyrethroid insecticide impregnated bednets and indoor insect repellents [2], the loss of life from malaria has been halved. For the last 72 years, from the time chloroquine was introduced as a substitute/alternative to quinine in malaria treatment, the disease has been contained by the use of five classes of individual pharmaceuticals (aminoquinolines, aryl-alcohols, including quinolines alcohols, antifolates, hydronaphthoquinone, and endoperoxides) and their combinations. However, malarial parasites have developed genetic resistance against most (perhaps all) of the effective antimalarials and their combinations. Besides, resistant parasites have become geographically widespread. The vector mosquitoes have also developed resistance to insecticides used to impregnate bed nets. The new affordable antimalarial chemical compounds and vaccines undergoing tests and trials are thought to be at least a decade away [3]. All these factors have posed a grave challenge for the control of malarial disease worldwide in the coming years. Discussion is in progress on ways to increase the life span of currently available pharmaceuticals by employing them in alternate combinations, to resist resistance in parasites and to combat parasite transmission. At this time when new effective and affordable malarial treatments are being eagerly awaited, a botanical treatment that appears to clear (artemisinin) resistant malaria has been recently described. Daddy *et al.*, (2017) have reported success in curing 18 cases of severe malaria by administering to the patient tablets made of dry leaves of *Artemisia annua* (the natural rich source of the pharmaceutical artemisinin) plants. This treatment called *Artemisia annua dry leaf therapy* (ALT) was found to have cured malaria caused by parasites resistant to currently used antimalarials, including artemisinin derivatives. ALT has been proven to be a safe, efficacious, and affordable antimalarial treatment, with multi-repurposing possibilities [4].

2. Kinds of malaria and symptoms

There are about 200 different unicellular eukaryotic apicomplexans obligate narrow host-range parasite species of the genus *Plasmodium*, transmitted by dipteran insect species, whose infection can cause various kinds of malarial diseases in a wide range of vertebrates. The five major species of *Plasmodium* that cause malaria in humans are *falciparum* (Pf), *knowlesi* (Pk), *malariae* (Pm), *ovale* (Po), and *vivax* (Pv). The important properties of these human malarial parasites are comparatively summarized (and the references concerned with this section are also given) in **Table 1**. Among the human malarial parasites, Pk is known to be a zoonotic species whose infection in several species of macaque monkeys produce malaria-like symptoms. Recently another zoonotic species—*Plasmodium simium* (Ps)—has been found to cause malaria in humans in the Atlantic forest area of Brazil. The natural hosts for Ps are monkeys of the genera *Aloulta, Brachyteles, Cebus,* and *Sapajus* [14].

The insect hosts of *Plasmodium* species are anopheline mosquitoes. Out of about 515 known species of *Anopheles*, about 70 are vectors of human malaria [15]. Each of Pf, Pk, Pm, Po, Pv, and Ps are transmitted to humans by several to many *Anopheles* species, in geographical areas of their occurrence. The genomes of the human malarial *Plasmodium* species and of the major *Anopheles* vector species have been sequenced. The vector for Ps has been identified as *Anopheles kertezsia cruzii*. Phylogenetic distance-wise the parasite species are related to each other as follows: Pf → Po → Pm → Pk, Pv, and Ps [14]. In terms of the frequencies of malaria infections caused by

S. No.		Characters	*Plasmodium falciparum (Pf)*	*Plasmodium vivax (Pv)*	*Plasmodium ovale*		*Plasmodium malariae (Pm)*	*Plasmodium knowlesi (Pk)*
					curtisi (Poc)	*wallikeri (Pow)*		
1	(A) Features of (n=14) genome	Size (Mb)	23.3	29.1	33.5	33.5	33.6	24.4
2		Estimated gene number	5355	6671	7165	6340	6559	5284
3		G+C content (%)	19	40	29	29	24	39
4	(B) Features of life cycle in human host	Pre-erythrocytic growth in hepatocytes (hepatic schizogony) (number of days = d)	5–7	6–9	8–9		14–16	6–9
5		Whether relapse causing hypnozoites are formed in liver?	No	Yes	Yes		No	No
6		Incubation period (d)	8–15	10–21	12–20		18–60	10–12
7		Fever cycle (erythrocytic schizogony) (number of hours = h)	Tertian (48)	Tertian (48)	Tertian (48)		Quartan (72)	Quotidian (24)
8		Nature of red blood cells affected	All types of erythrocytes	Reticulocytes	Reticulocytes		Mature erythrocytes	All kinds of erythrocytes
9		Size of parasitemia (number of parasites per μL of blood ($x10^3$)	20–500	20–50	9–10		5–10	0.5–10

S. No.	Characters		*Plasmodium falciparum* (*Pf*)	*Plasmodium vivax* (*Pv*)	*Plasmodium ovale* curtisi (*Poc*) wallikeri (*Pow*)	*Plasmodium malariae* (*Pm*)	*Plasmodium knowlesi* (*Pk*)
10		Whether cytoadherence of parasite cause microvascular dysfunction?	Yes	Rarely (if at all)	Rarely (if at all)	Rarely (if at all)	Yes
11		Whether severe malaria develops?	Yes	Yes	No	No	Yes
12		Whether recrudescence occurs?	Yes (when treatment fails)	Yes (when treatment fails)	Rare	Yes (sometimes after 30 to 50 y from the primary attack)	Yes
13		Time of appearance of gametocytes (d after the start of parasitemia)	8–14	0	0	0	Not known
14	(C) Features of life cycle in mosquito host	Transmission causing *Anopheles* mosquito vector species	Many species (≥ 70), most prominent are: *gambiae*, *culicifacies* and *stephensi*	Many species (≥ 71), most prominent are: *aquasalis*, *culicifacies*, *stephensi*, *darlingi* and *dirus*	Several species (≈ 10), most prominent are *funestus*, *gambiae*, *stephensi*, *freeborni*, *dirus*, *farauti* and *atroparvus*	Many species (≥ 30), most prominent are: *culicifacies*, *aconitus*, *arabiensis*, *atroparvus* and *freeborni*	Several species, including *craceus*, *hackeri*, *latens* and *bala-bacensis*
15		Time period of sporogony at 28°C (d)	7–12	8–10	12–14	18	12–13
16	(D) Major geographical areas of prevalence		Worldwide tropical and subtropical areas (especially in Africa, Asia, and Mediterranean)	Worldwide subtropical areas (especially in Asia, Latin America, and Africa)	Tropical regions of Africa and Asia and in Pacific islands, sympatrically (subspecies)	Worldwide tropical and subtropical areas (including Pacific islands)	Southeast Asia and South Asia

DOI: http://dx.doi.org/10.5772/intechopen.106736

S. No.	Characters	*Plasmodium falciparum* (*Pf*)	*Plasmodium vivax* (*Pv*)	*Plasmodium ovale*		*Plasmodium malariae* (*Pm*)	*Plasmodium knowlesi* (*Pk*)
				curtisi (*Poc*)	*wallikeri* (*Pow*)		
17	(E) Remarks	*Pf* is the preponderant cause of malaria. The falciparum malaria is the deadliest and if not treated timely the acute (or un-complicated) malaria turns into cerebral (or complicated) malaria.	*Pv* can cause severe disease and death due to splenomegaly. The Duffy blood group deficient in Africa when infected are often symptomless	In some cases, relapse can occur as late as 4–5 years from the initial inoculation		It is less life-threatening than *vivax* and *falciparum* malaria. However, it can cause chronic lifetime infection	This parasite is zoonotic, also causes malaria in the monkeys *Macaca fascicularis, M. nemestrina* and *Presbytis melalophos*. The disease in humans is mild, but can be lethal (mortality≈2%). The Duffy blood group people in West Africa are often insensitive to this parasite. Transmission occurs from humans to monkey and vice versa. Human-to-human transmission is rare (perhaps via the vector *A. dirus*)

Table 1.
Properties of malaria caused in humans by infection of different species of the alveolate parasite. Plasmodium *(Phylum: Apicomplexan; Family: Plasmodiidae) [5–13].*

them in humans, the parasites fall in the following order: Pf > Pv > Po, Pm > Pk > Ps. The malaria caused by Pf, Pv, and Pk can be fatal if not treated. The Po and Pm-caused malaria are less severe and generally not lethal. Pv, Ps, and Po-caused infections can remain dormant in the liver for up to many months. Pm infection can remain latent for years. The Duffy blood group deficient (*ackr1* = atypical chemokine receptor 1) humans (who are largely the inhabitants of west Africa) are resistant to infection by Pv and Pk because the parasites are unable to invade their $Fy\ a^{-}b^{-}$ erythrocytes [16].

The Pf, Pv, Po, Pm, Pk, and Ps malaria have differential distribution. Pv is the most widespread malaria; it is the major malaria causal parasite in subtropical areas of Asia, America, and Africa. Nearly half of the malaria cases that occur outside of Africa are related to Pv infection. More dangerous than Pv malaria, Pf malaria is predominant in Africa, but also occurs in tropical regions of Asia and in the middle east. Pf malaria is responsible for 90% of the malarial deaths in Africa. The distribution of Pm malaria is similar to that of Pf malaria except that it is much less frequent. Both Po and Pm are the cause of malaria in Pacific islands. There are two subspecies of Po called *P. curtisi* and *P. wallekeri*, both are cause of malaria in Africa and Asia, sympatrically. Together, Po and Pm account for about 10 million cases of new malaria each year. Malaria caused by Pk occurs largely in southeast- and south Asia. The Ps malaria is limited to Brazil. In areas where the frequency of occurrence of malaria infections is high, mixed infections of more than one Plasmodium species have been observed [17]. Recently, a rare case of malaria caused by infection of Pf, Pv, Po, and Pm has been reported from a forest area in central India, which has a high incidence of mixed infection [18].

Initial symptoms of malaria are often as nonspecific as one or more of the following types of sickness: fever, chills, sweating, fast heart rate, sore throat, cough, pneumonia, headache, muscular pain, joint pain, fatigue, difficulty in swallowing, hypersalivation, jaundice, nausea, weakness, vomiting, constipation, and enlargement of the spleen. Laboratory diagnosis is essential to confirm malaria. The most reliable diagnosis is the detection of parasite-infected red blood cells through microscopic examination of thick and thin blood films. The rapid diagnostic tests (RDTs), based on the detection of parasite antigens, can be used, but should not substitute for the needed microscopic tests [19]. Once diagnosed, a confirmed malaria patient should immediately begin receiving the WHO-prescribed treatment at the earliest.

The findings of the microscopic test are helpful in classifying malaria as uncomplicated or severe. In cases of noncomplicated malaria, the parasitemia (% of parasitized red blood cells) is lower than 2%. If parasitemia is 10%, the malarial patient is facing a severe form of the disease. The symptoms of severe malaria include high fever and one or more of the following conditions: renal impairment (dark urine and limited output) acidosis, hypoglycemia, spontaneous bleeding, breathing difficulties, severe anemia, prostration, or coma. Young children and pregnant women are not only more vulnerable to malarial infection but also prone to developing severe malaria. Consequences of severe malaria in a pregnant woman include miscarriage, stillbirth, premature birth, and birth defects in neonates. Generally, all kinds of malaria cause bone loss due to chronic bone inflammation and adversely affect the functioning of skeletal and heart muscles due to poor supply of nutrients and oxygen [20]. There occurs macrovascular dysfunction in Pf and Pk malaria due to adherence of infected cells to walls of blood vessels [21]. The above kinds of deficits imposed by malaria, span of morbidity, possibility of death can all be checked by antimalarial drug treatment, which also aims to clear malarial parasites from the body of a malarial patient such that malaria does not relapse and transmission to mosquitoes is blocked.

Antimalarial drugs are also used as chemoprophylaxis, in mass drug administration campaigns to limit the spread of malaria in endemic areas, and for travelers visiting the malaria-endemic areas.

3. Currently used antimalarial drugs

The antimalarial drugs are: quinine, mefloquine, halofantrine, and lumefantrine (aryl aminoalcohols); chloroquine, amodiaquine, and piperaquine (4-aminoquinolones); primaquine (8-aminoquinoline); pyronaridine (mannich base); atovaquone (naphthoquinone); proguanil, pyrimethamine and sulfadoxine (antifolates); tetracycline, doxycycline, and clindamycin (antibiotics); and artesunate, dihydro-artemisinin and artemether (artemisinin-derived endoperoxides). **Table 2** gives the chemical structures, purpose and regimen of administration to malaria patients, biological effects on *Plasmodium* parasites, and prescription properties. There is large difference in interclass and intraclass properties of the drugs. *In vivo* half-life of artemisinins is short (0.5 to few hours) as compared to that of lumefantrine, pyronaridine, pyrimethamine, sulfadoxine, piperaquine, and chloroquine (3 to 60 days). Quinine and artemether are highly insoluble in water and are usable for parenteral application. Artemisinins are very fast-acting drugs. Quinine, chloroquine, piperaquine, and artemisinins are able to block the transmission of parasites to mosquitoes. Primaquine too blocks transmission but also prevents Pv and Po malaria relapses. Quinine, mefloquine, lumefantrine, atovaquone, and artemisinins do not allow the multiplication of parasites in mosquitoes. Unlike proguanil, pyrimethamine, sulfadoxine, and atovaquone target singular but different parasite functions, whereas artemisinin derivatives, chloroquine, and quinine exemplify antimalarials, which target multiple functions in parasites.

To overcome deficiencies of individual chemotherapeutics and to slow down resistance development, antimalarials are now used in combinations. The following combinations have been recommended by WHO to cure various kinds of malaria (**Table 2**): chloroquine + primaquine (against Po and Pv malaria); quinine + tetracycline or clindamycin (against severe malaria); ACTs = artemether + lumefantrine or mefloquine, dihydroartemisinin + piperaquine, artesunate + pyronaridine or sulfadoxine + pyrimethamine or artesunate + amodiaquine (against uncomplicated malaria, especially those caused by Pf). Primaquine or alternatively tafenoquine is given additionally to stop relapses and transmission; both are contraindicated for G6PD deficient patients. Tertian malaria caused by Ps is curable by chloroquine + primaquine treatment [14]. The combinations used for chemoprophylaxis in endemic areas are atovaquone + proguanil and proguanil + chloromycetin. For chemoprophylaxis mefloquine and doxycycline are also used preferably singly.

4. Treatments based on currently used antimalarial drugs

Table 3 presents a summarized account of the first-line treatments for acute and severe malaria caused by different species of malaria parasites in adults, pregnant women, and young children, as recommended by WHO. The recommendations are a result of scores of trials carried out, for the cure of a different kind of malaria in endemic areas of their occurrence in Africa, America, Pacific islands, southeast and south Asia, on adult men and women, pregnant and lactating women and young

S. No.	Antimalarial compound (drug)				Prescription-cum-administration	Malarial parasite lifecycle stage(s) on which known to be active	Current knowledge about mechanism of action on parasite (s) and indication (purpose) of usage	Genetic markers, in *Plasmodium falciparum* (*Pf*) and *P. vivax* (*Pv*) parasites, for the resistance that has developed against the antimalarial	Remarks	Reference (s)
	Chemical class	Name	Structure	Biological half-life (hours = h; days = d)						
I	II	III	IV	V	VI	VII	VIII	IX	X	XI
1	(A) Aryl amino-alcohols	Quinine	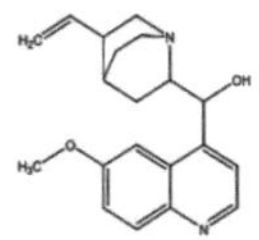	10–12 h	Parenteral or oral	Blood schizonticidal, gametocytocidal, and sporontocidal	Inhibits heme detoxification; used to treat malaria unresponsive to other drugs and to control transmission	Single nucleotide poly-morphisms (SNPs) in *Pfmdr1*[a], *Pfcrt*[b], *Pfnhe1*[c], *Pfmrp1*[d] and gene amplification in *Pfmdr1*	The drug is not to be given to patients with tinnitus and optic neuritis	[22, 23]
2		Mefloquine	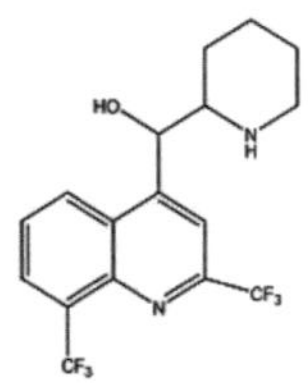	14–18 d	Oral 250 mg tablets (Larium; is relatively expensive)	Blood schizonticidal and sporontocidal against *Pf, Pv, Po,* and *Pm* malaria	Inhibits heme detoxification and parasite's ribosomes; used in the treatment of acute uncomplicated malaria	SNPs and copy number increase in *Pfmdr1*; SNPs in *Pvmdr1*	It is not to be given to pregnant women and neuropsychiatric patients	[24, 25]
3		Halofantrine	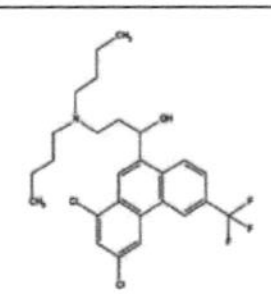	10–90 h	Oral 250 mg tablets (Halfan; is relatively expensive), 1500 mg in six doses over 18 h period	Blood schizonticidal in *Pf, Pv, Po,* and *Pm* malaria	As above	As above	It is contraindicated for cardiac disease patients	[26]
4		Lumefantrine	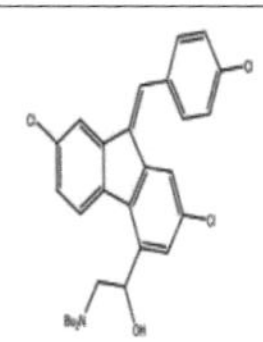	3–6 d	Oral (artemisinin-based combination therapy = ACT) tablets of 120 mg lumefantrine and 20 mg of artemether (Coartem); four tablets to be taken twice a day for 4 days	Blood schizonticidal and sporontocidal	Inhibits heme de-toxification; used together with artemether to treat acute malaria	SNPs and copy number increase in *Pfmdr1*	Safe medicine, including for children of 5 kg body weight	[27, 28]

DOI: http://dx.doi.org/10.5772/intechopen.106736

S. No.	Antimalarial compound (drug)				Prescription-cum-administration	Malarial parasite lifecycle stage(s) on which known to be active	Current knowledge about mechanism of action on parasite (s) and indication (purpose) of usage	Genetic markers, in *Plasmodium falciparum* (*Pf*) and *P. vivax* (*Pv*) parasites, for the resistance that has developed against the antimalarial	Remarks	Reference (s)
	Chemical class	Name	Structure	Biological half-life (hours = h; days = d)						
I	II	III	IV	V	VI	VII	VIII	IX	X	XI
5	(B) 4-Aminoquinolines	Chloroquine	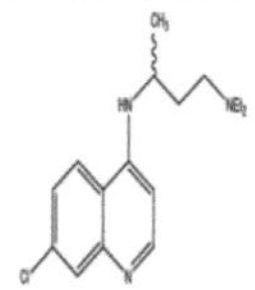	30–60 d	Oral tablets of 250 and 500 mg (Aralen; is the cheapest antimalarial drug); 2.5 g is administered in 48 h	Blood schizonticidal in *Pf*, *Pv*, *Po*, and *Pm* malaria, and gametocytocidal in *Pv* malaria	Inhibits heme detoxification; used to treat acute uncomplicated malaria and along with Primaquine as first line cure for *Pv* malaria	SNPs in *Pfcrt*, *Pfmdr1*, and *Pfmrp1*; and *Pvmdr1*, and *Pvcrt1*	Contraindicated for the patients with hepatic disease	[29, 30]
6		Amodiaquine	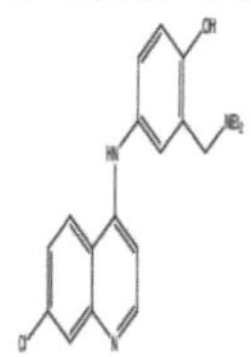	5 h	Oral tablets of 200 mg; 25–35 mg/kg body weight over 3 d period	Blood schizonticidal	Inhibits heme detoxification; treatment of acute uncomplicated malaria and along with sulfadoxine plus pyrimethamine for prophylaxis in travelers	SNPs and copy number increase in *Pfmdr1* and SNPs in *Pfcrt*	Contraindicated in patients with kidney and liver diseases and pregnant and breastfeeding women	[31, 32]
7		Piperaquine	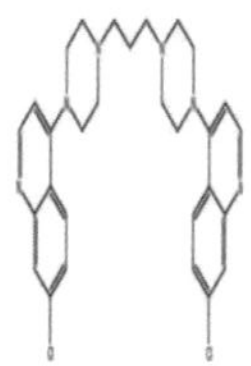	30 d	Oral 18 mg/kg body weight of Piperaquine plus 4 mg/kg body weight of dihydroartemisinin (ACT) for 3 d	Blood schizonticidal; given in combination with dehydroartemisinin to treat acute malaria and for transmission control and prophylaxis	Inhibits heme detoxification; the ACT is safe and effective against acute malaria in adults and children	*Pf plasmepsin-2,-3*[e] gene amplification	Contraindicated in pregnancy	[33, 34]

S. No.	Antimalarial compound (drug)				Prescription-cum-administration	Malarial parasite lifecycle stage(s) on which known to be active	Current knowledge about mechanism of action on parasite (s) and indication (purpose) of usage	Genetic markers, in *Plasmodium falciparum* (*Pf*) and *P. vivax* (*Pv*) parasites, for the resistance that has developed against the antimalarial	Remarks	Reference (s)
	Chemical class	**Name**	**Structure**	**Biological half-life (hours = h; days = d)**						
I	**II**	**III**	**IV**	**V**	**VI**	**VII**	**VIII**	**IX**	**X**	**XI**
8	(C) 8-Aminoquinoline	Primaquine	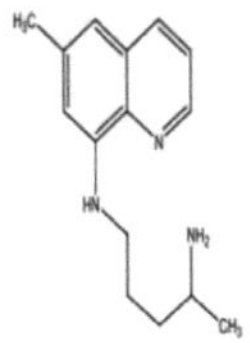	7 h	Oral 15 mg and 26.3 mg tablets	Eliminates hypnozoites, liver stage schizonts, and gametocytes and has very weak blood stage activity against *Pf* malaria	Impairs mitochondrial functions; to cure and prevent relapse of *Pv* and *Po* malaria and prevention of *Pv* malaria; stops transmission from humans to mosquitoes	Resistance is known but not the markers	Contraindicated for pregnant and breastfeeding women and glucose 6 phosphate dehydrogenase (G6PD) deficient individuals	[35, 36]
9	(D) Mannich base	Pyronaridine	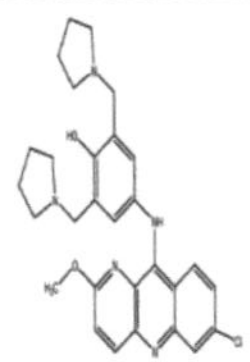	≤3–8 d	Oral (ACT) tablets of 180 mg Pyronaridine tetraphosphate plus 60 mg of Artesunate (Pyramax); given one/d for 3 d	Blood schizonticidal	Inhibits β-hematin formation	SNPs in *Pfmrp1*	Not to be given to patients with liver disease	[37, 38]
10	(E) Naphthoquinone	Atovaquone	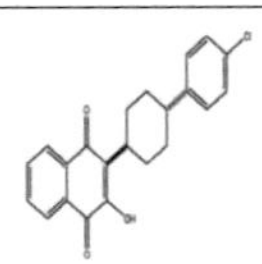	59 h	Oral tablet of 1 g Atovaquone and 400 mg Proguanil (Malarone); one tablet/d for 3 d, lower doses for children, and 25% strength tablet for prevention	Liver stage and blood stage schizonticidal, and sporonticidal	Acts against mitochondrial bc1 complex and inhibits parasite's respiration process; given in combination with Proguanil to treat acute malaria and for prophylaxis	SNPs in *Pfcytb*[b]	Not to be given to patients with hypersensitive reactions and renal impairment	[39, 40]

S. No.	Antimalarial compound (drug)				Prescription-cum-administration	Malarial parasite lifecycle stage(s) on which known to be active	Current knowledge about mechanism of action on parasite (s) and indication (purpose) of usage	Genetic markers, in *Plasmodium falciparum* (*Pf*) and *P. vivax* (*Pv*) parasites, for the resistance that has developed against the antimalarial	Remarks	Reference (s)
	Chemical class	**Name**	**Structure**	**Biological half-life (hours = h; days = d)**						
I	II	III	IV	V	VI	VII	VIII	IX	X	XI
11	(F) Antifolates	Proguanil	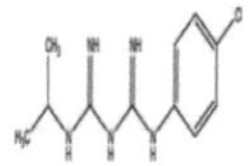	24 h	As above	Mild liver stage schizonticidal and blood stage schizonticidal for *Pf*, *Pv*, *Po* malaria	Inhibits dihydrofolate reductase (DHFR) synthesis or folate synthesis; the drug is administered together with Atovaquone or Chloroquine to treat acute malaria and for prophylaxis	SNPs in *Pfdhfr*[g] and *Pvdhfr*	As above	[41, 42]
12		Pyrimethamine	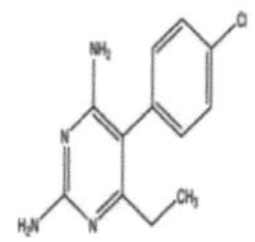	≤3–≥4 d	Oral tablet of 25 mg Pyrimethamine and 500 mg of Sulfadoxine (Fansidar; is a cost-effective drug); adults to take 2–3 tablets/week	Mild liver stage schizonticidal, blood stage schizonticidal, and sporontocidal	Inhibits dihydrofolate reductase (DHFR) synthesis and thereby folate synthesis; it is given along with sulfadoxine to cure acute malaria, even in pregnant women	As above	Not to be given to patients with megaloblastic anemia and folate deficiency	[43–45]
13		Sulfadoxine	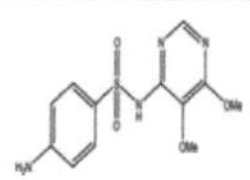	≤4–≥8 d	As above	Blood stage schizonticidal in *Pf* malaria but relatively ineffective in *Pv* malaria	Inhibits the dihydropteroate synthesis (DHPS) and thereby folate synthesis; indication as above	SNPs in *Pfdhps*[h] and *Pvdhps*	As above and also not to be given in patients with sulfur allergy	[43–45]

S. No.	Antimalarial compound (drug)				Prescription-cum-administration	Malarial parasite lifecycle stage(s) on which known to be active	Current knowledge about mechanism of action on parasite (s) and indication (purpose) of usage	Genetic markers, in *Plasmodium falciparum* (*Pf*) and *P. vivax* (*Pv*) parasites, for the resistance that has developed against the antimalarial	Remarks	Reference (s)
	Chemical class	Name	Structure	Biological half-life (hours = h; days = d)						
I	II	III	IV	V	VI	VII	VIII	IX	X	XI
14	(G) Antibiotics	Tetracycline	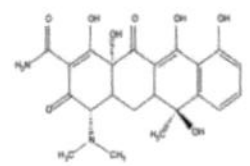	8–11 h	Oral 250 mg tablets (Sumycin and other brands; is cost-effective	Slow-acting liver and blood stage schizonticidal	Protein synthesis inhibitor; given along with Quinine	Resistance is not known	Not to be given to children of ≤ 8 y age	[46, 47]
15		Doxycycline	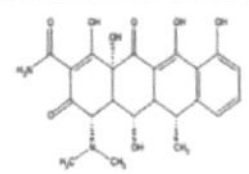	15–25 h	Oral 250 mg tablets; is highly cost-effective	As above	Inhibitor of protein synthesis; given along with fast-acting antimalarial to cure acute malaria and as prophylaxis for travelers	As above	Not to be given to pregnant women	[48, 49]
16		Clindamycin	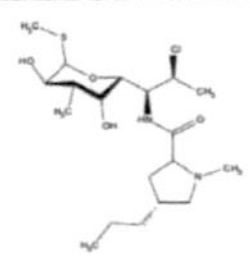	3 h	Oral 75 mg to 900 mg capsules; is cost-effective	Blood schizonticidal	Inhibition of protein synthesis, given along with Quinine to patients unable to tolerate Tetracycline	As above	Not to be given to patients with intestinal disease	[50, 51]
17	(H) Endoperoxides	Artesunate	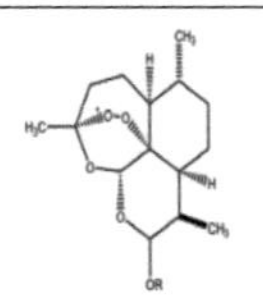 R=-CO-CH$_2$-CH$_2$-CO$_2^-$	0.5–1.4 h	Oral as ACT@ 4 mg/kg body weight of Artesunate with 10 mg/kg body weight of Amodiaquine or 25 mg/kg body weight of Mefloquine or 25 mg/kg body weight of each of Sulfadoxine and	Fast acting liver and blood stage schizonticidal, incomplete gametocytocidal, and sporontocidal; given along with combination ACT in acute malaria; parenterally and as a suppository in cerebral malaria	Fe (II) present in heme proteins clears the peroxide bond, and the free radicals thus generated react with essential parasite proteins inactivating them, such as sarcoplasmic endoplasmic reticulum calcium	SNPs in *Pf kelch-13*[i]; (the haptotype *C580Y* is undergoing a hard selective sweep in Southeast Asia); amplification of *Pfmdr1*	Not to be given to patients of respiratory disease, and pregnant and lactating women	[52, 53]

S. No.	Antimalarial compound (drug)				Prescription-cum-administration	Malarial parasite lifecycle stage(s) on which known to be active	Current knowledge about mechanism of action on parasite (s) and indication (purpose) of usage	Genetic markers, in *Plasmodium falciparum (Pf)* and *P. vivax (Pv)* parasites, for the resistance that has developed against the antimalarial	Remarks	Reference (s)
	Chemical class	Name	Structure	Biological half-life (hours = h; days = d)						
I	II	III	IV	V	VI	VII	VIII	IX	X	XI
					Pyrimethamine; all for 3 d; or Artesunate as suppository		ATPase and heme metabolism; prescribed to cure acute malaria as ACT partner and in severe malaria			
18		Dihydroartemisinin	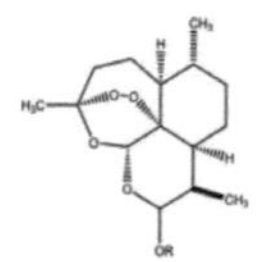 R=Me	0.5–0.75h	As shown at serial no. 7	Fastest acting Artemisinin derivative that does not allow trophozoite formation and is gametocytocidal and sporontocidal	Mode of action as above; treatment of acute malaria as an ACT component	As above	As above	[54, 55]
19		Artemether	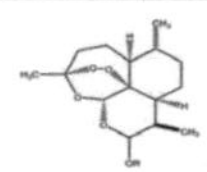 R=H	4–11h	As shown at serial no. 4; the drug is lipid soluble and is used orally, rectally, and intramuscularly	Mode of action like Artesunate; As an ACT it is a frontline drug for acute malaria	As above	As above	As above	[56, 57]

a–i = Antimalarial resistant drug alleles: a, mdr1 *= Multi-drug resistance gene on chromosome 5; b,* crt *= Chloroquine resistance transporter gene on chromosome 7; c,* nhe1 *= Sodium/hydrogen exchanger gene on chromosome 13; d,* mrp1 *= Multi-drug resistance-associated proteins gene on chromosome 1; e,* plasmepsin-2, -3 *= Aspartyl (protease plasmepsin gene located on chromosome 4; f,* cyt b *= cytochrome B gene on mitochondrial genome; g,* dhfr *= Dihydrofolate reductase gene on chromosome 8; h,* dhps *= Dihydropteroate synthetase gene on chromosome 4; i,* kelch-13 *= Kelch 13 propeller gene located on chromosome 13, (the gene product has three domains: an apicomplex domain, a BIB/POZ domain, and a β-propeller Kelch domain).*

Table 2.
Structure, activity, and related features of different classes of antimalarials, that are presently in use against various developmental stages of Plasmodium falciparum *(Pf),* Plasmodium vivax *(Pv),* Plasmodium ovale *(Po),* Plasmodium malariae *(Pm), and* Plasmodium knowlesi *(Pk) caused human malaria(s) and genetic markers of resistance detected against the antimalarials in* P.falciparum *and* P.vivax.

S. No.	Indicative malarial condition	Malaria caused by		
		Plasmodium falciparum	***Plasmodium vivax, P.ovale*, or of these mixed with *P. falciparum***	***P.vivax, P. ovale, P. malariae* or *P.knowlesi***
1	(A) Uncomplicated malaria: (i) in adults	Oral: Artemether + Lumefantrine (the drug(s) of choice)[a] ; Dihydroartemisinin + Piperaquine (not to be administered to patients suffering from cardiac condition(s))[b]; Atovaquone + Proguanil (known to produce pronounced gastrointestinal side effects)[c]; Quinine + Doxycycline[d]; and a single dose of 0.25 mg/kg body weight of Primaquine on the first day or 15 mg/Kg of methylene blue for 3 days	Oral: Artemether + Lumefantrine[a]; Dihydroartemisinin + Piperaquine[b] or Chloroquine[m]	Oral: Chloroquine[m]
2	(ii) in pregnant women	Oral: Quinine + Clindamycin (in: all trimesters)[e]; or Artemether + Lumefantrine (in all trimesters)	As in column 2; item 2; or Chloroquine[m]	As in column 3; item 2
3	(iii) in children (< 12 years)	Oral: Quinine + Clindamycin[e]; Atovaquone + Proguanil[f]; Artemether + Lumefantrine[g]; or Dihydroartemisinin + Piperaquine[h]	Chloroquine[n]	Chloroquine[n]
4	(B) Severe or complicated malaria: (i) in adults	Intravenous Artesunate for 24h or more (or until the patient can swallow tablets, but not more than 5 days)[i], followed by a full course of Artemether + Lumefantrine[a] or of Dihydroartemisinin + Piperaquine[b] or Intravenous Artesunate treatment[i] followed by a full course of Quinine + Doxycycline[d]; or alternatively Intravenous Quinine[j] for 48 hours or until the patient is able to swallow tablets, followed by oral Quinine + Doxycycline[k]	As in column 2; item 4; or intravenous artesunate treatment followed by the full course of Chloroquine	As in column 2, item 4
5	(ii) in pregnant women	Intravenous Artesunate[i], followed by Artemether + Lumefantrine or Dihydroartemisinin + Piperaquine as in item 4 above; or Intravenous Quinine followed by a course of Quinine + Clindamycin[l]	Oral: Chloroquine (in all trimesters); Artemether + Lumefantrine (in all trimesters)	As in column 2, item 4
6	(iii) in children (≤ 12 years)	A rectal suppository dose of upto 100 mg (10 mg/kg body weight) Artesunate followed by intravenous Artesunate or Quinine and thereafter dihydroartemisinin + Piperaquine	As in column 2	As in column 2

S. No.	Indicative malarial condition	Malaria caused by		
		Plasmodium falciparum	***Plasmodium vivax, P.ovale,* or of these mixed with *P. falciparum***	***P.vivax, P. ovale, P. malariae* or *P.knowlesi***
		or Quinine + Clindamycin; as for adults with dosage adjusted as per body weight		
7	Relapse (prevention): (i) in adults	Not applicable	Primaquine[o] (not to be administered to Glucose-6-phosphate dehydrogenase = G6PD deficient) [p]	As in column 3
8	(ii) in pregnant and breastfeeding women	As above	Chloroquine[q] followed by Primaquine upon withdrawal of breastfeeding	As in column 3

a = 4 tablets (such as of Coartem) followed by 4 tablets at 0, 8, 24, 36, 48, and 60 hours; b = 3 or 4 tablets (such as of Eurartesim) daily for 3 days; c = 4 tablets (such as of Malarone) daily for 3 days; d = 600 mg Quinine sulfate every 8 h for 5–7 days and 200 mg doxycycline daily; e = 600 mg quinine sulfate every 8 h plus 450 mg clindamycin every 8 hours for 7 days; f = 1 to 4 Malarone pediatric tablets (as per body weight from ≤ 10 kg to ≥ 40 kg); g = 1–4 tablets at 0, 8, 24, 36, 48, and 60 hours (as per body weight from ≤ 15 kg to ≥ 35 kg); h = ½ to 3 tablets, followed by equal amount at 24 and 48 hours (as per body weight ≤ 10 kg to ≥ 60 kg); i = 2.4 mg/kg body weight injection of artesunate at 0, 12, and 24 h and thereafter daily; j = starting dose of 20 mg/kg body weight of quinine hydrochloride in 5% dextrose over a 4 h period, followed by 10 mg/kg body weight of Quinine hydrochloride every 8 h for upto 48 h and later every 12 h; k = 600 mg quinine sulfate three times a day for 5 to 7 days from the start of quinine therapy, plus oral 200 mg of doxycycline each day for 7 days; l = intravenous quinine therapy to be followed by oral quinine, like, except in place of doxycycline, clindamycin (450 mg) will be administered three times a day for a period of 7 days; m = 620 mg at 0 h, 310 mg at 8 h and 310 mg on day 2 and 3; n = 10 mg starting dose, then 5 mg/kg at 8 h and also on day 2 and 3; o = 15 to 30 mg/day or 0.2–0.5 mg/kg body weight/day for 14 days depending on body weight; p = The G6PD deficiency may be administered by 0.75 mg/kg of primaquine per week for 8 weeks; q = 500 mg each week.

Table 3.
The prevalent antimalarial treatment regimens against un-complicated and complicated malaria(s) in adults, pregnant and breastfeeding women, and children [5, 28, 58–67].

children. Some of the references on which the WHO recommendations are based are given at the bottom of **Table 3**. The dosages of drugs for children are to be adjusted to body weight. Some drugs are prescribed when malarial patients suffer from concurrent ailments or inherited metabolic deficiencies, the proscriptions for each of the antimalarial drugs are given in **Table 2**. Importantly, primaquine is not to be administered to pregnant and/or breastfeeding women. Because severe malaria patients can suffer from a blockage in blood flow, filling up of fluid in lung's air sacks, clotting in blood vessel, renal failure, and/or seizures, etc., they must be treated in intensive care environment. Any concurrent bacterial infection in malaria patients should receive immediate attention, along with malaria treatment.

The options for the treatment of uncomplicated malaria in adult men and women are artemether + lumefantrine; dihydro-artemisinin + piperaquine; atovaquone +proguanil; quinine + doxycycline. Along with a drug combination, a dose of primaquine ensures control of the transmission. The treatment for Pv, Po or mixed malaria is one of the following: artemether + lumefantrine; dihydro-artemisinin + piperaquine; chloroquine. For Pm and Pk malaria, the drug recommended is chloroquine. The drug options for children against Pf malaria are: artemether + lumefantrine; dihydroartemisinin + piperaquine; atovaquone + proguanil;

quinine + clindamycin. Chloroquine is the drug recommended for children against Pv, Po, Pm, and Pk malaria. Pregnant women afflicted with any kind of malaria are recommended to use quinine + clindamycin or artemether + lumefantrine, and those having non- Pf malaria are also recommended chloroquine. The treatment options for patients with severe malaria in adult men and women caused by all kinds of parasites are intravenous artesunate for one or more days until the patient can swallow tablets, but not more than 5 days, followed by a full course of artemether + lumefantrine, dihydro-artemisinin + piperaquine or quinine + tetracycline; or intravenous quinine for 2 days or until the patient can begin to swallow tablets, followed by a full course of quinine + doxycycline. In the severe malaria cases caused by Pv or Pk, the intravenous treatments are to be followed by a full course of chloroquine. Pregnant women patients with severe Pf malaria are to be given intravenous artesunate or quinine treatments, like that for adult men and women. Whereas artesunate-treated pregnant women patients are to be given a full oral course of artemether + lumefantrine or dihydro artemisinin + piperaquine, those who received intravenous quinine will be given a full oral course of quinine + clindamycin. The severely ill pregnant women, with any non-Pf malaria, will be given a full course of oral chloroquine or artemether plus lumefantrine, irrespective of the trimester of pregnancy. Young children with complicated malaria are to be first treated with artesunate given rectally followed by the treatments (with dose adjustment according to the patient's body weight) recommended for severely ill adult patients.

5. Strategies proposed to treat and control multidrug-resistant malaria

The studies summarized in **Table 2** shows that resistance has developed against the antimalarial drug in current use singly or in two-drug combinations. It is visualized that in the absence of new drugs and vaccines in the near future, there is an urgent need to use the existing drugs in better ways and in new combinations. The two treatments advised for chloroquine-resistant Pv malaria are: (a) dihydroartemisinin + piperaquine with a dose of primaquine [66], and (b) administration of verapamil, the calcium channel blocker which serves as a chemo sensitizer, along with chloroquine to improve drug efficiency. The possible treatments advised for ACT-resistant Pf malaria are (a) A new ACT combination of artesunate + pyronaridine to be introduced as a treatment. (b) ACTs, such as dihydroartemisinin + piperaquine and artesunate + mefloquine be used rotationally (c) The period of use of prevalent ACTs be extended from 3 days to up to 7 days. (d) ACTs be used as combinations of artemisinin drugs with two partner drugs, such as artemether + lumefantrine + amodiaquine, and dihydroartemisinin + piperaquine + mefloquine. (e) The double and triple drug ACTs be used sequentially. (f) The combination of fosmidomicin and piperaquine serves as a sure cure. Another important suggestion is the administration of a dose of the drug ivermectin in the endemic areas along with the ACT or singly periodically on a mass scale. Ivermectin taken by mosquitoes along with the blood meal of ivermectin administered to humans will have a killing effect on them, thereby drastically controlling malaria transmission [67–69].

An entirely new strategy to treat multi-drug (ACT) resistant malaria has been developed wherein tablets made of dried leaves of the *A. annua* plant (natural resource of artemisinin drugs) are used [4]. The origin and essential features of this highly affordable malaria therapy are discussed below.

6. Artemisia annua dry leaf antimalarial therapy (ALT)

The ALT has been earlier called the whole Plant based artemisinin combination therapy (pACT). pACT was called a combination therapy because of the involvement of artemisinin and other metabolites present in the leaves of *A. annua* in the antimalarial therapeutic effect of *Artemisia annua* dry leaves [70, 71]. ALT is unlike the conventional ACTs (mentioned in **Tables 2** and **3**), in which the artemisinin component, extracted from *A. annua* or artemisinin synthesizing transgenic tobacco or *Physcomitrella patens* whole plant [72], or semi synthesized from *Artemisia annua* produced natural precursor(s) [73] is present in its derived pharmaceutical forms, such as artesunate, artemether, and dihydroartemisinin. ALT is a non-pharmaceutical antimalarial treatment that depends on artemisinin and many other metabolites naturally biosynthesized and present in the leaves of the *Artemisia annua* plant, but for many of which the mode(s) of antimalarial action remains to be revealed. To get WHO recommendation, ALT has to go through extensive and essential fundamental and clinical research which needs to demonstrate that ALT is safe, efficacious, and would not promote the development of resistance to artemisinin in malarial parasites.

ALT uses standardized tablets (**Figure 1**) as the antimalarial drug prepared by compressing the dried pulverized leaves, harvested from cultivated plants of a specific variety(ies) of *Artemisia annua*, which contain ≥1% artemisinin.

The origin of ALT, as a dependable medicine against multi-drug-resistant malaria, is based on information from historical texts and a number of experimental findings. Some of the important empirical basis for ALT is annotated below:

a. There is recorded evidence that the Chinese people have been using *A. annua* material as a remedy for fever and chills, such as those associated with malaria. One of the effective materials consumed in traditional medicine was the consumption of the juicy extract of water-soaked *A. annua* leafy stems. The

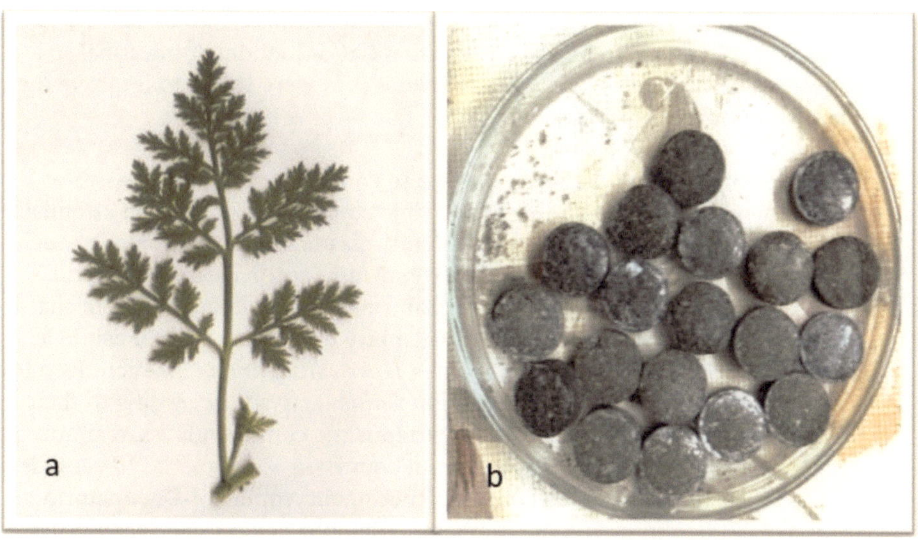

Figure 1.
ALT tablets made from dry Artemisia annua *cv Sanjeevani leaves. a =* A. annua *freshly harvested leaf; and b = Tablets made by compressing the dried* A. annua *leaves.*

Chinese traditional medicine literature does not report any case of resistance development against *A. annua* treatment used [74].

b. The *A. annua* plant material has been used by human populations in various parts of the world where the species existed naturally for various purposes, including for medicinal uses and as an item of food for livestock and humans without notice of any harmful effects [75] and therefore the species has been granted the GRAS (Generally Recognized As Safe) rating. Accordingly, *A. annua* leaves in amounts ≤ 30 g dry weight/day can be safely consumed [76].

c. In a study batch of healthy mice were orally fed on the one hand with an amount of artemisinin in its pure form, and on the other hand, were fed an equal amount of artemisinin in the form of *A. annua* dried leaves. The blood stream of mice fed with dry leaves contained > 40 times more artemisinin as compared to mice fed with pure artemisinin. Mice were required to be fed with > 45-fold more pure artemisinin (as a component of the normal mouse food) than artemisinin in dry *A. annua* leaves, so that artemisinin could be detected in the mouse bloodstream [77].

d. In another study, it was observed that oral administration of the *Artemisia annua* leaves to the *Plasmodium chabaudi*—infected mice killed the parasite without causing toxicity to mice. It was further found that parasitemia in the infected mice was reduced at least five-fold more by a single dose of *A. annua* leaves as compared to an equivalent dose of pure artemisinin, and the effect of dry leaves lasted longer than that of pure artemisinin (Elfawal *et al.*, 2012). The experiments at c and d above suggested that the presence of metabolites other than artemisinin in the dry leaves of *A. annua* improved both the bioavailability of artemisinin in the bloodstream and the therapeutic efficacy of artemisinin in infected red blood cells. These possibilities were evidenced by correlating the phytochemistry of *A. annua* leaves with the response of healthy and parasite-infected mice to the feeding of pure artemisinin versus *A. annua* leaves, as above and below in e and f. Recently, using CaCo-2 model of intestinal transport, the digestates of *A. annua* dried leaves were found to improve the artemisinin transport by 37% [78].

e. The leaves of *A. annua* plants are known to contain a number of classes of secondary metabolites including artemisinic compounds other than artemisinin. Many of these possess varying levels of anti-plasmodial activity, albeit much weaker than in artemisinin. The non-artemisinin, antimalarial compounds affect the survival of parasites via mechanisms that are independent of that for artemisinin or which determine the availability or activity of artemisinin at its site(s) of action. Some of the metabolites of *Artemisia annua* characterized for possession of their own kind of anti-*Plasmodium* activity, according to their chemical class, are as follows [79, 80]: artemisinic compounds = arteannuin B, artemisinic acid, dihydroartemisinic acid; coumarin = scopoletin; flavonoids = artematin, casticin, circilineol, chrysoplenetin, chrysophenol-D, eupatorin, kaempferol, luteolin, myrcetin, quercetin; phenolic acids = chlorogenic and rosmarinic acids; saponins; sulfated polysaccharides; terpenes = artemisia alcohol, artemisia ketone, borneol, camphene, camphor, caryophyllene, 1, 8-cineole, germacrene D, limonene, myrcene, nerolidol, α-pinene, phytol, sabinene, spathulenol, α-terpineol. The flavonoids and phenolic acids in general inhibit the cytochrome enzymes, present in the liver and intestine, that metabolize artemisinin to deoxyartemisinin, thereby increasing the bioavailability of artemisinin in the bloodstream [81].

f. ALT was shown to be effective against artemisinin-resistant malarial infections and its treatment was resilient to resistance development in animal model systems. Administration of a single oral dose of *A. annua* dry leaves (24 mg artemisinin/kg body weight) to rodents infected with artemisinin-resistant *P. yoelli* cured their parasitemia, whereas an equivalent dose of pure artemisinin proved to be ineffective on corresponding animals. It was further shown that the stable resistance to *A. annua* dry leaf treatment, in *P. chabaudi* infected mice, occurred 2.7 times slower than the acquirement of resistance to pure artemisinin. Achievement of resistance to dry *A. annua* leaf treatment in *P. chabaudi*-infected mice was found to be 1.6 times lower than that for the treatment with artesunate + mefloquine (ACT) [82].

g. The clinical use of ALT treatment on human patients with severe Pf malaria in the Democratic Republic of Congo proved the efficacy of ALT. For ALT treatment, tablets of 500 mg weight, each containing 5.5 mg artemisinin, were prepared by compressing powdered dry leaves of Anamed-A3 variety of *A. annua*. The patients given the ALT treatment were 6 males and 12 females, from 14 months to 60 years of age, whose malaria did not cure from treatment with artemether + lumefantrine, nor from intravenous artesunate treatment. The malaria patients had entered the severe phase which included symptoms, such as loss of consciousness, convulsions, frustration, shock, respiratory distress, pulmonary edema, bleeding, gastric distress, and jaundice. Among the patients, the adults were administered one tablet twice daily for 5 days, children of 5–15 kg body weight and 15–30 kg body weight, were given quarter and half tablet twice daily for 5 days, respectively, and those in a coma or too young to swallow tablets, the tablet-dose was crushed, mixed with water and delivered via nasogastric tube. All the patients got cured of their malarial disease and there were no adverse side effects. In ALT treatment on another set of patients, rectal administration of dried pulverized leaves of *Artemisia annua* was found effective in curing Pf malaria [83, 84]. More extensive studies are needed that will cover 28 days of follow-up after treatment with ALT.

From the evidence described above, about the roles of diverse phytochemicals present in the leaves of *A. annua* in augmenting the inhibitory/lethal effects of artemisinin in ALT on infections of *Plasmodium* species on animal model systems and about clinical efficacy and safety of ALT on human malaria patients, it is possible to conclude that ALT is an inexpensive but safe and effective option for treating acute and severe malaria. Since multiple secondary metabolites with the independent lethal mode of action on malarial parasites are involved in the efficacy of ALT, it is possible to further conclude that it will take a considerable time period before any resistance evolves against ALT treatment in malarial parasites or via it against artemisinin. It has been advised that the safety of ART treatment in pregnant women be evaluated and that nausea resulting from oral intake of dry leaf tablets may be controlled by encapsulation or use of anthelmintics or sweet substances [85]. Should there be recrudescence, the ALT treatment may be repeated or alternatively a triple ACT treatment be given.

7. ALT: establishment of the compositional consistency of tablets

Like for pharmaceuticals, stringent control over the quality of *A. annua* dry leaf tablets, during their manufacturing process, is essential for ALT's inclusion in the first line of antimalarial therapeutics. To achieve this objective in practice all the individual steps of the process must be standardized. To obtain leaves of high artemisinin content, only the identified genotypes of *A. annua* be grown under consistent and specified cultivation conditions. To retain the secondary metabolites in high concentrations, the harvested shoots of field-grown plants must be dried under clean and ambient conditions [86] to retain the secondary metabolites present in them in high concentrations. From the dry shoots, leaves are to be mechanically separated from the stem on clean surface, the dry leaves produced from different fields should be homogenized, sieved, pulverized using a blade cutter or equivalent instrument, characterized, and converted into tablets of standard weight, size, and content of artemisinin and a few flavonoids and terpenes, under hygienic conditions [80].

The *A. annua* crops can be cultivated in temperate and subtropical agroenvironments, such as those available in the countries of central and southern Europe, central Asia, southeast Asia, south Asia, east Africa, South America, and in Australia. Several genetically improved and bred varieties of wide adaptability, whose leaves upon drying contain 0.7 to 1.2 % artemisinin, are readily available, including Anamed (A3), Artemis, CPQPA, Jeevanraksha, Arogya, and Sanjeevani [87]. Besides, several to many seed industry-bred varieties of *A. annua* are also available.

In India, Jeevanraksha was developed as a product of a polycross hybrid of Asha variety x a Chinese accession followed by back crossing with Chinese parent, selected for ≥ 0.5% artemisinin content in vegetative stage leaves in subsequent generations. Arogya was a selection of globular-shaped hyper-branched segregants from Jeevanraksha lines that had adapted to the temperate agroclimate of Kashmir having ≥ 0.8% artemisinin content in vegetative stage leaves. Sanjeevani was developed as a polycross product of Arogya x Jeevanraksha selected for ≥ 1.0% artemisinin content in leaves of the vegetative stage (Sushil Kumar, personal communication).

A. annua is a short day-flowering, open-pollinated annual shrubby species that completes its life cycle in upto one year time. The sowing and harvesting times of *A. annua* crops to obtain high-quality produce of leaves has been prescribed according to the agro-climates of country-wise geographical locations of cultivation and variety (ies) [87]. The nursery-grown plants of one month or more of age are transplanted in fields @ 20–70 thousand plants/ ha, depending on the plant architecture and average field duration of plant population of the variety used. Nursery plants are raised by spreading the seeds on a wet soil surface, in farmyard manure fertilized field. The number of seeds required for planting 1 ha of the crop is 3–5 g. Fields of sandy-to-sandy loam soil type are used and fertilized with manure and fertilizers @ N:P: K: 60:40:40 kg/ha. The transplanted *A. annua* crop, to produce dry leaves for ALT, is harvested before flowering occurs on plants. The plant shoots are dried at temperatures ≤ 40 °C, in the field, under shade, or in specially designed temperature-controlled chambers. The desirable moisture content in the dried leaves is 10–12%. Dry leaves are stored and transported in the form of large blocks by compressing the leaves in molds.

Artemisia annua has been in commercial cultivation by farmers in India for more than 15 years, under the public-institution (CSIR-CIMAP) assisted farmer-company (IPCA) partnerships. In recent years such farmer-company partnerships have covered 2500 h/y, largely in north-west India and in this region preponderantly in the

Indo-Gangetic plains area. *A.annua* is also being cultivated in central and southern India. As a result, India has become a major resource of artemisinin and its derivatives. According to the agroclimate of the Indo-Gangetic plains, the most suitable time for the sowing of the nursery is 15 December to 15 January. Seedlings are transplanted in to the fields vacated by potato crops between 20 February and 1 March. This summer crop of *A. annua* is harvested between May 28 and June 5 (several weeks before the onset of monsoon rains) and shoots are dried under shaded conditions. Alternatively, or additionally, the plants growing in the nursery are transplanted in fields vacated by wheat crop from 15 May onwards, and the resulting crop is harvested between 21 September and 1 October (after the withdrawal of monsoon rains and with the onset of inflorescence development, but before flowering occurs). The autumn crop is dried in temperature-controlled chambers. The yield of dry leaves from the summer and autumn, harvested crop is 2.5 and 3.5 T/ha, with 0.8 to 1.2% artemisinin content, respectively, depending on the variety used; the highest levels of ART (1–1.4%) are present in the leaves harvested from the crops of Sanjeevani variety (Sanjay Kumar, Ramesh Srivastava, and Anil Gupta, personal communication).

Need is felt internationally for new genotypes of *A. annua* and for methodologies of plant population propagation such that the individual plants under cultivation have the same genotype or largely similar genotypes. Since *A. annua* is an open-pollinated crop, individual plants in populations of its registered varieties Anamed (A3), Jeevanraksha, Sanjeevani, and others demonstrate phenotypic differences arising from the segregation of alleles of thousands of genes which are present in heterozygous condition. A genomic study has confirmed the presence of heterozygosity at a large number of protein-coding genes, among 63226 genes identified in *A. annua*. The quality of dry leaf tablets from any available variety is the result of an average phenotype of its cultivated populations. In the future it is desirable to have ALT tablets from plants of a single genotype. There are several possibilities to pursue this aim. One of these is to develop elite inbred lines through selfing in existing varieties for 6 or more generations. The seeds of the chosen inbred line will be always produced in isolation. Second, F1 hybrids of two selected inbred lines, selected for heterosis, may be chosen for cultivation. Again, F1 seeds will be produced from co-cultivation in isolation of the parental inbred lines whose own seeds will be produced in isolation. Special genotypes, an important one being photo-period independent early flowering, could be developed in the background of chosen singular genotype(s). When suitable genotype(s) have become available for mono-genotype-culture, an alternative method to produce planting material on a mass scale could be the deployment of micro-propagation procedures [88, 89]. Any one selected plant from Jeevanraksha, Sanjeevani, or Anamed (A3) could become a clonal variety with the use of micropropagation for genotype multiplication.

8. Cost-effectiveness of ALT treatment

The ALT treatment in comparison to ACT treatment is highly cost-effective. In the Indo-Gangetic plains area, the cost of cultivation, harvesting, and processing of harvested shoots to obtain dry leaves of *A. annua* var Jeevanraksha, Arogya or Sanjeevani (all genetically related), and profit for farmers, under the farmer-private company partnership scheme, for two hectares of crop yield of 50 tons of dry leaves is ~ Rs. 2, 00, 000 (or ~US$ 3,500). The cost of producing 10 million tablets of 500 mg dry leaves each can therefore be speculated as ~ Rs 5,00,000 (or ~ US$ 8500).

Considering the expenditure of all kinds on the supply chain of ALT tablets, the cost of a 10 tablets treatment for an adult is estimated as less than Rs 1 (or less than US Cents 17). The ALT treatment in India will be at least 60 to 150-fold less costly than an ACT treatment. It is possible to conclude that large-scale adoption of ALT treatment as advised above can tremendously advance the aim of WHO and 97 malaria-endemic countries, including India, to significantly reduce or eliminate the burden of malaria by 2030. ALT capsules have the added advantage of being used as suppositories.

9. Possibilities of using ALT beyond malaria

A variety of disease conditions in humans and livestock are known to respond curatively to artemisinic-, terpenoid-, and flavonoid-compounds present in *A. annua* leaves. There is thus a strong possibility that ALT tablets may prove to be of therapeutic value against many diseases beyond malaria. There is robust evidence that demonstrates that many viruses-, bacteria-, fungi-, protozoa-, and helminths- caused infectious diseases on the one hand and autoimmune-, and digestive systems/ metabolic- disorders, and cancers on the other hand are attenuated/ prevented by treatment with artemisinins and *A. annua* leaves [90].

The drugs artemisinin and artesunate have been found to inhibit replication/ multiplication of hepatitis causing hepatitis B (HBV) and C (HCV) viruses and sore-inducing herpes virus and it is close relative cytomegalovirus in cultured human cells [91]. The *in vitro* growth of *Mycobacterium tuberculosis* (the bacterium which causes tuberculosis in humans), as well as the tubercular bacterial growth in infected mice, has been found to be arrested by artesunate. The addition of artemisinin to the culture of *Aspergillus fumigatus* (which causes aspergillosis in human) has been observed to stop the growth of fungus. Artemether and extracts of *A. annua* leaves have proved lethal to *in vitro* growing *Acanthamoeba castellani* (a cause of amoebiasis in humans) [92]. Treatment of mice infected with *Acanthamoeba* with water-, alcohol- or chloroform- extract of *Artemisia annua* leaves was observed to have increased the life span of diseased animals. Feeding of *A. annua* leaves to the broiler chickens infected with *Eimeria tenella* parasites saved the infected animals from the development of coccidiosis disease [93]. Growth of both visceral and cutaneous leishmaniasis causing *Leishmania* parasites, in human macrophage cultures, was found to be attenuated by the treatment of artemisinin. Analogously, the leishmania infections in model animals were also observed to have been arrested by treatment with artemisinin or *A. annua* leaf powder. Artesunate was observed to inhibit the *Toxiplasma gondii* infection of cultured human cells and of mice *in vivo.* Trypanosomiasis (human African sleeping sickness) like disease caused by *Trypanosoma brucci* infection in experimental mice and rats were found to have been cured by artemether treatment. Artemisinin and artesunate treatments given individually inhibited the growth of *T. brucci* and *T. cruzi* (the cause of chagas disease in humans) in cultured human cells. Infection in humans and in experimental mice of *Schistosoma mansoni*, as well as S. japonicum (both the species are cause of schistosomiasis disease), was observed to get inhibited by treatment with each of the drugs- artemether, dihydroartemisinin, and artesunate [94].

In different studies, artesunate was found to cure/suppress and relieve symptoms of collagen-induced rheumatoid arthritis, Crohn's disease, ovalbumin-induced asthma, and lipopolysaccharide-induced uveitis, all in model animals. Obesity and fatty liver diseases caused by consumption of a high fat/ nutrition diet in experimental animals were found to be cured by treatment with *A. annua* leaf extracts. The *A.*

annua leaf extract also cured alloxan-induced diabetes in rats. It was found that artemether treatment, to type1 diabetic zebrafish, mice and rats, and human pancreatic islets, transformed the pancreatic α cells into β cells such that insulin synthesis started relieving the type 1 diabetes symptoms [95]. Cells of human cell lines of pancreatic-, hepatocellular-, gastric-, colorectal- and renal- cancer stopped proliferating and got killed by an oncosis-like process upon treatment with artesunate. Also, the xenographs of pancreatic-, hepatocellular-, gastric- and renal-cancers in animal models were found to regress upon treatment with artesunate. The artemisinin treatment produced analogous results in *in vitro* and *in vivo* gall bladder cancer and in *in vitro* cervical cancer. The experimental findings that artemisannua controlled obesity and diabetes in model animals strongly suggest that ALT as a treatment for these diseases in humans [87].

Clearly, the above discussion suggests that the mechanisms of biological actions of artemisinins and artemisannua are such that these agents serve as broad-spectrum therapeutics, such as to cure a variety of human diseases. These observations raise the possibility that perhaps ALT can substitute for artemisinins and artemisannua and ALT can be a therapy for multiple diseases beyond malaria. In view of the above, the need for pilot studies and clinical trials on quality-controlled ALT tablets for studying the response of their administration to patients of each of the different nonmalarial, as well as malarial diseases, that respond to artemisinins and artemisannua, cannot be overemphasized.

10. Concluding remarks

In the last ten years, the incidence of malaria disease was reduced by 20% and mortality among malaria patients by 30%. This was in the main achieved by the use of two-drug ACTs and chloroquine in the treatment of falciparum and vivax malaria, respectively, and by the use of primaquine treatment to block the transmission of parasites from humans to mosquitoes (**Table 3**). However, the falciparum and vivax malarial parasites have developed genetic resistance against a large majority of the approved antimalarial pharmaceuticals in some of their populations in malaria-endemic areas, thereby making the drugs ineffective (**Table 2**). There has been independent development of artemisinin resistance in southeast Asia and Africa; consequently, ACT treatments too have become ineffective in parts of these geographical areas. To meet the challenge of multi-drug resistant falciparum malarial strains, treatment with three-drug ACTs has been advised. This year a new treatment (ALT) has been added to cure the acute and complicated malaria caused by ACT-resistant falciparum parasites. The ALT treatment comprises capsules filled with or tablets made from *A. annua* dry leaf powder, derived from cultivated plants of specific variety(ies) bred for ≥ 1% artemisinin content and a combination of other therapeutically active metabolites naturally present. A regimen of two 500 mg leaf powder tablets a day for 5 days was found to cure adults suffering from ACT-resistant complicated falciparum malaria that was unresponsive to ACT or iv artesunate (most likely artemisinin-resistant). The ALT treatment's malaria curing property has been related to antimalarial activities of artemisinin, several other artemisinic compounds, many terpenes and flavonoids, and other types of molecules present in the dry *A. annua* leaves. ALT is safe and seems resilient against artemisinin drug resistance development. The cost of an ALT treatment was estimated to be about 100-fold lower than that of an ACT treatment. Extensive putative use of ALT has gained importance since a recent policy statement of WHO emphasizes the importance of affordability for everyone of safe, efficacious, and quality medical products. The ALT, besides being an efficacious antimalarial treatment has properties that raise possibilities of its multi-repurposement as a treatment against all those diseases which respond curatively to artemisinin, its derivatives and *A. annua* leaf powder or its extracts. This list includes diseases as diverse as hepatitis, tuberculosis, leishmaniasis, toxoplasmosis, trypanosomiasis, schistosomiasis, asthma, rheumatoid arthritis, diabetes, and cancers of various body organs. There is now an urgent need for (a) further evaluation of artemisinin efficacy against several of the listed diseases in vivo models, and (b) pilot studies and clinical trials to attest ALT treatment for varied malaria and diseases beyond malaria for which artemisinin efficacy has been experimentally established, for the benefit of billions of patients of above-listed diseases.

Acknowledgements

The author is highly grateful to the Director KIET Group of Institutions, Dr. (Col) A. Garg; Joint Director KIET Group of Institutions, Dr. Manoj Goel and Principal KIET School of Pharmacy, Dr. K. Nagarajan; Emeritus Scientist, Prof. Sushil Kumar for their continuous inspiration, guidance, and support.

Author details

Richa Goel
Department of Pharmacognosy, KIET School of Pharmacy, KIET Group of Institutions, Ghaziabad, UP, India

*Address all correspondence to: richagoel06@gmail.com

References

[1] WHO. Artemisinin and artemisinin based combination therapy resistance Status report [Internet]. April 2017. WHO-HTM-GMP-2017.9-eng.pdf [Accessed: July 22, 2022]

[2] Landier J, Parker DM, Thu AM, Carrara VI, Lwin KM, et al. The role of early detection and treatment in malaria elimination. Malaria Journal. 2016;**15**:363

[3] Dondorp AM. New genetic marker for piperaquine resistance in *Plasmodium falciparum*. The Lancet Infectious Diseases. 2017;**17**:119-121

[4] Daddy NB, Kalisya LM, Bagire PG, Watt RL, Towler MJ, Weathers PJ. *Artemisia annua* dried leaf tablets treated malaria resistant to ACT and i.v. artesunate: Case reports. Phytomedicine. 2017;**32**:37-40

[5] Antinori S, Corona A, Castelli A, Rech R, Borghi B, et al. Severe *Plasmodium falciparum* malaria in the intensive care unit: A 6-year experience in Milano, Italy. Travel Medicine and Infectious Disease. 2017; **17**:43-49

[6] Rutledge GG, Bohme U, Sanders M, Reid AJ, Cotton JA, et al. *Plasmodium malariae* and *P. ovale* genomes provide insights into malaria parasite evolution. Nature. 2017;**542**:101-104

[7] York A. Seasonal malaria chemoprevention in the Sahel. The Lancet Infectious Diseases. 2017;**17**:588

[8] Anvikar AR, Shah N, Dhariwal AC, Sonal GS, Pradhan MM, et al. Epidemiology of *Plasmodium vivax* malaria in India. The American Journal of Tropical Medicine and Hygiene. 2016; **95**:108-120

[9] Doctor SM, Liu Y, Anderson OG, Whitesell AN, Mwandagalirwa MK, et al. Low prevalence of *Plasmodium malariae* and *Plasmodium ovale* mono-infections among children in the Democratic Republic of the Congo: A population-based, cross-sectional study. Malaria Journal. 2016;**15**:350

[10] Sutherland CJ. Persistent Parasitism: The adaptive biology of malariae and ovale malaria. Trends in Parasitology. 2015;**32**:808-819

[11] Laurent S, Miller B, Burton TA, Amaratunga C, Men S, et al. Artemisinin-resistant *Plasmodium falciparum* clinical isolates can infect diverse mosquito vectors of Southeast Asia and Africa. Nature Communications. 2016;**6**:8614

[12] Tainchum K, Kongmee M, Manguin S, Bangs MJ, Chareonviriyaphap T. Anopheles species diversity and distribution of the malaria vectors of Thailand. Trends in Parasitology. 2015;**31**:109-119

[13] Singh B, Daneshvar C. Human infections and detection of *Plasmodium knowlesi*. Clinical Microbiology Reviews. 2013;**26**:165-184

[14] Brasil P, Zalis MG, de Pina-Costa A, Siqueira AM, Júnior CB, Silva S, et al. Outbreak of human malaria caused by *Plasmodium simium* in the Atlantic Forest in Rio de Janeiro: A molecular epidemiological investigation. The Lancet Global Health. 2017;**5**:e1038-e1046

[15] Sinka ME, Bangs MJ, Manguin S, Rubio-Palis Y, Chareonviriyaphap T, et al. A global map of dominant malaria vectors. Parasites & Vectors. 2012;**5**:69

[16] De Carvalho GB, de Carvalho GB. Duffy Blood Group System and the malaria adaptation process in humans. Revista Brasileira de Hematologia e Hemoterapia. 2011;**33**:55-64

[17] Mayxay M, Pukrittayakamee S, Newton PN, White NJ. Mixed-species malaria infections in humans. Trends in Parasitology. 2004;**20**:233-240

[18] Krishna S, Bhandari S, Bharti PK, Basak S, Singh N. A rare case of quadruple malaria infection from the highly malaria-endemic area of Bastar, Chhattisgarh, India. PLOS Neglected Tropical Diseases. 2017;**11**:e0005558

[19] Kakkilaya BS. Rapid diagnosis of malaria. Laboratory Medicine. 2003;**8**: 602-608

[20] Lee MSJ, Maruyama K, Fujita Y, Konishi A, Lelliott PM, et al. Plasmodium products persist in the bone marrow and promote chronic bone loss. Science Immunology. 2017;**2**:eaam8093

[21] White NJ. Malaria parasite clearance. Malaria Journal. 2017;**16**:88

[22] Dondorp AM, Fanello CI, Hendriksen IC, Gomes E, Seni A, et al. Artesunate versus quinine in the treatment of severe *falciparum* malaria in African children (AQUAMAT): An open-label, randomised trial. Lancet. 2010;**376**:1647-1657

[23] Achan J, Talisuna AO, Erhart A, Yeka A, Tibenderana JK, et al. Quinine, an old anti-malarial drug in a modern world: Role in the treatment of malaria. Malaria Journal. 2011;**10**:144

[24] Sullivan DJ, Matile H, Ridley RG, Goldberg DE. A common mechanism for blockade of heme polymerization by antimalarial quinolines. The Journal of Biological Chemistry. 1998;**273**: 31103-31107

[25] Grigg MJ, William T, Menon J, Barber BE, Wilkes CS, et al. Efficacy of artesunate-mefloquine for chloroquine-resistant *Plasmodium vivax* malaria in Malaysia: An open-label, randomized, controlled trial. Clinical Infectious Diseases. 2016;**62**:1403-1411

[26] Croft AM. Developing safe antimalaria drugs: Key lessons from mefloquine and halofantrine. The International Journal of Risk & Safety in Medicine. 2007;**19**:153-161

[27] Ezzet F, Van Vugt M, Nosten F, Looareesuwan S, White NJ. Pharmacokinetics and pharmacodynamics of lumefantrine (benflumetol) in acute *falciparum* malaria. Antimicrobial Agents and Chemotherapy. 2000;**44**:697-704

[28] Plucinski MM, Talundzic E, Morton L, Dimbu PR, Macaia AP, et al. Reply to "no robust evidence of lumefantrine resistance". Antimicrobial Agents and Chemotherapy. 2015;**59**: 5867-5868

[29] Krafts K, Hempelmann E, Skorsha-Stania A. From methylene blue to chloroquine: A brief review of the development of an antimalarial therapy. Parasitology Research. 2012;**111**:1-6

[30] Mwanza S, Nambozi M, Chileshe J, Joshi S, Malunga P, Kabuya JB, et al. Chloroquine-sensitive *Plasmodium falciparum* in a high burden malaria area after over a decade of its withdrawl as first-line antimalarial medicine: Case of Nchelenge District. BMJ Global Health. 2017;**2**:A17

[31] Sa JM, Twu O, Hayton K, Reyes S, Fay MP, et al. Geographic patterns of *Plasmodium falciparum* drug resistance

distinguished by differential responses to amodiaquine and chloroquine. Proceedings of the National Academy of Sciences USA. 2009;**106**:18883-18889

[32] Cairns M, Cisse B, Sokhna C, Cames C, Simondon K, et al. Amodiaquine dosage and tolerability for intermittent preventive treatment to prevent malaria in children. Antimicrobial Agents and Chemotherapy. 2010;**54**:1265-1274

[33] Davis TME, Hung TY, Sim IK, Karunajeewa HA, Ilett KF. Piperaquine: A resurgent antimalarial drug. Drugs. 2005;**65**:75-87

[34] Witkowski B, Duru V, Khim N, Ross LS, Saintpierre B, et al. A surrogate marker of piperaquine-resistant *Plasmodium falciparum* malaria: A phenotype–genotype association study. The Lancet Infectious Diseases. 2017;**17**: 174-183

[35] Hill DR, Baird JK, Parise ME, Lewis LS, Ryan ET, Magill AJ. Primaquine: Report from CDC expert meeting on malaria chemoprophylaxis. The American Journal of Tropical Medicine and Hygiene. 2006;**75**:402-415

[36] Graves PM, Gelband H, Ribeiro I. Primaquine for reducing transmission of *Plasmodium falciparum* malaria. The Lancet Infectious Diseases. 2009;**16**: 674-684

[37] Auparakkitanon S, Chapoomram S, Kuaha K, Chirachariyavej T, Wilairat P. Targeting of hematin by the antimalarial pyronaridine. Antimicrobial Agents and Chemotherapy. 2006;**50**:2197-2200

[38] Croft SL, Duparc S, Arbe-Barnes SJ, Craft J, Shin CS, et al. Review of pyronaridine anti-malarial properties and product characteristics. Malaria Journal. 2012;**11**:270

[39] Srivastava IK, Vaidya AB. A mechanism for the synergistic antimalarial action of atovaquone and proguanil. Antimicrobial Agents and Chemotherapy. 1999;**43**:1334-1339

[40] Fowler RE, Sinden RE, Pudney M. Inhibitory activity of the anti-malarial atovaquone (566C80) against ookinetes, oocysts, and sporozoites of *Plasmodium berghei*. The Journal of Parasitology. 1995;**81**:452-458

[41] Staines HM, Burrow R, Teo BH, Chis Ster I, Kremsner PG, Krishna S. Clinical implications of Plasmodium resistance to atovaquone/proguanil: A systematic review and meta-analysis. Journal of Antimicrobial Chemotherapy. 2018;**73**: 581-595

[42] Boggild AK, Parise ME, Lewis LS, Kain KC. Atovaquone-proguanil: Report from the CDC expert meeting on malaria chemoprophylaxis. The American Journal of Tropical Medicine and Hygiene. 2007;**76**:208-223

[43] Gutman J, Slutsker L. Intermittent preventive treatment with sulfadoxine-pyrimethamine: More than just an Antimalarial? The American Journal of Tropical Medicine and Hygiene. 2017;**11**: 9-10

[44] Gatton ML, Martin LB, Cheng Q. Evolution of resistance to sulfadoxine-pyrimethamine in *Plasmodium falciparum*. Antimicrobial Agents and Chemotherapy. 2004;**48**:2116-2123

[45] Ayubu MB, Kidima WB. Monitoring compliance and acceptability of intermittent preventive treatment of malaria using sulfadoxine pyrimethamine after ten years of implementation in Tanzania. Malaria Research and Treatment. 2017; **2017**:1-5

[46] Dahl EL, Shock JL, Shenai BR, Gut J, DeRisi JL, Rosenthal PJ. Tetracyclines specifically target the apicoplast of the malaria parasite *Plasmodium falciparum*. Antimicrobial Agents and Chemotherapy. 2006;**50**:3124-3131

[47] Gaillard T, Madamet M, Tsombeng FF, Dormoi J, Pradines B. Antibiotics in malaria therapy: Which antibiotics except tetracyclines and macrolides may be used against malaria? Malaria Journal. 2016;**15**:556

[48] Gaillard T, Briolant S, Madamet M, Pradines B. The end of a dogma: The safety of doxycycline use in young children for malaria treatment. Malaria Journal. 2017;**16**:148

[49] Tan KR, Magill AJ, Parise ME, Arguin PM. Doxycycline for malaria chemoprophylaxis and treatment: Report from the CDC expert meeting on malaria chemoprophylaxis. The American Journal of Tropical Medicine and Hygiene. 2011;**84**:517-531

[50] Obonyo CO, Juma EA. Clindamycin plus quinine for treating uncomplicated *falciparum* malaria: A systematic review and meta-analysis. Malaria Journal. 2012;**11**:2

[51] Burkhardt D, Wiesner J, Stoesser N, Ramharter M, Uhlemann AC, et al. Delayed parasite elimination in human infections treated with clindamycin parallels "delayed death" of *Plasmodium falciparum in vitro*. International Journal of Parasitology. 2007;**37**:777-785

[52] Barber BE, William T, Grigg MJ, Menon J, Auburn S, et al. A prospective comparative study of *knowlesi, falciparum,* and *vivax* malaria in sabah, Malaysia: High proportion with severe disease from *Plasmodium knowlesi* and *Plasmodium vivax* but No mortality with early Referral and artesunate therapy. Clinical Infectious Diseases. 2013;**56**:383-397

[53] Gopalakrishnan AM, Kumar N. Antimalarial action of artesunate involves DNA damage mediated by reactive oxygen species. Antimicrobial Agents and Chemotherapy. 2015;**59**:317-325

[54] Rijken MJ, McGready R, Phyo AP, Lindegardh N, Tarning J, Laochan N, et al. Pharmacokinetics of dihydroartemisinin and piperaquine in pregnant and nonpregnant women with uncomplicated *falciparum* malaria. Antimicrobial Agents and Chemotherapy. 2011;**55**:5500-5506

[55] Agarwal A, McMorrow M, Onyango P, Otieno K, Odero C, et al. A randomized trial of artemether-lumefantrine and dihydroartemisinin-piperaquine in the treatment of uncomplicated malaria among children in western Kenya. Malaria Journal. 2013;**12**:254

[56] Esu E, Effa EE, Opie ON, Uwaoma A, Meremikwu MM. Artemether for severe malaria Cochrane database. Systematic Reviews. 2014;**9**:CD010678

[57] Rutledge GG, Marr I, Huang GKL, Auburn S, Marfurt J, et al. Genomic characterization of recrudescent *Plasmodium malariae* after treatment with artemether/lumefantrine. Emerging Infectious Diseases. 2017;**23**:1300-1307

[58] Abraham G. Malaria in pregnancy: Is artemisinin-based treatment safe. Evidence-Based Medicine. 2017;**15**:63-65

[59] Dellicour S, Sevene E, McGready R, Tinto H, Mosha D, et al. First-trimester artemisinin derivatives and quinine treatments and the risk of adverse

pregnancy outcomes in Africa and Asia: A meta-analysis of observational studies. PLoS Medicine. 2017;**14**:e1002290

[60] Phuc BQ, Rasmussen C, Duong T, Dong L, Loi M, Ménard D, et al. Treatment failure of dihydroartemisinin/piperaquine for *Plasmodium falciparum* malaria. Emerging Infectious Diseases. 2017;**23**:715-717

[61] Tine RC, Sylla K, Faye BT, Poirot E, Fall FB, et al. Safety and efficacy of adding a single low dose of primaquine to the treatment of adult patients with *Plasmodium falciparum* malaria in senegal, to reduce gametocyte carriage: A Randomized controlled trial. Clinical Infectious Diseases. 2017;**65**: 535-543

[62] Kremsner PG, Adegnika AA, Hounkpatin AB, Zinsou JF, Taylor TE, et al. Intramuscular artesunate for severe malaria in African children: A multicenter randomized controlled trial. PLoS Medicine. 2016;**13**:e1001938

[63] Lalloo DG, Shingadia D, Bell DJ, Beeching NJ, Whitty CJM, Chiodini PL. UK malaria treatment guidelines. The Journal of Infection. 2016;**72**:635-649

[64] Pekyi D, Ampromfi AA, Tinto H, Traoré-Coulibaly M, Tahita MC, et al. Four artemisinin-based treatments in African pregnant women with malaria. Malawi Medical Journal. 2016; **28**:139-149

[65] Sirima SB, Ogutu B, Lusingu JPA, Mtoro A, Mrango Z, et al. Comparison of artesunate-mefloquine and artemether-lumefantrine fixed-dose combinations for treatment of uncomplicated *Plasmodium falciparum* malaria in children younger than 5 years in sub Sahara Africa: A randomized, multicentre, phase 4 trial. The Lancet Infectious Diseases. 2016;**16**:1123-1133

[66] White NJ. Can new treatment developments combat resistance in malaria? Expert Opinion on Pharmacotherapy. 2016;**17**:1303-1307

[67] Kumar S, Kumari R, Pandey R. New insight-guided approaches to detect, cure, prevent and eliminate malaria. Protoplasma. 2015;**251**:717-753

[68] Verlinden BK, Louw A, Birkholtz LM. Resisting resistance: Is there a solution for malaria? Expert Opinion on Drug Discovery. 2016;**11**: 395-406

[69] Dondorp AM, Smithuis FM, Woodrow C, von Seidlein L. How to contain artemisinin- and multidrug-resistant falciparum malaria. Trends in Parasitology. 2017;**33**:353-363

[70] Weathers PJ, Towler M, Hassanali A, Lutgen P, Engeu PO. Dried-leaf *Artemisia annua*: A practical malaria therapeutic for developing countries? World Journal of Pharmacology. 2014;**3**: 39-55

[71] Elfawal MA, Towler MJ, Reich NG, Golenbock D, Weathers PJ, Rich SM. Dried whole plant *Artemisia annua* as an antimalarial therapy. PLoS One. 2012;**7**: e52746

[72] Malhotra K, Subramaniyan M, Rawat K, Kalamuddin M, Qureshi MI, et al. Compartmentalized metabolic engineering for artemisinin biosynthesis and effective malaria treatment by oral delivery of plant cells. Molecular Plant. 2016;**9**:1464-1477

[73] Paddon CJ, Keasling JD. Semi-synthetic artemisinin: A model for the use of synthetic biology in pharmaceutical development. Nature Reviews. Microbiology. 2014;**12**: 355-367

[74] Dhingra V, Rao KV, Narasu ML. Artemisinin: Present status and perspectives. Biochemical Education. 1999;**27**:105-109

[75] Yimer S, Sahu O. Traditional medicines for treatment of African diseases by *Artemisia annua*. International Journal of Medical Science and Public Health. 2016;**4**:22-32

[76] Duke JA. Handbook of Phytochemical Constituents of GRAS Herbs and Other Economic Plants. London: CRC Press; 2001

[77] Weathers PJ, Arsenault PR, Covello PS, McMickle A, Teoh KH, Reed DW. Artemisinin production in *Artemisia annua*: Studies in planta and results of a novel delivery method for treating malaria and other neglected diseases. Phytochemistry Reviews. 2011; **10**:173-183

[78] Desrosiers MR, Weathers PJ. Effect of leaf digestion and artemisinin solubility for use in oral consumption of dried *Artemisia annua* leaves to treat malaria. Journal of Ethnopharmacology. 2016;**190**:313-318

[79] Bhakuni R, Jain D, Sharma R, Kumar S. Secondary metabolites of *Artemisia annua* and their biological activity. Current Science. 2001;**80**:35-48

[80] Goel R, Singh V, Gupta AK, Mallavarapu GR, Kumar S. Constituents of the essential oil of *Artemisia annua* variety Sanjeevani compared with those of its parental varieties Arogya and Jeevanraksha: Selection for high artemisinin content co-selected high sesquiterpene content in essential oil. Journal of Essential Oil-Bearing Plants. 2018;**21**(5):1336-1348

[81] Weathers PJ, Towler MJ. Changes in key constituents of clonally propagated *Artemisia annua* L. during preparation of compressed leaf tablets for possible therapeutic use. Industrial Crops and Products. 2014;**62**:173-178

[82] Elfawal MA, Towler MJ, Reich NG, Weathers PJ, Rich SM. Dried whole-plant *Artemisia annua* slows evolution of malaria drug resistance and overcomes resistance to artemisinin. Proceedings of the National Academy of Sciences. 2015; **112**:821-826

[83] Abolaji GT, Olooto FM, Williams FE. Development of value added tea bags and capsules of *Artemisia annua* Anamed (A3) whole plant for malaria treatment. Agrosearch. 2016;**16**:69-73

[84] Onimus M, Carteron S, Lutgen P. The surprising efficiency of *Artemisia annua* powder capsules. Medicinal and Aromatic Plants. 2013;**2**:125

[85] Yarnell E. *Artemisia annua* (Sweet Annie), other Artemisia species, artemisinin, artemisinin derivatives, and malaria. Journal of Restorative Medicine. 2014;**3**:69-84

[86] Ferreira JFS, Janick J. Production and detection of artemisinin from *Artemisia annua*. International Symposium on Medicinal and Aromatic Plants. 1995;**209**:41-49

[87] Goel R, Singh V, Pandey R, Kumari R, Srivastava S, Kumar S. Perspectives of the *Artemisia annua* dry leaf therapy (ALT) for malaria and of its re-purposement as an affordable cure for artemisinin-treatable illnesses. Proceedings of the Indian National Science Academy. 2018;**84**(3):731-780

[88] Goel R, Singh V, Srivastava S, Mallavarapu GR, Goel D, Kumar S. *Artemisia* (Asteraceae) essential oils: Compositional variation and mechanisms of its origin, biosynthesis of

constituents, correspondence between biological activities and ethnomedicinal usage and repurposement prospects. Proceedings of the Indian National Science Academy. 2019;**85**(4):723-790

[89] Gopinath B et al. In vitro propagation of an important medicinal plant *Artemisia annua* L. from axillary bud explants. Advances in Applied Science Research. 2014;**5**:254-258

[90] Goel R, Singh V. Rajkumari. Cost effective natural treatment against infestation by *Tribolium castaneum* in stored food products. International Journal of Green Pharmacy. 2018;**12**(2): S394-S400

[91] Paeshuyse J, Coelmont L, Vliegen I, Hemel J Van, Vandenkerckhove J, et al. Hemin potentiates the anti-hepatitis C virus activity of the antimalarial drug artemisinin. Biochemical and Biophysical Research Communications 2006;348:139–144

[92] Deng Y, Ran W, Man S, Li X, Gao H, et al. Artemether exhibits amoebicidal activity against *Acanthamoeba castellanii* through inhibition of the serine biosynthesis pathway. Antimicrobial Agents andChemotherapy. 2015;**59**: 4680-4688

[93] Dragan L, Gyorke A, Ferreira JF, Pop IA, Dunca I, et al. Effects of *Artemisia annua* and *Foeniculum vulgare* on chickens highly infected with *Eimeria tenella* (Phylum Apicomplexa). Acta Veterinaria Scandinavica. 2014;**56**:22

[94] Akande F, Fagbemi B. *In vivo* and *in vitro* effects of artemisinin group of drugs on trypanosomosis in mice. Journal of Natural Sciences Engineering and Technology. 2011;**10**:73-80

[95] Song Y, Lee SJ, Jang SH, Kim TH, Kim HD, et al. Annual wormwood leaf inhibits the adipogenesis of 3T3-L1 and obesity in high-fat diet-induced obese rats. Nutrients. 2017;**9**:E554

Chapter 10

Combating Antimalarial Drug Resistance: Recent Advances and Future Perspectives

Samuel Uzondu, Adaeze Echezona, Chinekwu Nwagwu, Adaeze Onugwu, Lydia Ugorji, Chinazom Agbo, Franklin Kenechukwu, John Ogbonna, Paul Akpa, Petra Nnamani, Audu Momoh and Anthony Attama

Abstract

This chapter X-rayed antimalarial drug resistance (ADR) by plasmodium species with a particular focus on *P. falciparum*, which is the most deadly species of the malaria parasite responsible for over 90% of the global malaria burden domiciled in Sub-Saharan Africa. The introduction intently looked at malaria therapeutics across the decades and the development of drug resistance by the parasite. With the malaria parasite (*P. falciparum*) as the focal point, the mechanisms by which they develop resistance to antimalarial drugs was looked at, including factors affecting drug resistance development. Armed with this knowledge, the chapter also highlighted the therapeutic interventions taken against this hydra-headed monster together with their limitations and recent advances towards addressing those limitations or opening new frontiers for research exploration. Future perspectives that will provide research strategy and direction as possible tools for combating drug resistance development by the malaria parasite were also discussed.

Keywords: antimalarial drug resistance (ADR), *P. Falciparum*. Malaria, mutation

1. Introduction

Malaria is a public health concern which has ravaged majorly Sub-Saharan Africa which accounts for over 90% of the global malaria burden [1]. This disease is caused by Plasmodium species, five of them are known to cause the disease in man. They *are Plasmodium falciparum, Plasmodium vivax, Plasmodium ovale, Plasmodium malariae, Plasmodium knowlesi. Plasmodium falciparum* is the responsible for the most deadly form of the disease found in Sub-Saharan Africa causing the highest global morbidity and mortality rates in Africa. Children from 0 to 5 years and pregnant women are the most vulnerable to this disease. There has been a lot of therapeutic interventions by way of drugs targeted at eliminating or eradicating malaria. Prior to the introduction of the first synthetic drug chloroquine, cinchona alkaloids, quinine and quinidine have been used for the treatment of malaria. Chloroquine was introduced in 1940 as the mainstay for malaria treatment for about a decade plus until the parasite developed resistance to it. This led to the development and introduction of other drug classes consecutively as follows.

a. 4-Aminoquinolines (e.g. chloroquine, amodiaquine and piperaquine)

b. Aminoalcohols (e.g. mefloquine, halofantrine and lumefantrine)

c. Antifolates (e.g. sulphadoxine, pyrimethamine, proguanil)

d. Hydroxynaphthoquinone (e.g. atovaquone)

e. Endoperoxides (e.g. artemisinin and derivatives with their combination with other antimalarial drugs (ACTs) [2].

The following classes of drugs consecutively have been used clinically in the treatment of malaria; (1)4-aminoquinolines (e.g. chloroquine, amodiaquine and piperaquine) (2) aminoalcohols (e.g. mefloquine, halofantrine and lumefantrine) (3) antifolates (e.g. Sulphadoxine, pyrimethamine, proguanil) (4) hydroxynaphthoquinone (e.g. atovaquone) and (5) endoperoxides [e.g. artemisinin and derivatives with their combination with other antimalarial drugs (ACTs.)] Classes 1–4 are no longer used as first lines as a result of resistance development to them by the malaria parasite. Currently the endoperoxides' clinical efficacy against the malaria parasite is being threatened by emergence of artemisinin-resistant and ACT-resistant strains of the parasite particularly in the Greater Mekong Subregion (GMS) and recently in Africa [3].

The phenomenon of Antimalarial Drug Resistance (ADR) has led to the clinical retirement of Drug Classes 1–4 and is threatening the clinical efficacy of Drug Class 5-endoperoxides e.g. Artemisinins and their combinations. This is shown in the **Figure 1** below.

A critical look at **Figure 1** shows ADR as shown by the brown band generally causes a reduction in the clinical lifespan of the antimalarial drug as one moves interclass. This reduction in clinical lifespan has led to the retirement of drug classes 1–4 as first line treatment for malaria. Drug class 5; the Artemisinins and their combinations (ACTs) are currently under threat of resistance by the malaria parasite. ACTs are the WHO-recommended firstline and lastline (of some sorts) treatment for malaria. ACTs are one of the major factors responsible for the global successes recorded in the fight against malaria for about two decades now. The recent emergence of ACT-resistant strains of the malaria parasite in GMS and Africa has underlined the need for the discovery and development of novel therapeutic agents with novel mechanisms of action as one of the ways of tackling this hydra-headed monster. In tackling ADR, it is pertinent to zoom in on it and take a close look at it.

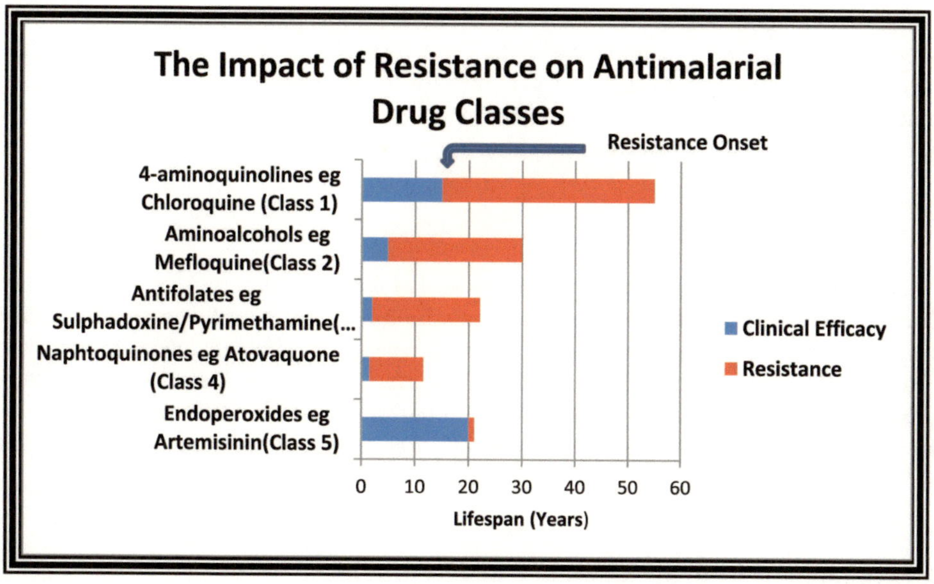

Figure 1.
The impact of resistance on antimalarial drug classes. (adapted from a journal article, drawn with Microsoft excel).

2. What is antimalarial drug resistance (ADR)?

Antimalarial Drug Resistance (ADR) can be best described as resistance to antimalarial drugs by the malaria parasite; Plasmodium species particularly *P. falciparum* which is responsible for the most deadly form of malaria - Falciparum malaria. *P. falciparum* is responsible for over 90% of the global malaria burden domiciled in Sub-Saharan Africa. It is the most virulent plasmodium species responsible for high morbidity and mortality rates of malaria observed in Africa particularly Sub-Saharan Africa. ADR has rendered most of the antimalarial drug classes clinically ineffective; these drug classes include 4-aminoquinolines, antifolates, mefloquine and atovaquone etc.

2.1 Development of ADR

When the malaria parasite is exposed to antimalarial drugs, initially it succumbs to the pharmacological action of the drug, over time develops resistance to it. Resistance development by the parasite is its adaptation to the new environment (with the presence of the drug) a complete departure from the old environment (absence of the drug). Continuous use of antimalarial drugs particularly at sub-therapeutic doses exposes them to the malaria parasite leading to the development of resistant strains of the parasite with several resistance phenotypes, some of these resistance genotypes might not necessarily have the resistance phenotypes. In Africa, the most frequent PfKelch13 mutation is A578S, this mutation does not confer Artemisinin resistance in vivo or in vitro [4]. The period between the first introduction of the antimalarial drug and the emergence of resistant strains of the parasite is laden with a variety of adaptive activities which may include genetic mutations which may include Gene Copy Number variations (CNV), Point mutations etc. An example of point mutation is the substitution of the Amino acid lysine with threonine at position 76 on the protein

(K76T). Gene copy number variants are deletions and amplification of a gene or a set of continuous genes and contribute to the great diversity of P.falciparum genome. *In vitro* studies have revealed their roles in parasite fitness phenotypes which include transmissibility, drug resistance, red cell invasion [5]. Resistance can also be imported into sensitive parasitic cells from neighboring resistant cells by R-plasmids transfer.

2.2 Resistance phenotypes

ADR by *P. falciparum* manifests with several resistance phenotypes which include; delayed parasite clearance, increased transmissibility, decreased schizont susceptibility, decreased gametocyte susceptibility, Ring stage resistance. Clinically, delayed parasite clearance is the phenotype used to establish resistance to antimalarial drugs. Parasite clearance rate can be used to measure delayed parasite clearance. It is quantified as the time taken by the antimalarial drug to reduce parasitaemia by half: for sensitive strains of *P. falciparum*, it is usually between 1 and 3 h, for resistant strains >5 h [6].

3. Mechanisms of drug resistance development

ADR by *P. falciparum* occurs through various mechanisms which include;

a. Reduction of the drug concentration at the site of action (Efflux mechanism): This is the mechanism of resistance by *P. falciparum* to chloroquine, a 4-aminoquinoline. Point mutation in the *P.falciparum* chloroquine resistance transporter gene (PfCRT) results in the transporter effluxing more of the chloroquine out of the digestive vacuole reducing its effective intravacuolar concentration. Point mutation in the *P. falciparum* multidrug resistance-1 transporter (Pfmdr1) gene is responsible for the resistance of *P. falciparum* to amodiaquine, piperaquine and pyronaridine [7].

b. Structural changes in the drug-binding receptors which could be part of an enzyme or enzymes or part of a cascade system-electron transport chain. Mutations in two key enzymes of the parasite"s folate synthesis pathway - Dihydropteroate Synthethase (DHPS) and Dihydrofolate Reductase (DHFR) is responsible for resistance to the antifolates - sulphadoxine, pyrimethamine etc. A single point mutation in the cytochrome b (CYTb) subunit of the bc1 complex confers resistance to atovaquone [7]. Mutations in Kelch-13(K13) Propeller domains are responsible for resistance to the artemisinins and Artemisinin Combination Therapy (ACTs).

3.1 Factors affecting drug resistance development

Having looked at the mechanisms of drug resistance, it is pertinent to also look at the enabling factors which include:

3.1.1 Spontaneous mutations

This occurs as a natural survival strategy of the parasite independent of the presence of the drug, Mutations occur *de novo*. The parasite's genome replication rate,

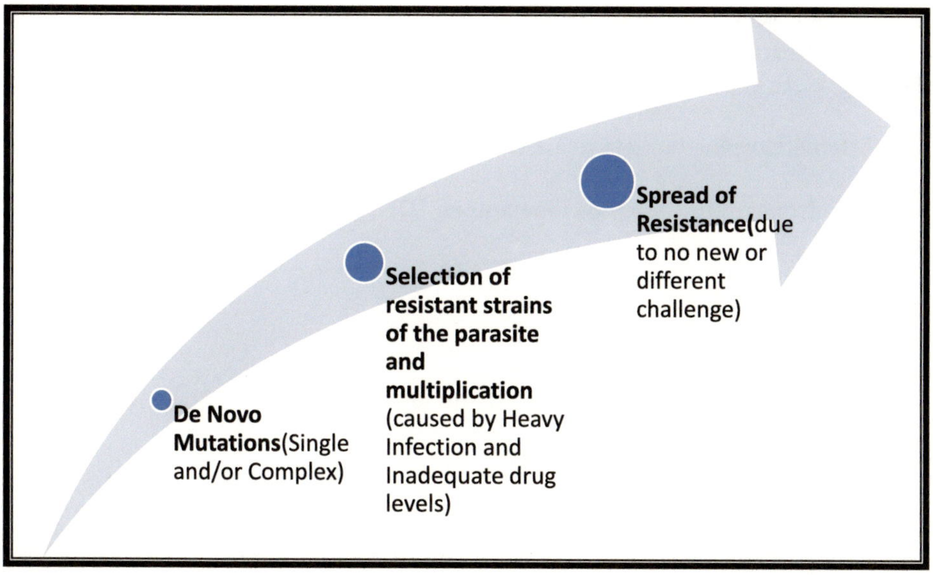

Figure 2.
Showing factors enabling resistance development and spread (adapted from www.malariasite.com with the aid of www.biorender.com).

mutation rate per base pair per parasite generation are the principal determinants of spontaneous mutation [8].

3.1.2 The antimalarial drug pharmacokinetics

The selection of resistant mutants in the presence of the drug as shown in **Figure 2** is principally dependent on its pharmacokinetics (Slowly eliminated drugs with a long tail of sub-lethal dose generally select faster) and magnitude of drug use within the parasite population (the higher the drug pressure per parasite the faster the selection).

4. Measures to tackle antimalarial drug resistance (ADR)

ADR has retired drug classes 1–4 (**Figure 1**) clinically. Currently Drug class 5 (**Figure 1**) faces a big threat of being retired too by ADR. What measures has been taken to checkmate this hydra-headed monster and their limitations?

4.1 Combination therapy

The advent of chloroquine resistance led the World Health Organization (WHO) to approve some combination therapies which included various combinations of Antifolates e.g. Sulphadoxine 500 mg + Pyrimethamine 25 mg (SP), SP + Chloroquine (CQ), SP + Amodiaquine etc. The rationale for combination therapy is combining at least two drugs with different mechanisms of action against the malaria parasite. The aforementioned combination therapies are no longer in use as a result of resistance development to one or both drugs in the combination by the malaria parasite, secondly due to adverse effects of one or both drugs in the combination. With the introduction of Artemisinins as the mainstay for the treatment of uncomplicated *P. falciparum* malaria and the subsequent development of resistance to artemisinin monotherapy, WHO approved Artemisinin-based Combination therapy (ACT) as the first line of treatment for uncomplicated and resistant *P. falciparum* malaria. The following ACTs approved by WHO are currently in clinical use;

a. Artemether plus Lumefantrine (AL)

b. Dihydroxyartemisinin plus Piperaquine (DHA-PPQ)

c. Artesunate plus Amodiaquine (AS-AQ)

d. Artesunate-Pyronaridine (AS-P)

e. Artesunate-Sulphadoxine-pyrimethamine (AS-SP)

f. Artesunate-Mefloquine (AS-MF).

The rationale for ACTs is combining a short-acting artemisinin with a long-acting partner drug whose duration of action provides the much-needed antimalarial cover long after the action of artemisinins has withered. This strategy was meant to overcome the phenomenon of ADR but sadly in 2009, there were reports of a deadly strain of *P. falciparum* (artemisinin-resistant P. *falciparum*) in the Greater Mekong Subregion (GMS) comprising Laos, Cambodia, Vietnam, Thailand, Myanmar and Yunnan Province in Southern China. The magnitude of this resistance threat in the GMS was to the extent of resistance to four out of the five WHO-approved ACTs for use in the region. This led to the setting up of the Regional Artemisinin-resistance Initiative (RAI) by the Global fund to address this emerging global health threat in the GMS in 2013. The outcomes of the RAI strategy in the GMS will be discussed under the section; Recent Advances against ADR.

4.2 Continuous discovery of chemically and mechanistically novel antimalarial agents

The need for unrelenting search for chemically and mechanistically novel antimalarial agents has been underscored by the growing threat of ACT-resistant malaria in the GMS. The past decade has seen an unprecedented renewed focus on the discovery of new antimalarial entities through extraordinary collaboration between academia (parasitologists, medicinal chemists, pharmacologists, clinicians) and industrial/private partnerships e.g. Medicines for Malaria Venture (MMV). The following promising antimalarial drug leads are products of such collaborations and are in the product development (patient exploratory) stages (**Figure 3**).

4.3 Limitations

Despite the above measures taken against ADR, limitations abound and they include development of resistance by *P. falciparum* to ACTs which presents as delayed parasite clearance. The huge cost involved in drug discovery and development projects is a great limitation to the search for novel antimalarial agents with novel mechanism(s) of action [9]. Some of the candidates have not gone beyond Phase II clinical trials because of safety concerns. The ones that crossed Phase II clinical trials do not

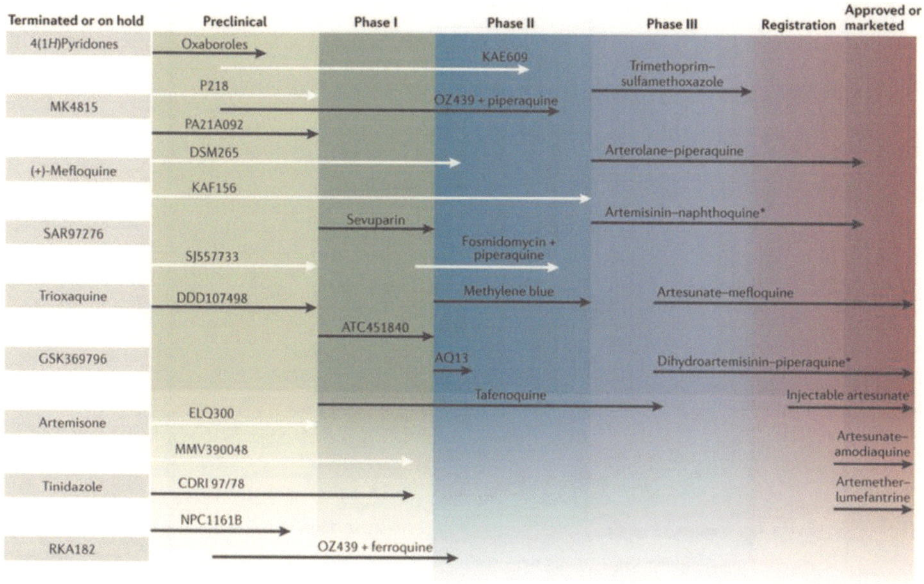

Figure 3.
Showing progression of the clinical development of new antimalarial candidates over the past five years (source: www.researchgate.net, date accessed: 28th June, 2022).

have significant antimalarial action due to resistance development and may exhibit unexplained loss of potency necessitating stoppage of such multi-billion dollar drug discovery and development projects.

5. Recent advances

Advances in the fight against ADR should among other challenges and areas of need address major limitations mentioned above. There has been renewed drive in terms of research to tackle head-on ADR using a multi-pronged approach, this has led to some recent advances which includes but not limited to the following:

5.1 Regional artemisinin-resistance initiative (RAI)

Launched in 2013 by the Global Fund to tackle Artemisinin resistance in the GMS (with the exception of Yunnan province in Southern China) [10] using a multi-pronged approach which included treatment and prophylactic strategies resulted in 88% reduction in indigenous malaria cases and 95% reduction in *P. falciparum* cases [1]. Partly responsible for the success story of malaria control in the GMS is the policy of Drug Rotation-exposure of the malaria parasite to different cycles of ACTs.

5.2 Nanomimics

This era of an emerging global threat (ACT-resistant malaria), an emerging, very promising strategy is the concept of nanomimics, an ingenious strategy developed by Najer et al. [11]. Researchers in Switzerland have successfully designed and tested host cell nanomimics. They developed a single procedure to produce polymer

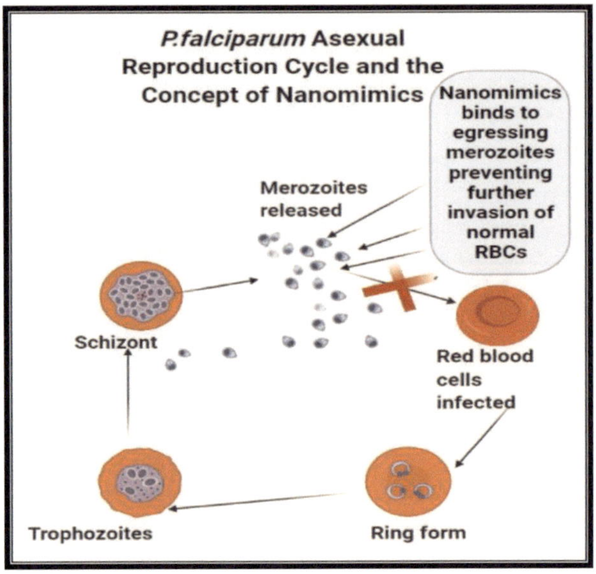

Figure 4.
Polymer-based RBC membrane nanomimics (source: Self-drawn with www.biorender.com).

vesicles-small artificial bubbles with host cell receptors on the surface [11]. The concept of nanomimics is shown in **Figure 4**.

In **Figure 4**, an infected red blood cell undergoes various stages of the life cycle of the malaria parasite, mature schizonts rupture to release merozoites (light-blue) which are bound by nanomimics (nanoscaled polymer vesicles) preventing them from further invading normal red blood cells trapping them within the blood which exposes them to the immune system of the host.

Usually, the malaria parasites destroy their host cell after 48 h and then infect new red blood cells. At this stage they have to bind to specific cell receptors. Nanomimics as a result of their size and composition bind egressing parasites thus blocking the invasion of new cells [11]. The parasites are no longer able to invade cells and are consequently exposed to the host immune system, which kills them. Nanomimics exhibit a dual action; a therapeutic-like and vaccine-like effects. By preventing further invasion of red blood cells, it stops the progression of the disease (therapeutic-like action) and by exposing the bound merozoites to the host immune system for destruction (vaccine-like action) [12]. The intelligence of this strategy is that there is no payload (drug), malaria parasites are not exposed to any payload (exposure is key for resistance development). Non exposure of malaria parasites to drugs using this strategy could bring back exposure-caused, resistance-retired antimalarial drugs like chloroquine, SP, etc. as frontline antimalarial drugs [13]. This strategy is potentially resistance-proof and should be explored for possible translation into products for clinical trials.

5.3 Targeted drug delivery

This is one approach that inhibits resistance development by ensuring that adequate concentration of the antimalarial drug is delivered at the desired site of action ensuring rapid clearance of the parasite. The majority of antimalarial drugs under development are lipophilic with poor plasma solubility and large biodistribution volumes which ultimately results in low accumulation in RBCs [9, 10]. This buttresses the need for targeted drug delivery to deliver optimum concentrations of drug within RBCs.

Targeted drug delivery using antibodies is a promising strategy that could be harnessed to combat resistant malaria. Antibodies have successfully been used to target pRBCs [14]. Antibody-targeted liposomes having on their surface $F(ab)_2$ fragments of mouse monoclonal antibody raised against *P. berghei*-infected mouse erythrocytes significantly increased the therapeutic efficacy of chloroquine implying that target-specific liposomes can cure CQ-resistant malarial infections [15]. A tenfold increase in the therapeutic effect of CQ was observed when delivered in liposomes covalently functionalized with oriented, specific half antibodies against *P. falciparum* late form-infected RBCs [14]. Antibody-functionalized liposomes can discriminate pRBCs from non-infected RBCs specifically delivering antimalarial drugs to pRBCs in sufficient concentration to clear parasitaemia, however their use as targeting molecule in antimalarial therapy is limited by their high cost of production [16], high immunogenicity and the potential decrease in targeting efficiency due to variability in plasmodium protein expressed on the surface of pRBCs [17].

An interesting alternative to antibody-mediated targeted delivery is the use of certain glycosaminoglycans like heparin, heparan sulphate and chondroitin sulphate [18], which are found in the human body and are being recognized as one of the main pRBC-binding molecules [17]. Heparin bound to liposomes has a dual action as a pRBC-targeting molecule acts mainly on trophozoites of some pfEMP1-expressing lines [19] and on schizont stages [20] and as an antimalarial drug (Nanomimic polymer constructs) blocks the merozoites from invading red blood cells [21]. Heparin is cheaper than monoclonal antibodies resulting in heparin-bound liposomes having ten times less cost than immunoliposomes of similar targeting activity [18]. In addition, resistance to heparin as antimalarial drug have not been reported [21]. Heparin when covalently bound to liposomes has substantially reduced anticoagulant activity [18]. Heparin maybe limited in its application as a targeting ligand as a result of its anticoagulant actions but when used at non-anticoagulant concentration, it increased the efficacy of encapsulated primaquine threefold in *in vitro P. falciparum* cultures [18]. Heparin when compared with immunoliposomes for targeted drug delivery is cheaper, has lower or no immunogenicity and may potentiate the effect of the payload when used at non-anticoagulant concentrations. Heparin-related polysaccharides such as heparan sulphate, chondroitin sulphate can be used as targeting moieties, in comparison with heparin have much lower anticoagulant action [18].

5.4 Triple artemisinin-based combination therapy (TACT)

This is a combination of an artemisinin with two partner drugs as against the conventional one partner drug. This strategy is being proposed (in the face of the growing threat of artemisinin-resistant P.falciparum malaria which is causing delayed parasite clearance by ACTs) as a measure to tackle to artemisinin-resistant *P. falciparum* malaria. The result of a multicentre, open-label, randomized clinical trial of triple artemisinin-based combination therapy versus artemisinin-based combination therapy conducted in the GMS showed overall that 42-day Polymerase Chain Reaction (PCR) corrected efficacy of dihydroartemisinin-piperaquine plus mefloquine (97%; 95% CI 93–99) was higher than for dihydroartemisinin-piperaquine

(60%; 52–67) with a risk difference of 37%, 29–45; $p<0.0001$ [22]. There was no difference in efficacy between Artemether-Lumefantrine plus amodiaquine and Artemether-Lumefantrine-treated groups suggesting no relative advantage of having a triple combination of Artemether-Lumefantrine in treating resistant P.falciparum malaria [22]. Parasite half-lives in patients with Pfkelch 13 C580Y mutated infections were shorter in those treated with dihydroartemisinin-piperaquine plus mefloquine [mean = 6.93, SD = 1.77] than those treated with dihydroartemisinin-piperaquine [7.39 h (1.46); $p = 0.019$] [22]. This suggests albeit strongly that dihydroartemisinin-piperaquine plus mefloquine as a promising TACT candidate against artemisinin-resistant *P. falciparum* malaria. Extensive clinical trials involving TACTs has to be done to really establish and justify a possible switch from ACTs to TACTs.

5.5 Drug development

There are promising drug candidates which are at various product development stages in researches conducted by some of the global pharmaceutical companies and some Research Institutions (Universities) or partnerships between the two resulting in drugs licensed for use with market authorization (refer to **Table 1**). The drug tafenoquine was recently licensed for radical cure of *P. vivax* malaria [23]. Medicines for Malaria Ventures (MMV) is at the forefront n novel drug discovery and development research.

6. Future perspectives

The way of the future is that of malaria eradication. The strategy to drive this should be anchored on the development of novel, smart, resistance-proof, antimalarial nanoformulations that with a single exposure lead to cure and prophylaxis (transmission-blocking ability). To this end, the application of nanotechnology in combating drug resistance in plasmodium species holds a lot of promises. Future strategies should target delivering antimalarial drugs via non-receptor-mediated pathways which are not under the genetic control of the parasite [24]. To this end, liposomal delivery holds a lot in stock since liposomes deliver drugs to their intracellular targets by fusing with the parasite's cell membrane. This technique can be used to deliver drugs whose resistance mechanisms are receptor-mediated e.g. chloroquine [25]. The parasite is less likely to modify the chemical composition of its cell membrane as that may affect its survival in terms of nutrient acquisition from its host. Future research should target what would be called a "Starving Strategy" whereby the parasite is starved of its nutrient supply from the red blood cell by developing Plasmodium surface anion channel blockers whose channel-blocking ability is by nanoadhesion - a phenomenon where nanocarriers block the nutrient pore channels by forming strong bonds with the negatively charged nutrient channels.

Nanomimics development and optimization is another smart move in beating the resistance trap of the parasite and should be explored [12]. Nanocarriers such as dendrimers present diverse opportunities of formulating combination drug products with novel mechanism of action that with a single exposure may possibly eradicate the parasite. Discovery and development of host-derived factors with therapeutic activity against the parasite are possible research options that will eradicate the parasite since the host-derived factors are not under the genetic control of the parasite.

Research		Translational		Product development			Access
Lead Optimization	**Candidate Profiling** →	**Preclinical**	**Human Volunteers** →	**Patient Exploratory**	**Patient Confirmatory**	**Regulatory Review** →	**Approved/ERP**
Phenotypic Lead Mitsubishi Tanabe	**MMV072** Eisai	**MMV371** Janssen	**Atoguanil** Ipca	**Ganaplacide-Lumefantrine** Novartis	**Dihydroartemisinin-piperaquine dispersible** Alfasigma	**Sulphadoxine-Pyrimethamine** Universal Corporation	**Artemether-Lumefantrine dispersible** Novartis
Pf Carl series Calibr		**MMV183** TropIQ	**MMV533** Sanofi	**Cipargamin** Novartis	**Artemether-Lumefantrine < 5 kg** Novartis	**Sulphadoxine-Pyrimethamine** Swipha/Biogaran	**Artesunate for Injection** Fosun Pharma
GWT 1 Eisai		**GSK 701** GSK	**INE963** Novartis	**ZY19489+ ferroquine** Zydus	**Sulphadoxine-Pyrimethamine** Emzor Pharmaceutical		**Artesunate for Injection** Ipca
Molecular Target DDU Dundee		**MMV609** Univ. of Kentucky		**M5717 + Pyronaridine** Merck KGaA/Shin Poong	**Primaquine dispersible** B & O Pharm.		**Dihydroartemisinin-Piperaquine** Alfasigma
Azabenzimidazole UNICAMP		**GSK 484** GSK			**Artemether-Lumefantrine-Amodiaquine FDC** Tridem/MORU		**Pyronaridine-artesunate** Shi Poong
Mini portfolio Novartis		**IWY 357** Novartis					**Pyronaridine-artesunate granules** Shi Poong
4-aminoquinoline LSTM and University of Liverpool							**Artesunate-Amodiaquine** Sanofi
Molecular target UCB							**Artesunate-Mefloquine** Cipla

Research		Translational		Product development			Access
Lead Optimization	**Candidate Profiling →**	**Preclinical**	**Human Volunteers →**	**Patient Exploratory**	**Patient Confirmatory**	**Regulatory Review →**	**Approved/ERP**
DHODH Broad							**Suphadoxine-Pyrimethamine + Amodiaquine dispersible** Fosun Pharma
DHODH UTSW/UW/ Monash							**Sulphadoxine-Pyrimethamine + Amodiaquine dispersible** S Kant
Phenotypic Lead Merck KGaA-UCT							**Artesunate rectal capsules** Cipla
Whole Cell Actives H3D							**Artesunate rectal capsules** Strides Pharma
Irresistibles GHDD1							**Tafenoquine** GSK
YRS Takeda							**Tafenoquine Pediatric** GSK
ATP 4 Series Drexel							

Table 1.
Showing drug candidates in clinical development and their progression, accessed from www.mmv.org/research-development/mmv-supported-projects, date accessed: 29th June, 2022.

In all, nano-smart delivery of antimalarial drugs is the key to tackling and preventing resistance development in plasmodium species bringing global efforts steps closer to the actualization of the WHO ideal goal of malaria eradication by 2030.

7. Conclusion

This chapter introduced malaria and Antimalarial Drug Resistance (ADR), its impact on global health, therapeutic interventions and their resistance by the malaria parasite. The mechanisms of resistance development by the parasite and factors causing it were discussed in detail. Armed with the knowledge of the foregoing, measures including nanotechnological approaches to combat the resistance trap of the parasite and their limitations were looked at and also the future perspectives in the fight against drug resistance by *P. falciparum.* It is envisaged that application of nanotechnology tools to develop antimalarial nanomedicines would help bring back antimalarial drugs that have been retired because of resistance of malaria parasites to these drugs and possibly lead to the development of novel, smart, resistance-proof formulations that will eliminate and possibly eradicate malaria globally.

Conflict of interest

The Authors declare no conflict of interest.

Nomenclature

ACT	Artemisinin-based Combination Therapy
CRT	Chloroquine Resistance Transporter
WHO	World Health Organization
TACT	Triple Artemisinin-based Combination Therapy

Author details

Samuel Uzondu*, Adaeze Echezona, Chinekwu Nwagwu, Adaeze Onugwu, Lydia Ugorji, Chinazom Agbo, Franklin Kenechukwu, John Ogbonna, Paul Akpa, Petra Nnamani, Audu Momoh and Anthony Attama
NanoMalaria Research Unit, Drug Delivery and Nanomedicines Research Laboratory, Department of Pharmaceutics, Faculty of Pharmaceutical Sciences, University of Nigeria, Nsukka, Nigeria

*Address all correspondence to: samuel.uzondu@unn.edu.ng

References

[1] WHO. Word Malaria Report 2021. 2021. pp. 2013-2015

[2] Baindara P. Mechanism of bacterial co-resistance. Singapore: Springer; 2019. pp. 191-210. DOI: 10.1007/978-981-13-8503-2_10

[3] Conrad M, Rosenthal P. Antimalarial drug resistance in Africa: The calm before the storm? The Lancet Infectious Diseases. 2019. DOI: 10.1016/S1473-3099(19)30261-0

[4] Uwimana A, Legrand E, Stokes B, et al. Emergence and clonal expansion of in vitro artemisinin-resistant plasmodium falciparum kelch13 R561H mutant parasites in Rwanda. Nature Medicine. 2020; **26**(10):1602-1608. DOI: 10.1038/s41591-020-1005-2

[5] Simam J, Rono M, Ngoi J, et al. Gene copy number variation in natural populations of Plasmodium falciparum in Eastern Africa. BMC Genomics. 2018;**19**(1). DOI: 10.1186/s12864-018-4689-7

[6] White L, Flegg J, Phyo A, et al. Defining the In Vivo Phenotype of Artemisinin-Resistant Falciparum Malaria: A Modelling Approach. PLoS Medicine. 2015;**12**(4). DOI: 10.1371/journal.pmed.1001823

[7] Blasco B, Leroy D, Fidock DA. Antimalarial drug resistance: Linking plasmodium falciparum parasite biology to the clinic. Nature Medicine. 2017. DOI: 10.1038/nm.4381

[8] Ross LS, Fidock DA. Elucidating mechanisms of drug-resistant plasmodium falciparum. Cell Host & Microbe. 2019;**26**(1):35-47. DOI: 10.1016/j.chom.2019.06.001

[9] Medicines for Malaria Venture. MMV-supported projects. Geneva, Switzerland: MMV; 2018

[10] The Global Fund. Focus on Regional Artemisinin-resistance Initiative (RAI) Eliminating Malaria in the Mekong

[11] Najer A, Wu D, Bieri A, et al. Nanomimics of host cell membranes block invasion and expose invasive malaria parasites. ACS Nano. 2014;**8**(12): 12560-12571. DOI: 10.1021/nn5054206

[12] Najer A, Thamboo S, Duskey JT, et al. Analysis of molecular parameters determining the antimalarial activity of polymer-based Nanomimics. Macromolecular Rapid Communications. 2015;**36**(21):1923-1928. DOI: 10.1002/marc.201500267

[13] Amato R, Lim P, Miotto O, et al. Genetic markers associated with dihydroartemisinin–piperaquine failure in plasmodium falciparum malaria in Cambodia: A genotype–phenotype association study. The Lancet Infectious Diseases. 2017;**17**(2):164-173. DOI: 10.1016/S1473-3099(16)30409-1

[14] Urbán P, Estelrich J, Cortés A, Fernàndez-Busquets X. A nanovector with complete discrimination for targeted delivery to plasmodium falciparum-infected versus non-infected red blood cells in vitro. Journal of Controlled Release. 2011;**151**(2):202-211. DOI: 10.1016/j.jconrel.2011.01.001

[15] Owais M, Varshney GC, Choudhury A, Chandra S, Gupta CM. Chloroquine encapsulated in malaria-infected erythrocyte-specific antibody-bearing liposomes effectively controls chloroquine-resistant plasmodium berghei infections in mice. Antimicrobial

Agents and Chemotherapy. 1995;**39**(1): 180-184. DOI: 10.1128/aac.39.1.180

[16] Agrahari V, Mitra AK. Therapeutic delivery. Therapeutic Delivery. 2016; **7**(2):117-138

[17] Marques J et al. Application of heparin as a dual agent with antimalarial and liposome targeting activities toward plasmodium-infected red blood cells. Nanomedicine Nanotechnology, Biology Medicine. 2014;**10**(8):1719-1728. DOI: 10.1016/j.nano.2014.06.002

[18] Marques J et al. Adaptation of targeted nanocarriers to changing requirements in antimalarial drug delivery. Nanomedicine Nanotechnology, Biology Medicine. 2017;**13**(2):515-525. DOI: 10.1016/j.nano.2016.09.010

[19] Barragan A, Spillmann D, Kremsner PG, Wahlgren M, Carlson J. Plasmodium falciparum: Molecular background to strain-specific rosette disruption by glycosaminoglycans and sulfated glycoconjugates. Experimental Parasitology. 1999;**91**(2):133-143. DOI: 10.1006/expr.1998.4349

[20] Glushakova S et al. Exploitation of a newly-identified entry pathway into the malaria parasite-infected erythrocyte to inhibit parasite egress. Scientific Reports. 2017;**7**(1):1-13. DOI: 10.1038/s41598-017-12258-x

[21] Boyle MJ, Richards JS, Gilson PR, Chai W, Beeson JG. Interactions with heparin-like molecules during erythrocyte invasion by plasmodium falciparum merozoites. Blood. 2010; **115**(22):4559-4568. DOI: 10.1182/blood-2009-09-243725

[22] van der Pluijm RW et al. Triple artemisinin-based combination therapies versus artemisinin-based combination therapies for uncomplicated plasmodium falciparum malaria: A multicentre, open-label, randomised clinical trial. Lancet. 2020;**395**(10233):1345-1360. DOI: 10.1016/S0140-6736(20)30552-3

[23] Tse EG, Korsik M, Todd MH. The past, present and future of anti-malarial medicines. Malaria Journal. 2019;**18**(1): 1-21. DOI: 10.1186/s12936-019-2724-z

[24] Wicht KJ, Mok S, Fidock D. Molecular mechanisms of drug resistance in plasmodium falciparum malaria. Annual Review of Microbiology. 2020. DOI: 10.1146/annurev-micro-020518-115546

[25] Deye N, Vincent F, Michel P, Ehrmann S, Da Silva D, Piagnerelli M, et al. (2016). Changes in cardiac arrest patientsâ€TM temperature management after the 2013 â€œTTMâ€ trial: Results from an international survey. Annals of Intensive et al.Polymer and lipid based drug delivery strategies for malaria treatment. Tropical Medicine & International Health. 2015;**6**(1):149-149. DOI: 10.1186/s13613-015-0104-6

Chapter 11

Purine and Pyrimidine Pathways as Antimalarial Targets

Yacoba V.T. Minnow and Vern L. Schramm

Abstract

Malaria continues to plague the endemic regions of sub-Saharan Africa and Southeast Asia. With the current development of artemisinin resistance and a risk of failure of the current first line therapies, there is a growing need for novel antimalarials. Purine and pyrimidine metabolism in *Plasmodium* is distinctly different from the human host, making these pathways valid targets for the development of novel antimalarials. Targeting key enzymes in these pathways with transition state analogs has provided high affinity inhibitors. Transition state mimicry can also provide selectivity for the parasite enzymes over the homologous enzymes of the human host. Resistance of *Plasmodium* parasites to current antimalarials will be compared to resistance development induced by transition state analogs inhibitors, a feature that may contribute to decreased resistance development. Tight binding and specificity of transition state analog inhibitors provide important features for novel antimalaria therapy with low toxicity and prevention of antibiotic resistance.

Keywords: purine salvage, pyrimidines, antimalarials, transition state analog inhibitors, resistance

1. Introduction

Malaria remains the leading cause of mortality in the endemic regions of Sub-Saharan Africa and Southeast Asia. The WHO estimates that in 2020, there were 241 million malaria cases globally with 627,000 associated deaths, an increase from years prior [1, 2]. Additionally, although progress continues to be made in some regions, such as Southeast Asia reporting a 78% reduction in malaria cases, Sub-Saharan Africa accounts for more than 90% of the global malaria incidence. Children 5 years and younger are highly susceptible to malaria with a 77% mortality rate [1, 3, 4].

Malaria is caused by the apicomplexan parasite, *Plasmodium sp*. The five main species able to cause disease in humans are *Plasmodium falciparum, Plasmodium vivax, Plasmodium ovale, Plasmodium knowlesi* and *Plasmodium malariae. Plasmodium falciparum (P. falciparum)* is the most prevalent and the most lethal of these [5]. Malaria infection is established when an infected female anopheles mosquito takes a blood meal from humans and introduces sporozoites into the bloodstream which invade human liver hepatocytes. The sporozoites replicate in the hepatocytes for 5–8 days and can generate thousands of merozoites which are released to infect the erythrocytes [6, 7]. Asexual replication occurs in the erythrocytes where parasites undergo several nuclear divisions and generate between 6 and 30 daughter merozoites per infected erythrocyte [6]. Symptomatic malaria is characterized by the sustained parasitization and destruction of red blood cells as well as the host immune responses. Thus, drug development efforts are directed toward the intra-erythrocytic asexual stage of the parasite.

Over the centuries-long battle with malaria, treatment has been developed from both natural product and chemical synthetic sources. Quinine, originally isolated from the bark of the cinchona tree, gave way to its synthetic counterparts, chloroquine, amodiaquine, and mefloquine, among others [8, 9]. Likewise, artemisinin was isolated from the Chinese herb, *Artemisia annua* (Qinghao), and gave way to the synthetic artemisinin derivatives now used in the first line malaria treatment, artemisinin-based combination therapy (ACT) [10]. However, resistance to these antimalaria treatments, have slowed global efforts toward the eradication of malaria [11–15]. Resistance development has led to increased efforts to identify novel antimalarials, including the recent development of the RTS,S malaria vaccine, providing a potential positive outlook for malaria control [16, 17]. New drug development efforts for malaria must identify novel targets, their mechanisms of action, and must be well tolerated with minimal side effects. Short treatment periods are essential to promote compliance and to minimize resistance development.

Transition state mimicry is a promising approach to malaria drug discovery. The technique utilizes features of transition state structure of essential target enzymes to produce tight binding and highly selective analogs [18]. Transition state analogs (TSAs) against the purine and pyrimidine pathway enzymes of *P. falciparum* have resulted in inhibitor molecules with the potential for new antimalarial combination therapies.

Rapid nucleic acid synthesis during intra-erythrocytic parasitic growth makes purine and pyrimidine synthesis in *Plasmodium* parasites an important target for novel drug development. Although both host and parasite share some enzymes in these pathways, key differences allow for *Plasmodium*-specific and selective molecules.

2. Purine metabolism

Plasmodium parasites are purine auxotrophs as they do not express the enzymes necessary to perform *de novo* purine synthesis [19, 20]. Substantial new DNA and RNA synthesis occurs during the asexual cycle of *Plasmodium*, requiring large amounts of purine and pyrimidine nucleotide precursors and the energetic contribution from ATP. Parasites therefore rely completely on the host erythrocytes for the salvage of purine nucleosides and nucleobases for the synthesis of adenylate and guanylate compounds. Hence the parasite genome contains highly expressed genes corresponding to purine transporters and purine salvage enzymes [21]. Human erythrocytes contain high (millimolar) concentrations of adenylate nucleotides, but *Plasmodium* parasites have no kinase to phosphorylate adenosine molecules or ribosyltransferases to salvage adenine from the host. Therefore, purine salvage in *Plasmodium* requires ATP catabolism, through hypoxanthine formation, by essential enzymes making up the purine salvage pathway (**Figure 1**) [22]. The central concept in targeting purine salvage pathways for *Plasmodium* involves prevention of hypoxanthine and inosine formation in both erythrocytes and parasites and/or prevention of hypoxanthine or inosine conversion to purine nucleotides in the parasites.

Purine precursors formed in erythrocytes must gain entry to the parasite for conversion to nucleotides. Pathways proposed to facilitate the uptake of purine

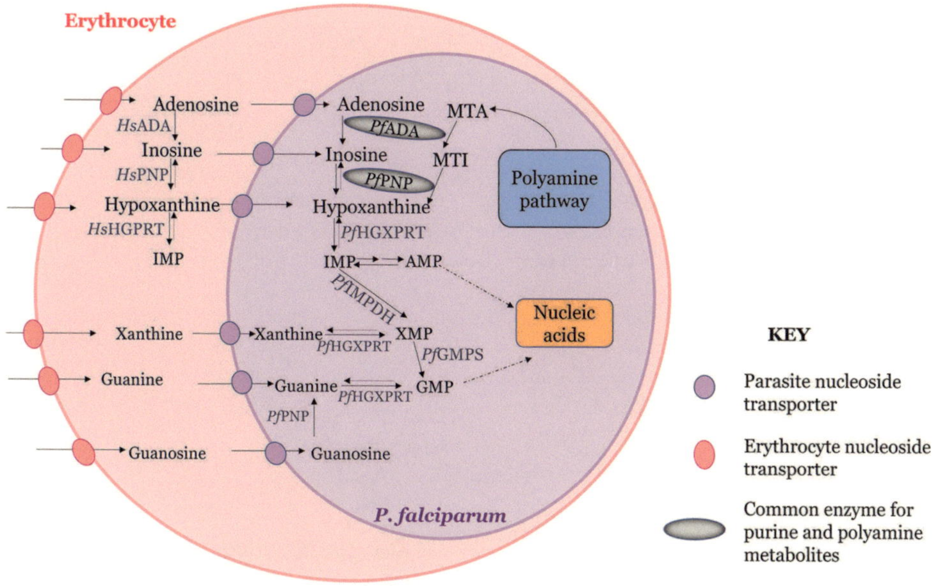

Figure 1.
Purine salvage pathway in P. falciparum and human erythrocytes. In P. falciparum, but not in humans, there is a link to the polyamine pathway via MTA.

nucleosides and nucleobases across the parasite membrane include; (1) saturable or facilitated transport of adenosine, (2) non-saturable, channel like transport and (3) the tubovesicular membranes induced by parasitization of the host erythrocytes [23, 24]. A major path for purine uptake is known to be the equilibrative nucleoside transporters (ENTs) that promote nucleoside and nucleobase transport into the parasite. Four classes of ENTs have been identified in *Plasmodium falciparum* and *Plasmodium vivax* (*Pf*ENT 1-4, *Pv*ENT 1-4) [24–28]. Inhibitors designed against *Pf*ENT1 prevent the uptake of purines and inhibit the growth of parasites in culture [29, 30]. The essentiality of the purine salvage pathway to the survival of *Plasmodium* parasites, makes targeting the component enzymes attractive for novel antimalarial therapies. These include adenosine deaminase (ADA), purine nucleoside phosphorylase (PNP) and hypoxanthine-guanine-xanthine phosphoribosyltransferase (HGXPRT). Antimalarial validation of these targets has been confirmed by potent inhibitors that cause purine starvation and death of the parasites.

2.1 Adenosine deaminase (ADA, EC 3.5.4.4)

Plasmodium falciparum ADA (*Pf*ADA) catalyzes the zinc-dependent irreversible deamination of adenosine and deoxyadenosine to form inosine and deoxyinosine. *Pf*ADA can also catalyze the hydrolysis of 5′-methylthioadenosine (MTA) to 5′-methylthioinosine (MTI), a reaction that is distinctly absent from the mammalian ADA [31]. MTA is a product of the polyamine biosynthetic pathway, establishing that polyamine synthesis also plays a role in the purine salvage pathways for *Plasmodium* parasites. Parasites must metabolize MTA to prevent feedback inhibition of the polyamine biosynthetic pathway. Polyamine synthesis is also critical to the parasites since they cannot salvage polyamines from the host erythrocytes [see below]. Coformycin and 2′-deoxycoformycin are transition state or intermediate-like powerful inhibitors

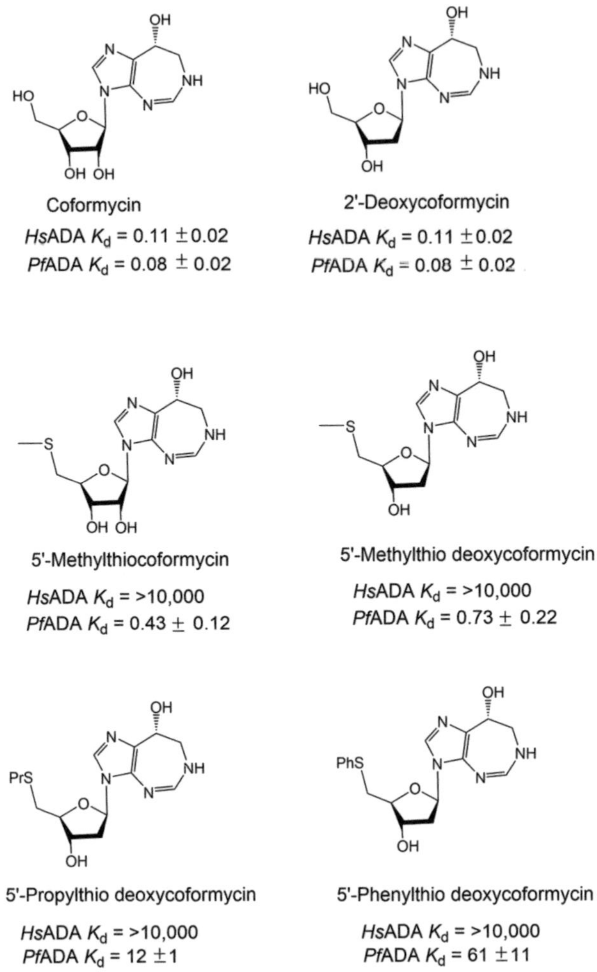

Figure 2.
Transition state analogs of HsADA and PfADA. The 5′-functionalized inhibitors provide improved selectivity for the parasite enzyme over the human enzyme. 5′-methylthio inhibitors are more potent thant the 5′-propylthio and 5′-phenylthio inhibitors.

of ADA. They were originally identified as natural products and inhibit both human and parasite enzymes with picomolar affinities (**Figure 2**) [32]. 2′-Deoxycoformycin (Pentostatin) is an FDA-approved treatment for hairy cell leukemia, where the accumulation of adenosine or 2′-deoxyadenosine, leads to an unbalanced nucleotide pool, initiating apoptosis in B and T cells [32]. Unfortunately, there is insignificant inhibition of *Plasmodium* parasite growth by these inhibitors.

The dual specificity of *Pf*ADAs serves to guide the synthesis of novel *Pf*ADA inhibitors with a high degree of selectivity for the parasite enzyme. In addition, the transition state structures of *Pf*ADA and human ADA (*Hs*ADA) are similar but distinct, with *Pf*ADA displaying an early transition state and a more intermediate-like transition state for *Hs*ADA, corresponding to their distinct catalytic turnover numbers (k_{cat}) (**Figure 3**). These differences are reflected by the state of protonation at N1 of the purine ring and the N1-H bond distances. The differences permit the design and synthesis of *Plasmodium*-specific transition state analogs [33]. Earlier work

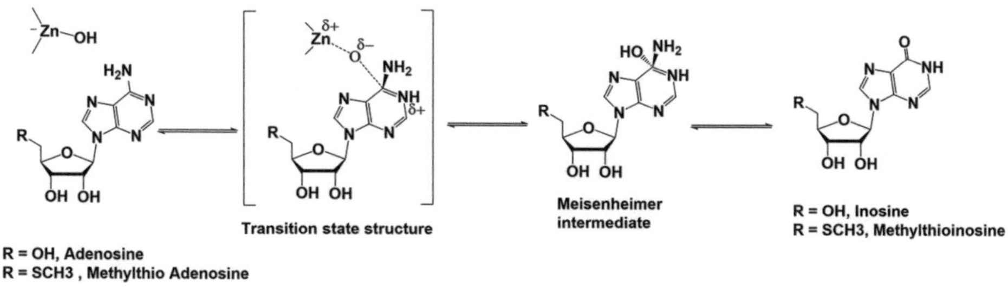

Figure 3.
Reaction scheme and transition state structure of ADA.

reported the synthesis of 5′-methythiolcoformycin (MT-coformycin), a sub nanomolar (K_i^* = 0.43 nM) transition state analog inhibitor of *plasmodium* ADA with over a 20,000-fold selectivity over the human ADA. Other functionalized 5′- and 2′-deoxy-coformycin molecules also retained selectivity for the *Plasmodium* enzyme (**Figure 2**) [31, 32]. MT-coformycin and coformycin inhibited the growth of *plasmodium* parasites in culture when MTA is used as the sole purine source, clearly demonstrating the deaminase as an essential step in conversion of MTA toward hypoxanthine [31, 34]. This effect is not observed when adenosine or MTI is used as a purine source, demonstrating that an intact polyamine pathway is not required for purine salvage in *Plasmodium* species. The high degree of selectivity of the 5′-functionalized coformycins demonstrates the importance of utilizing substrate specificity and transition state analysis to design target-selective inhibitors.

2.2 Purine nucleoside phosphorylase (PNP, EC 2.4.2.1)

The enzyme responsible for forming purine bases from nucleosides in the purine salvage pathway is PNP, catalyzing the reversible phosphorolysis of inosine to hypoxanthine and ribose 1-phosphate [35]. *Plasmodium* PNP substrate specificity includes MTI, to generate hypoxanthine and 5-methylthioribose 1-phosphate [36]. MTI appears to be a parasite specific metabolite and has not been identified in mammalian pathways [37]. Hypoxanthine serves as a key precursor to nucleotide synthesis; therefore, the parasite adopts multiple pathways to generate hypoxanthine. PNP also converts guanosine and 2′-deoxyguanosine to form guanine and (2-deoxy) ribose 1-phosphate (**Figure 1**). PNP displays specificity for 6-oxopurines with adenine containing purine rings having no effect as substrates or inhibitors [31].

Plasmodium falciparum PNP (*Pf*PNP) and human PNP (*Hs*PNP) have distinct structures and catalytic sites and share only ~20% sequence similarity [38]. Structurally, *Pf*PNP is more similar to PNP from bacterial sources and is homohexameric, displaying a trimer of dimer structure, while *Hs*PNP like other mammalian PNP is trimeric (**Figure 4**). Like *Pf*ADA, *Pf*PNP displays a broad substrate specificity that includes 6-oxopurine nucleosides and 5′-methylthio 6-oxopurine nucleosides as substrates. These differences form the basis for generation of species-specific inhibitors with discrimination for the *Plasmodium* enzyme.

The transition state structures of *Pf*PNP and *Hs*PNP, reveal similar catalytic mechanisms involving the formation of an oxocarbenium ion at the transition state (**Figure 5**). However, the two catalytic site interactions differ in the hydrogen bond and van der Waals interactions formed with the leaving group. The result is a more constrained active site environment at the transition state for *Pf*PNP than for *Hs*PNP [39]. The

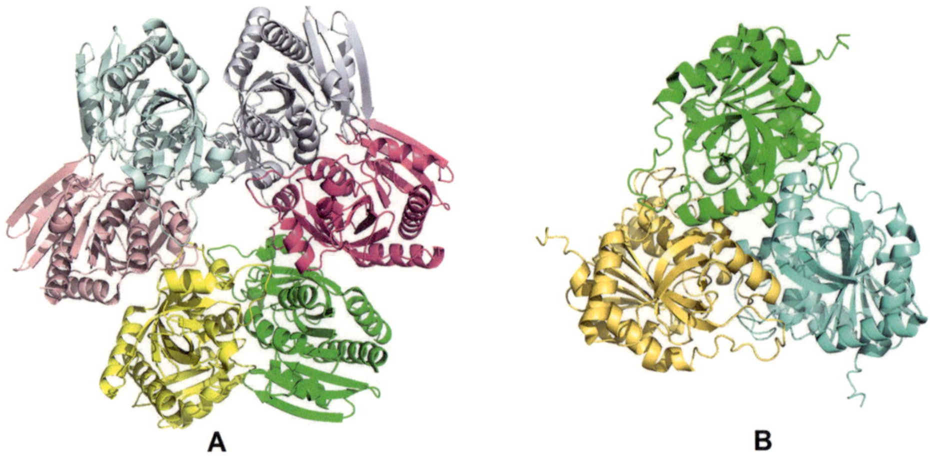

Figure 4.
A, Homohexameric structure of PfPNP displaying a trimer of dimer conformation (1NW4). B, trimeric structure of HsPNP (1PF7).

Immucillin-H (ImmH) transition state analog was designed to resemble the transition state structure of bovine PNP and inhibits that enzyme with a K_i^* of 23 pM. Although there are distinct differences between the transition state structures of *Hs*PNP, *Pf*PNP and bovine PNP, ImmH is a potent inhibitor of all three enzymes, with *Hs*PNP K_i^* = 56 pM and *Pf*PNP K_i^* = 600 pM [40, 41]. DADMe-ImmH and DADMe-ImmG were developed as second generation PNP inhibitors designed to mimic the fully dissociative transition state, and thereby more closely resemble the transition state structures of *Hs*PNP and *Pf*PNP [42]. The introduction of a methylene bridge increases the bond distance between the 9-deazahypoxanthine (DADMe-ImmH) or the 9-deazaguanine (DADMe-ImmG) and the riboxocarbenium mimic. Additionally, the 9-deazapurine scaffold increases the pK_a to permit protonation at N7 and the cation at N1′ mimics the cationic charge at this position of the transition state to more closely mimic the transition state. These features of the transition state translate to an improvement in the dissociation constant for *Hs*PNP from 56 pM for ImmH to 16 pM for DADMe-ImmH and to 2 pM for DADMe-ImmG. Transition state analogs bind tightly to their cognate enzymes by converting the catalytic potential into thermodynamic binding. The k_{cat} for *Hs*PNP is approximately 50 times greater than for *Pf*PNP, and this is reflected in the affinity of the inhibitors for the two enzyme species. Thus, the dissociation constant (K_i^*, the K_d after slow onset inhibition) for *Pf*PNP is 500 pM for DADMe-ImmH and is 670 pM for DADMe-ImmG, reflecting its lower catalytic potential [42–44].

Inhibition of both *Hs*PNP and *Pf*PNP is required to cause a purine-less death of *Plasmodium falciparum* parasites in culture, as formation of hypoxanthine in erythrocytes or in the parasite will meet the needs for purine base salvage. In cell cultures, *Hs*PNP inhibition occurs at low concentrations of PNP inhibitors with inhibition of *Pf*PNP occurring at higher concentrations. Inhibition of both PNPs is thus required for the antiparasitic effects of the immucillins, with the IC_{50} values corresponding to the molar concentration of PNP present [45, 46]. The purine-less death induced by PNP inhibitors targets hypoxanthine production. Confirmation of hypoxanthine starvation as the mechanism of action, and the lack of other targets from this therapy, comes from the full restoration of parasite growth when hypoxanthine is added to culture media [45].

The genetic deficiency of *Hs*PNP is known to cause a T cell immune deficiency by causing accumulation of 2′-deoxyguanosine (dGuo), a metabolite completely dependent on *Hs*PNP for its recycling. Without *Hs*PNP, activated T cells transport dGuo and convert it to dGTP which can reach toxic levels for DNA polymerase. In humans, activated T cells are therefore sensitive to the loss of *Hs*PNP function with no effect observed in naive T cells, B cells, and other mammalian cells [47, 48]. The selective toxic effects of *Hs*PNP inhibition in human T cells is slow to develop, taking a year or more to be symptomatic in newborns. The more rapid effect in *Plasmodium* suggests that inhibiting both human and parasite PNPs for antimalaria therapy will have minimal side effects. Furthermore, oral administration of DADMe-ImmG clears *Plasmodium falciparum* parasites from infected *Aotus* monkeys [49]. Although not yet tested in clinical trials for malaria, the companion compound, DADMe-ImmH, is also a powerful inhibitor of both *Hs*- and *Pf*PNPs and has been in extensive phase 2 clinical trials for gout [50]. PNP inhibitors as an antimalarial therapy block hypoxanthine formation in both erythrocytes and parasites. Human blood hypoxanthine is present at approximately 1 μM, while *Aotus* blood was found to have approximately 40 μM hypoxanthine [49]. Therefore, PNP inhibition as an antimalarial therapy is expected to be a more effective in humans than in the *Aotus* test animal where several days of oral drug therapy were required to clear the parasites [49]. This hypothesis remains to be tested.

Other selective inhibitors remain an attractive option when developing novel antimalarial therapeutics. Therefore, using the dual specificity of *Pf*PNP for MTI, the transition state analog, 5′-methylthio-immucillin-H (MT-ImmH) was synthesized [46]. MT-ImmH has a 100-fold specificity for *Pf*PNP over *Hs*PNP, underscoring the importance of exploring transition state chemistry and substrate specificity to develop selective inhibitors (**Figure 5**) [46].

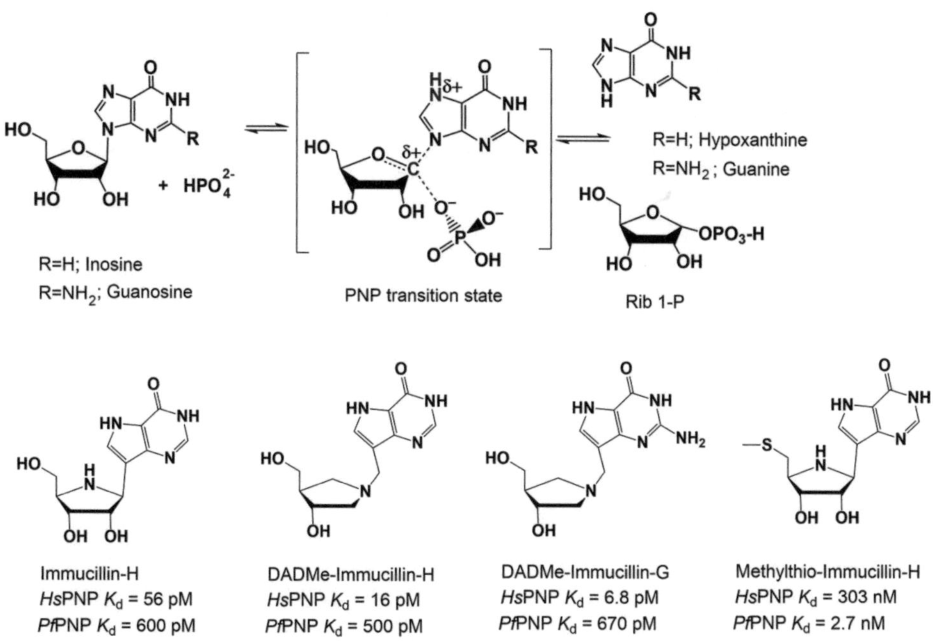

Figure 5.
Reaction scheme and transition state structure of PNP (upper panel). Lower panel; transition state analogs of PNP with dissociation constants for HsPNP and PfPNP. Methylthio-Immucillin-H provides over 100-fold selectivity for the parasite enzyme.

2.3 Hypoxanthine-guanine-xanthine phosphoribosyltransferase (HGXPRT, EC 2.4.2.8, EC 2.4.2.22)

Hypoxanthine is the essential purine precursor for *Plasmodium* and HGXPRT is an essential enzyme in the *Plasmodium* purine salvage pathway, as the only enzyme to incorporate hypoxanthine into the parasite nucleotide pool. HGXPRT catalyzes the phosphoribosylation of hypoxanthine, guanine, and xanthine using 5-phosphoribosyl-α-D-1-pyrophosphate (PRPP) to generate inosine 5′-monophosphate (IMP), guanosine 5′-monophosphate (GMP) and xanthine 5′-monophosphate (XMP) respectively [51]. Pyrophosphate (PPi) is generated as the second product of the reaction (**Figure 6**). IMP serves as the precursor for the synthesis of both adenine and guanine-based nucleotides. The single distinction in substrate specificity between the *Plasmodium* HGXPRT (*Pf*HGPRT) and the human HGPRT (*Hs*HGPRT) is the inability of the human homolog to use xanthine as a substrate [52]. Xanthine in humans is converted to uric acid by xanthine oxidase and is the terminal end of purine metabolism, followed by its excretion into the urine [53, 54].

*Pf*HGXPRT has been identified as the most highly expressed purine salvage enzyme in *P. falciparum* and has been reported to have the highest activity compared to other enzymes of purine salvage identified by Reyes and coworkers [55]. Parasites may have evolved to use hypoxanthine as a key nucleotide precursor because it is the end-product of purine catabolism in human erythrocytes, with subsequent oxidation to uric acid occurring in other tissues. The high amounts of intracellular phosphates in erythrocytes favors the activity of PNP to produce hypoxanthine [55, 56]. Since its identification, *Pf*HGXPRT has been the most targeted enzyme for purine salvage in *P. falciparum*. Detailed kinetic and structural analyses have led to the design of many inhibitors of *Pf*HGXPRT activity. Challenges in targeting *Pf*HGXPRT include its similarities to *Hs*HGPRT and the need for the anionic phosphate group, making cell access a problem [57–60].

*Pf*HGXPRT and *Hs*HGPRT share 76% sequence similarity and 44% sequence identity [61]. Active site residues in contact with substrates and inhibitors are conserved (**Figure 7**). Purine nucleoside analogs and transition state analogs have been investigated and many prove to be good inhibitors of both *Pf*HGXPRT and *Hs*HGPRT.

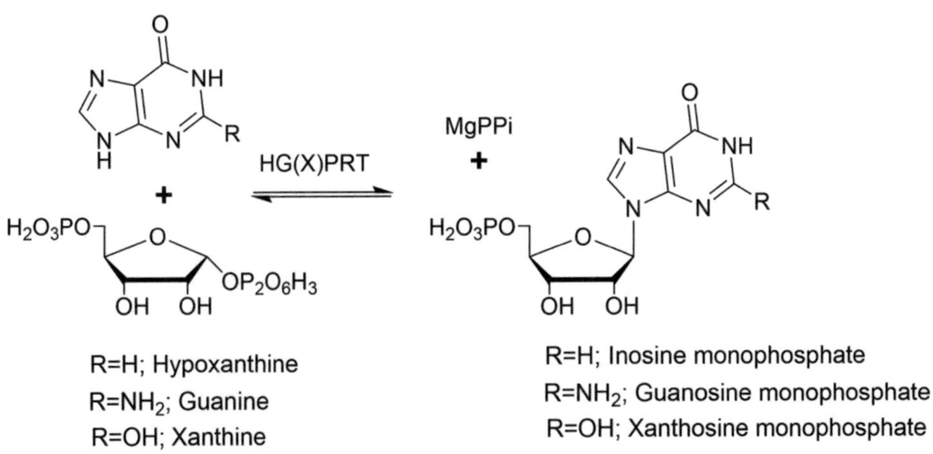

Figure 6.
Reaction scheme for HG(X)PRT. PfHGXPRT has a unique substrate specificity for xanthine. HsHGPRT does not.

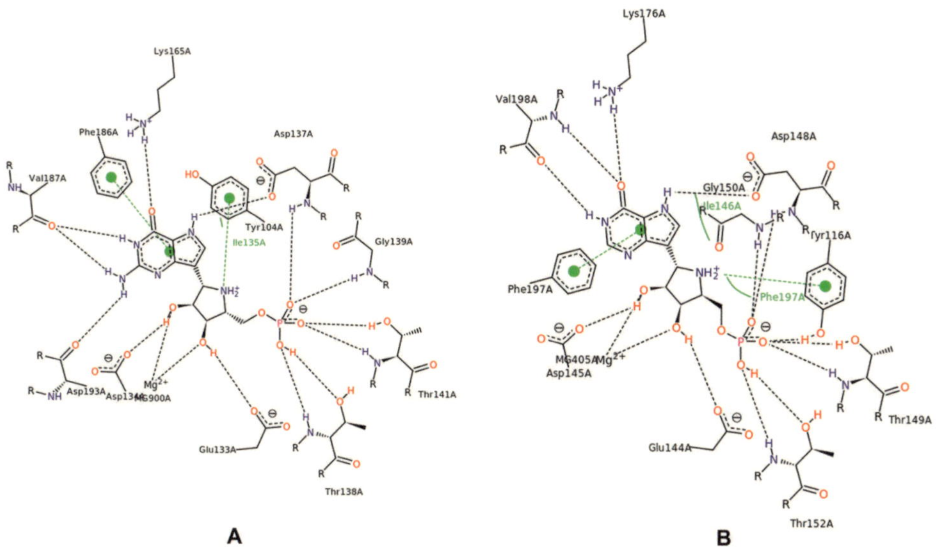

Figure 7.
Two-dimensional ligand interaction map showing A, Immucillin-G phosphate bound to HsHGPRT (1BZY) and B, Immucillin-H phosphate bound PfHGXPRT (1CJB). Active side residues that make contact with inhibitors are similar in both enzymes.

Acyclic nucleoside phosphonates (ANPs) however provide the greatest selectivity for the *Plasmodium* enzyme compared to phosphate-based compounds (**Figure 8**) [62, 63]. Crystal structures of *Hs*HGPRT in complex with ANP and free *Pf*HGXPRT suggest that the increased in selectivity when the phosphate groups are replaced with phosphonates is attributed to tighter hydrogen bonding around the phosphonate group and flexibility of the 6-oxo binding pocket [60].

TSAs are the tightest binding HG(X)PRT inhibitors reported to date. Although the first-generation transition state analogs, immucillin-G phosphate (ImmGP) and immucillin-H phosphate (ImmHP) were designed based on the proposed similarity of the transition state structure to other phosphoribosyltransferases, they bind potently but without discrimination for parasite or human HG(X)PRT (**Figure 8**) [41] and are subject to host enzymatic degradation by phosphomonoesterases. Structural analysis of TSAs bound to both *Hs*HGPRT and *Pf*HGXPRT as well as downfield proton chemical shift differences observed by NMR of bound inhibitors suggested that selectivity for *Pf*HGXPRT may be achieved by substituting TSAs with electron-withdrawing or electron-donating groups to alter hydrogen-bonding distances [41]. Recently, the transition state structure of *Pf*HGXPRT has been solved and provides detailed information on bond distances in the transition state [61]. With this knowledge, serinol-based mimics of the riboxocarbenium with a methylene bridge linking the oxocarbenium mimic to the 9-deazapurine ring were designed to mimic the bond distances in the transition state structure and synthesized. These compounds have proven to be the tightest and most selective inhibitors of *Pf*HGXPRT, with K_i^* values as low as 650 pM and selectivity indices for *Pf*HGXPRT greater than 500-fold relative to *Hs*HGXPRT [64, 65].

HGXPRT TSAs are phosphate or phosphonate-based compounds with a net negative charge at physiological pH, making them impermeable to cell membranes. Prodrug approaches are therefore required for their biological activity. Prodrugs of *Pf*HGXPRT inhibitors involve ANPs with intramolecular esters in the form of lysophospholipid prodrugs, designed to be activated by intracellular phospholipase C,

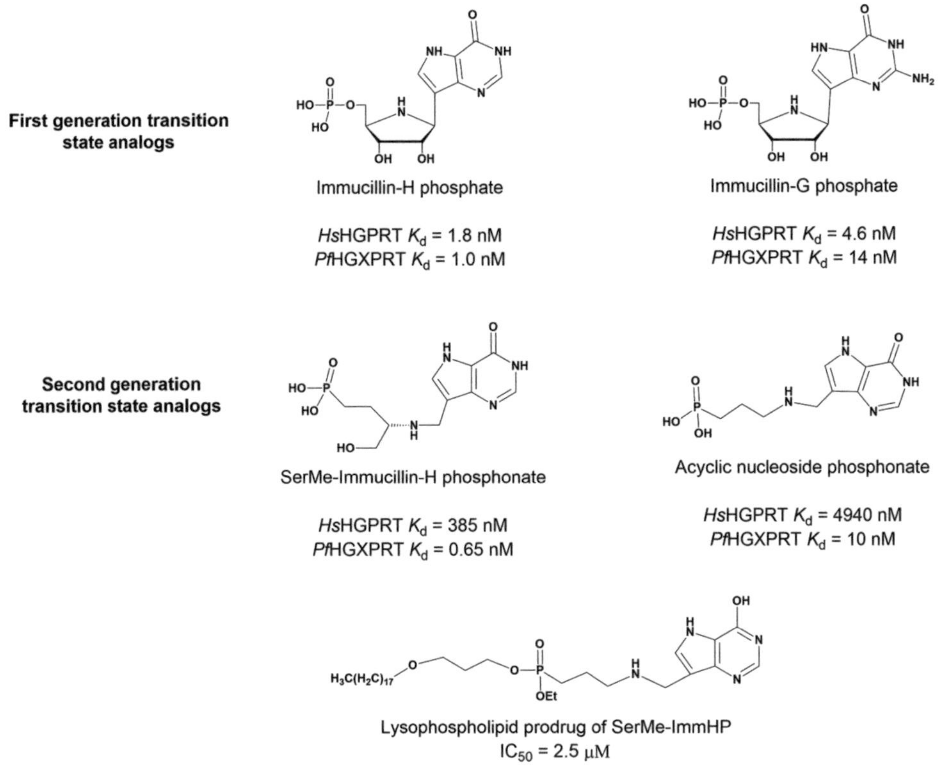

Figure 8.
First generation and second generation transtion state analogs for HG(X)PRT. Dissociation constants for HsHGPRT and PfHGXPRT are shown for each inhibitor. The second generation analogs provide greater selectivity for the PfHGXPRT. Lysophospholipid prodrug with biological activity against P. falciparum parasites in culture shown in lower panel.

or phosphoramidate prodrugs with a multistep activation mechanism [66]. Prodrug approaches have been validated in several FDA-approved nucleoside antiviral drugs [67]. The prodrug approaches improve the biological activities of TSAs of *Pf*HGXPRT to give anti-parasite IC_{50} values in the micromolar range (2–7 μM) against *P. falciparum* parasites cultured in human blood (**Figure 8**) [65]. With a K_i^* of 650 pM, disparity between the K_i^* for the enzyme and the micromolar IC_{50} values of lysophospholipid prodrugs suggests that more efficient prodrug approaches are needed to fully capture the tight-binding capabilities of TSAs intracellularly. *Pf*HGXPRT is a challenging target because of the multiple cellular and membrane barriers between an oral drug and the intracellular parasites. However, similar challenges have been overcome for antivirals and they provide a lesson for prodrug approaches. In summary, *Pf*HGXPRT is a challenging but valid target for the development of novel antimalarials and TSAs currently provide the most promising approach.

2.4 Downstream enzymes of purine salvage

Given how essential purine salvage is to the survival of *Plasmodium* parasites, it is remarkable that the pathway evolved to rely on only three major enzymes, ADA, PNP and HGXPRT, based on the genome interpretation and protein expression levels in the parasites [55]. As concentration of free guanine in human blood is very low, it is not feasible for *Plasmodium* spp. to synthesize guanosine monophosphate (GMP) using HGXPRT [51]. Two enzymes downstream of HGXPRT, inosine 5′-monophosphate dehydrogenase (IMPDH) and GMP synthetase (GMPS) work sequentially to synthesize GMP (**Figure 1**) [68]. These two enzymes control GMP synthesis in most organisms [69]. IMPDH catalyzes the NAD^+ dependent reaction that coverts IMP to xanthine monophosphate (XMP) and NADH [70]. GMPS is composed of two domains, an ATP pyrophosphatase domain and a glutamine amidotransferase (GAT) domain [68, 71]. By this mechanism, GMPS catalyzes the ATP-dependent irreversible amination of XMP on carbon 2 to form GMP. Inhibitors of both IMPDH and GMPS have been shown to have antimalaria properties and have been the subject of recent drug development [21, 68].

Mycophenolic acid is an IMPDH inhibitor and inhibits *P. falciparum* parasites in culture with an IC_{50} of about 5 μM [21, 72, 73]. Bredinin is an inhibitor that has been shown to inhibit both IMPDH and GMPS [68, 74] and suggest that both IMPDH and GMPS are targets to explore for novel antimalarials. Although the IMP to GMP pathway involves phosphorylated intermediates, both mycophenolic acid and bredinin are non-phosphorylated natural products (or derivatives) that provide orally available access to tissues. Both mycophenolic acid and bredinin are used in immune suppression, and they have not been useful as antimalarials.

2.5 Purine salvage and polyamine synthesis

Polyamines are synthesized by the transfer of propyl amino groups from decarboxylated S-adenosylmethionine to putrescine to form spermidine (one transfer) and spermine (two transfers) [75]. MTA is the product of each transfer in the polyamine biosynthetic pathway. MTA is also a substrate for *Pf*ADA, whereby it is deaminated to methylthioinosine. These steps provide a path for this abundant product of the polyamine pathway to be channeled into the into the purine salvage pathway [76]. Polyamines are present at high amounts in the intraerythrocytic stages of *Plasmodium* spp., which can perform both *de novo* synthesis and salvage of polyamines [76, 77]. Given that parasites can only perform salvage of purines, the valuable purines used in the polyamine pathway are economically recycled. MTA is converted by the action of *Pf*ADA to produce MTI. MTI is a substrate for *Pf*PNP to form hypoxanthine and methylthioribose 1-phosphate. MTI is not found in human metabolism and recent studies have suggested that MTI production by *Plasmodium falciparum* in infected humans leads to activation of human Toll-like receptor 8 (TLR8), a signal for the stimulation of host innate immunity [37]. This connection provides an interesting link to the potential use of *Pf*PNP inhibitors as a potential therapeutic in human malaria. MTI is removed from *P. falciparum* metabolism exclusively by *Pf*PNP as *Hs*PNP does not use MTI as substrate. Therefore, inhibition of purine salvage via *Pf*PNP will increase MTI, increase signaling from TLR8 and have an immune stimulatory effect for the clearance of infected erythrocytes. Crosstalk between the polyamine pathway and purine salvage in *Plasmodium* parasites, together with the potential immunostimulatory effect of polyamine metabolites, underscores the importance of the polyamine pathway to purine salvage in *Plasmodium* parasites [37]. Inhibition of either the polyamine or the purine salvage pathways in *Plasmodium* parasites will be detrimental to parasites by; (1) purine starvation and death and (2) immune stimulation to promote clearance by host immune cells.

3. Pyrimidine metabolism

Opposite to the purine requirements of *Plasmodium falciparum*, the parasites are incapable of pyrimidine salvage from host erythrocytes; and pyrimidine synthesis requires the *de novo* pathway. This requirement contrasts with host cells with pathways for *de novo* synthesis and salvage of pyrimidine nucleotides [78]. Pyrimidine synthesis occurs by the action of six sequential enzymes to produce uridine monophosphate (UMP) as the primary product and a precursor to the other pyrimidine nucleotides (**Figure 9**) [79]. The enzymatic steps following UMP synthesis in *P. falciparum* are not well characterized, however, pyrimidine biosynthesis is linked to folate metabolism via the action of thymidylate synthetase (TS) [80]. Differences in the pathway between the human host and *Plasmodium* are important for selective targeting of *Plasmodium* parasites. In humans, the first three enzymes of the pyrimidine biosynthetic pathway, carbamoylphosphate synthetase II (CPS II), aspartate transcarbamoylase (ATC) and dihydroorotase (DHO) are a single protein, multiple domains, multifunctional enzyme complex, the CAD complex. In *Plasmodium*, CPS II, ATC and DHO are encoded as distinct genes, produce independent proteins and are organized on different locations on chromosomes, Ch. 13 for CPS II and ATC, and Ch. 14 for DHO [78, 81].

CPS II and ATC in *P. falciparum* are poorly characterized despite the role of CPS II as a key regulator of the pathway [20, 82]. The most thoroughly characterized enzymes of *Plasmodium* pyrimidine biosynthesis are dihydroorotate dehydrogenase (DHODH) and orotate phosphoribosyltransferase (OPRT) [83]. The transition state

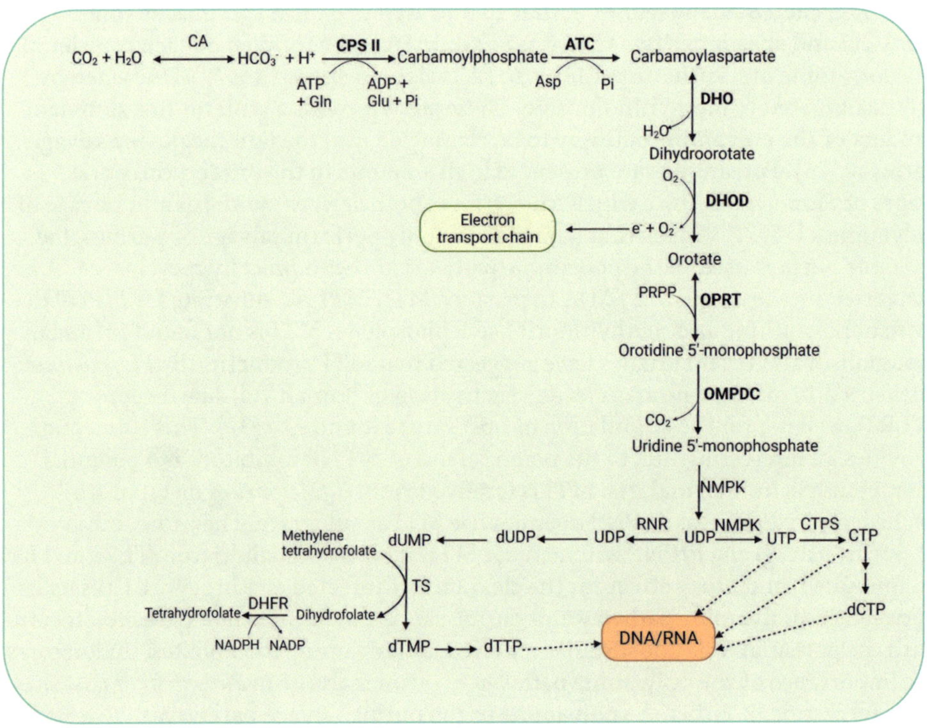

Figure 9.
De novo pyrimidine biosynthetic pathway. The pyrimidine biosynthetic pathway is conserved in Plasmodium and humans.

structures of human (*Hs*OPRT) and *Plasmodium falciparum* OPRT (*Pf*OPRT) have previously been solved and transition state analog inhibitors of both *Hs*OPRT and *Pf*OPRT have been designed (detailed below).

3.1 DHODH (EC 1.3.5.2)

DHODH is the fourth enzyme in the pyrimidine biosynthetic pathway and is expressed as two isozymes. The isozyme expressed from chromosome 7 codes for a mitochondria-associated DHODH and chromosome 9 expresses a cytosolic DHODH, where the mitochondrial form is essential for *Plasmodium* growth [84]. DHODH catalyzes the formation of orotate from dihydroorotate, a rate-limiting step for pyrimidine biosynthesis. *Plasmodium* spp., like the human host, express a type II DHODH, localized in the inner membrane of the mitochondrion [84, 85]. The electron transport chain provides quinone for the redox activity of DHODH. Recent studies have highlighted *Pf*DHODH as a potential antimalaria target, showing that inhibiting *Pf*DHODH leads to parasite death in culture and animal models [85–87].

Selective inhibition of *Pf*DHODH has been achieved with DSM265, a triazolopyrimidine with a 4000-fold selectivity over mammalian DHODH. DSM265 has resulted in phase II clinical trials for the treatment of malaria, a first for any inhibitor of the parasite pyrimidine biosynthetic pathway. DSM265 inhibits both blood and liver stages of the malaria parasite with a biological efficacy similar to chloroquine in murine malaria models [87–89]. The pharmacokinetic analysis of DSM265 supported single dose therapy for use as a once weekly prophylactic [87]. Single dose administrations are considered important for patient compliance. Since the discovery of DSM265, DSM421, an improvement on DSM265 in terms of compound solubility, plasma stability and equal targeting of *P. falciparum* and *P. vivax* has also been reported in preclinical development [90]. Other studies have followed suit, using pharmacophore screening and structure-guided virtual studies to identify *plasmodium* specific DHODH inhibitors with submicromolar IC_{50} values [91, 92].

Pyrimidine biosynthesis is coupled to the mitochondrial electron transport chain (ETC) by DHODH and its requirements of quinones for catalytic activity (**Figure 9**). This coupling results in indirect inhibition of DHODH by ETC inhibitors such as atovaquone, an approved antimalarial often used in combination with proguanil [93]. Although DHODH and the linked mitochondrial ETC were promising targets with extensive discovery and development programs providing powerful inhibitors, the rapid development of resistance in clinical trials has hindered their development toward approved drugs [94, 95].

3.2 OPRT (EC 2.4.2.10)

Reduction of dihydroorotate by DHODH produces orotic acid and the following step, catalyzed by *Pf*OPRT, catalyzes the production of the nucleotide orotidine monophosphate (OMP) from orotate and PRPP. OMP is subsequently converted to UMP by OMP decarboxylase (OMPDC). *Plasmodium* and human OPRTs differ in the early steps of the pyrimidine biosynthetic pathway. Thus, human OPRT is fused to OMPDC to form the single protein, bifunctional enzyme called UMP synthase [96]. In *Plasmodium*, OPRT and OPMDC have been purified as monofunctional enzymes however, there are recent reports suggesting that OPRT and OPMDC may exist as a heterotetrameric enzyme in *Plasmodium* with the potential for hydrolysis into the single enzymes during purification [83, 97, 98]. Detailed kinetic characterizations of both human and *P. falciparum* OPRTs (*Hs*OPRT and *Pf*OPRT respectively) have been reported and active site differences between the homologs have been characterized [83, 98].

The essential function of OPRT in pyrimidine biosynthesis and therefore for parasite proliferation has been demonstrated by the selective killing of cultured *P. falciparum* parasites by pyrazofurin, an inhibitor of OPRT with anti-parasite IC_{50} values of 6–20 μM [21, 99]. Additionally, 5-fluororotate and 5-aminouracil have inhibitory activity against *Pf*OPRT with IC_{50} values of 42 nM and 8 μM respectively [21]. 5-Fluororotate selectively targets *P. falciparum* parasites in culture with an IC_{50} of 6 nM [100]. The mechanism of action is proposed to arise from an indirect effect of the toxic 5-fluorodeoxyuridylate metabolite on TS [101]. *Plasmodium* express TS as a single protein, multi-domain bifunctional enzyme with dihydrofolate reductase (DHFR) whereas TS exists as a monofunctional enzyme in mammals [21, 99, 100].

Transition state analysis of *Pf*OPRT and *Hs*OPRT reported an S_N1 transition state with a partial dissociative orotate and riboxocarbenium ion character for both enzymes [102]. Despite differences in the enzyme organization, *Pf*OPRT and *Hs*OPRT possess similar transition state structures, where the ribocation is fully developed, the dianionic orotate is fully dissociated and there is weak participation of the pyrophosphate nucleophile (**Figure 10**) [102]. The transition state structures provided information for the design of several TSAs with nanomolar affinities for both *Hs*OPRT and *Pf*OPRT (**Figure 10**) [103]. Inhibition of *Hs*OPRT might have potential utility for the treatment of autoimmune diseases and some malignant neoplastic diseases. However, no anti-parasitic activity was observed for any of the TSAs in cultured *P. falciparum.* The lack of activity was attributed to permeability barriers and target

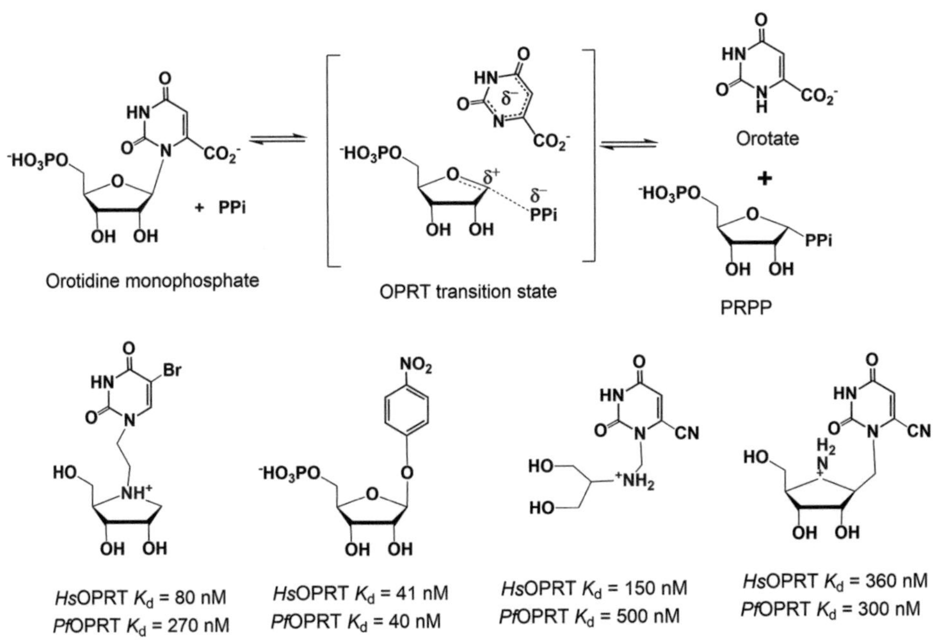

Figure 10.
Upper panel: OPRT reaction scheme and transition state structure. The transition state structure is similar for PfOPRT and HsOPRT. It features a fully developed ribocation and a fully dissociated dianionic orotate with weak participation of the pyrophosphate. Lower panel: Transition state analogs synthesized and tested on PfOPRT and HsOPRT.

access, but no permeability studies have been reported [103]. *Pf*OPRT remains a viable antimalarial target requiring further studies to elucidate and develop species-specific antimalarials.

3.3 OMPDC (EC 4.1.1.23)

The decarboxylation of OMP to form UMP is catalyzed by OMPDC, the sixth enzyme in the *de novo* pyrimidine biosynthetic pathway [78]. OMPDC has achieved catalytic notoriety as it has been considered the most proficient pure protein catalyst, giving a catalytic reaction rate enhancement of approximately 10^{17} [104, 105]. Unlike other decarboxylases, OMPDC requires no metal ions or cofactors for its catalytic activity [105]. Recent studies indicate that *Plasmodium falciparum* OMPDC may form a tight heterotetrameric complex with OPRT (*Pf*OMPDC$_2$-*Pf*OPRT$_2$) with properties distinct from the bifunctional human OPRT [106, 107]. Although both are expressed and encoded by two separate genes, unique amino acid insertions in both proteins not present in the homologous proteins of other organisms allow the formation of the heterotetrameric complex [98, 106]. Additional support comes from the kinetic characterization of fused *P. falciparum* OPMDC and OPRT, expressed in *Escherichia coli*, where the catalytic efficiency of the fused enzymes was enhanced several orders of magnitude relative to either enzyme acting as monofunctional proteins, leading the authors to call the fusion a 'super' enzyme [97].

Nucleoside 5′-monophosphate analogs, 6-azauridine 5′-monophosphate (AzaUMP), allopurinol-3-riboside 5′-monophosphate (allopurinol MP), pyrazofurin 5′-monophosphate (pyrazofuin MP), and xanthosine 5′-monophosphate (XMP) are potent inhibitors of both human and parasite OMPDCs (**Figure 11**) [108]. These display a strong preference for *Pf*OMPDC, with selectivity ranging from 11 to 150-fold preference for the parasite enzyme [108]. The differential binding of XMP has been investigated by comparing X-ray crystal structures of both enzymes. Few differences in active site residues were observed and specificity may be as a result in hydrogen bonding differences between ligand and active site residues (**Figure 12**). Another reported difference is the βα5-loop present at the dimerization interface, which displays different conformations and amino acid substitutions in *Pf*OMPDC compared to *Hs*OMPDC and is postulated to cause different active site rearrangements around the pyrimidine binding region [108]. The phosphate binding loop is also larger in *Hs*OMPDC than in *Pf*OMPDC [108]. Repositioning of the loop is a proposed requirement to bind XMP as observed for XMP-bound *Pyrococcus horikoshii* OMPDC [108]. Interestingly, the phosphate loop is the same size and shape in *P. horikoshii* OMPDC and *Pf*OMPDC, therefore, these enzymes may bind XMP similarly. XMP is a 150-fold more potent inhibitor of *Pf*OMPDC than of *Hs*OMPDC [108].

No crystal structures of inhibitor bound *Pf*OMPDC are available to understand the basis for inhibitor selectivity. However, the high preference of inhibitors for parasite OMPDC compared to the human enzyme indicates the possibility of developing potent and selective antimalarials. Inhibition of OMPDC has focused on nucleotide analogs, where the 5′-phosphate is a significant contributor to binding. A substantial barrier to drug development for nucleotide inhibitors is the anionic charge, as phosphoryl anions are membrane impermeable and phosphomonoesters are susceptible to phosphomonoesterases. Prodrug approaches, now being used in antiviral therapy for the delivery of phosphate nucleosides may be useful in development of OMPDC inhibitors.

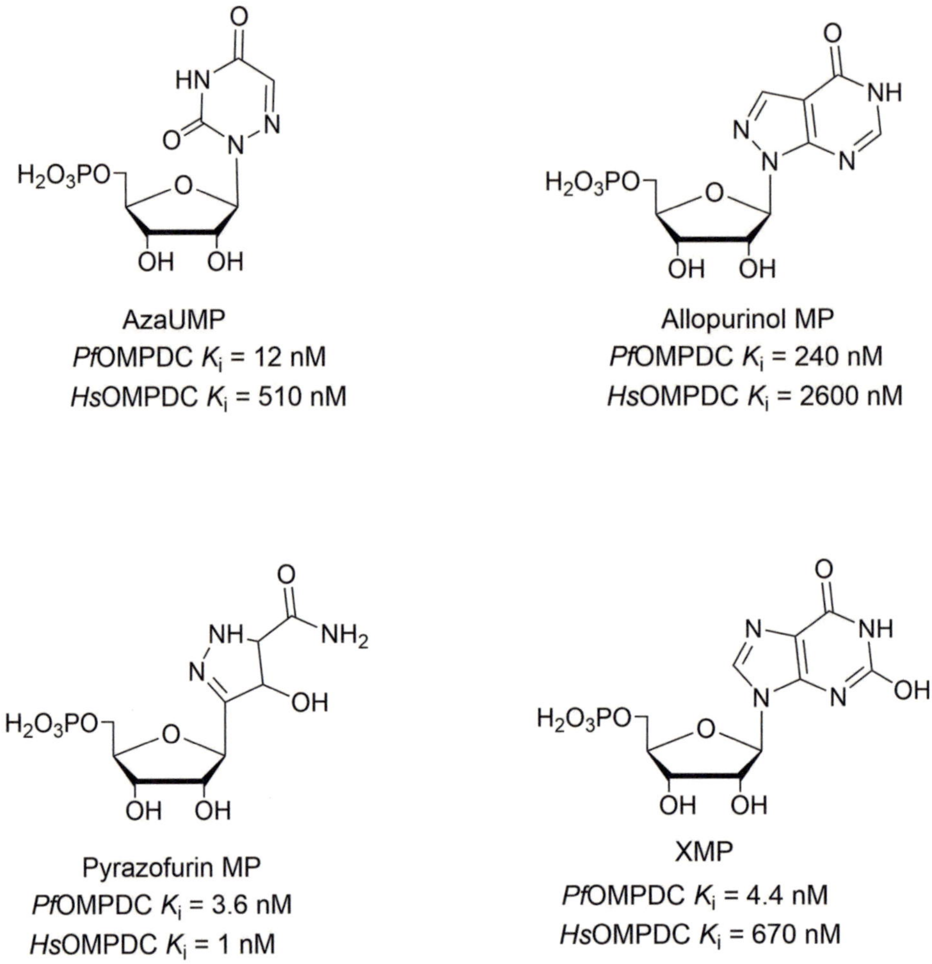

Figure 11.
Nucleoside 5′-analogs of OPMDC showing inhibitory constants for both PfOMPDC and HsOMPDC. Inhibitors are highly selective, 11–150-fold for PfOMPDC over HsOMPDC. Values are as reported in [108].

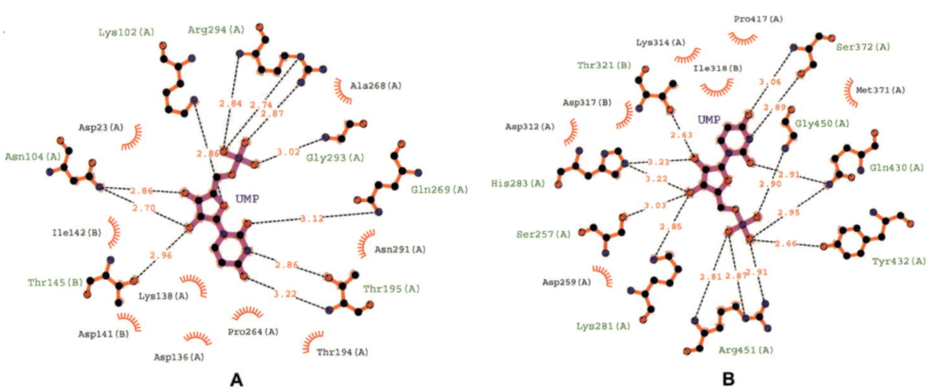

Figure 12.
2-dimensional ligand interaction map of UMP bound A, PfOPMDC (6DSR) and B, HsOMPDC (2V30). Similar active site residues make contact with UMP.

3.4 DHFR (EC 1.5.1.3) and TS (EC 2.1.1.45)

De novo purine synthesis in the host and pyrimidine synthesis in both host and parasites are dependent on folate metabolites for the donation of carbon units. The pyrimidine biosynthetic pathway is linked to folate metabolism by TS, which requires 5,10-methylene tetrahydrofolate as a methyl donor for its catalytic activity [109]. DHFR and TS are both targets for human cancers [110]. In *Plasmodium falciparum*, DHFR and TS are expressed as a single protein, two-domain bifunctional DHFR-TS enzyme system, catalyzing the synthesis of deoxythymidylate monophosphate (dTMP) from dUMP and the NADPH-dependent reduction of dihydrofolate (DHF) to tetrahydrofolate (THF) [80]. The bifunctional coupling of adjacent steps in the pathway is proposed to cause "substrate channeling", an efficient utilization of folate production for the synthesis of purines, pyrimidines, and amino acids [111, 112]. Since malaria parasites are unable to salvage pyrimidines, if metabolites or cofactors required by the folate pathway are cut off, thymidine biosynthesis is blocked, and parasites die from pyrimidine starvation [20, 80]. Thus, DHFR has been a frequently-drugged target for antimalaria therapy.

Pyrimethamine (PYR) and proguanil (PG) are approved antimalaria therapeutics which selectively target *Pf*DHFR by several hundred-fold compared to the human counterparts [20, 113]. Mutations in the *DHFR* gene conferring resistance to both PYR and PG have led to diminished clinical effectiveness as single therapeutics for malaria. However, the combination of pyrimethamine with sulfadoxine (SP), which blocks dihydropteroate synthase, a folate precursor, act synergistically in the treatment of severe malaria [114]. Despite the prevalence of molecular mutations causing resistance to SP, WHO still recommends SP for intermittent preventative treatment for pregnant women and, often, in combination with amodiaquine, an inhibitor of *Plasmodium* heme polymerase, for seasonal malaria prevention [115]. PG is also used in combination with atovaquone, an inhibitor of the mitochondrion electron transfer chain, which also directly impacts pyrimidine biosynthesis because of its coupling to DHODH [116, 117].

Recent searches for additional inhibitors of DHFR-TS identified the antimicrobial triclosan to inhibit the proliferation of intraerythrocytic *P. falciparum* and is a 775 nM inhibitor of *P. vivax* DHFR. Triclosan displays a 20-fold selectivity for *Plasmodium* enzymes relative to human DHFR [118]. To preempt the development of resistance, Tarnchompoo and coworkers have developed hybrid inhibitors of DHFR with both flexible and rigid side chains that target both wild-type and multiple resistance *P. falciparum* [119]. Hybrid inhibitors include sub-nanomolar inhibitors of *Pf*DHFR with 10-fold selectivity over *Hs*DHFR [119]. Flexible cycloguanil analogs have been characterized that are low nanomolar inhibitors of multiple mutant *Pf*DHFR [120]. Fragment-based screening approaches to inhibitor design have identified non-pyrimidine scaffolds that inhibit *Pf*DHFR-TS with IC_{50} in the range of 28–695 μM and are highly selective over *Hs*DHFR [121]. This approach offers a new avenue to tackle antifolate resistance and develop new antifolate antimalarials, but remains in development [121].

DHFR-TS is a validated target for antimalaria combination therapy by blocking synthesis of dTMP. The functional characteristics of DHFR-TS including its crystal structure and the structures of drug-resistant DHFR-TS allows for the identification and development of next-generation selective inhibitors of either catalytic domain that will address resistance to current antifolate drugs for malaria. New approaches are being explored, including peptide-based antagonists of *Pf*DHFR-TS in the quest for novel and potent antifolate/anti-pyrimidine drugs [122].

4. Transition state analogs and drug development

Transition state theory postulates that chemically stable mimics of the enzymatic transition state will bind tightly to the target [123, 124]. All chemical, including enzymatic reactions, proceed via a transition state, a transient high energy species that lies along the reaction coordinate between reactants and products [125, 126]. Transition states are the balance point of a catalytic reaction where bonds are partially broken or formed and the probability for product formation and return to reactants is equal. Enzymes have evolved to highly favor the transition state geometry, hence their very large rate enhancement factors, typically of 10^{10} to 10^{15}, a very large decrease in the activation energy of the reaction [18]. Chemically stable mimics of the transition state bind to and stabilize this favored enzymatic transition state geometry, capture part of the transition state energy and bind very tightly [18, 127–129]. Therefore, transition state analysis provides a powerful tool to develop molecules with high inhibitory potential for their target enzymes. Kinetic isotope effects (KIE) remain the best approach to study enzymatic transition states and together with quantum computational chemistry, allows the construction of electrostatic potential maps that provide information on the transition state structure [18]. This information enables the design of transition state analogs that bind with high fidelity to their cognate enzymes, millions of times tighter than substrates. Transition state analogs are some of the tightest binding enzymatic inhibitors and have the propensity to bind their target enzymes with dissociation constants in the nanomolar to femtomolar range (10^{-9} to 10^{-15} M) [123, 125, 126]. A feature of transition state analogs is the ability to convert the enzyme potential for catalysis into binding energy, therefore the more catalytically efficient the enzyme, the tighter the potential for transition state analog binding [127].

The immucillins are chemically stable transition state analogs that mimic the ribocation transition state of N-ribosyltransferases, enzymes that include *Pf*PNP and *Pf*HGXPRT, both important in purine salvage in *P. falciparum* [50]. Immucillin-H (also known as: BCX1777, Forodesine and Mundesine) (**Figure 5**) is an inhibitor of PNPs and has been approved in Japan for the treatment of resistant or relapsed peripheral T cell lymphoma (PTCL). Immucillin-A, as Galidesivir (also known as BCX4430) continues in phase I - II clinical trials for antiviral therapy. It is converted to the triphosphate form where it blocks RNA chain elongation in RNA viruses, including Yellow Fever and SARS-CoV2 [130]. DADMe-Immucillin-H (also known as: BCX4208, Ulodesine) has completed phase II clinical trials for gout, by virtue of its powerful inhibition of human PNP, an essential step in formation of uric acid in humans [50]. No immucillins or related transition state analogs for purine and pyrimidine pathways have yet entered clinical trials for antimalaria therapy though several are in preclinical testing [128].

The immucillins differ from traditional antibiotic discovery. Antibacterials are often discovered by cell wall screening or genomic targeting to inhibit cell wall synthesis [131]. Immucillins and related transition state analogs are designed to mimic the geometry of the transition state of their specific enzymes [129]. The resulting transition state analogs can be powerful tight-binding inhibitors with exquisite specificity for their targeted enzymes. Transition state inhibitor design is adding new candidates for drug development.

Immucillins in preclinical development as antimalaria drugs include the PNP-targeting DADMe-ImmG, a powerful inhibitor that is a picomolar inhibitor for both human and *Pf*PNPs. Administration at nanomolar concentrations to parasites cultured in human erythrocytes caused purine-less death of *P. falciparum*. Testing in *Aotus* primates infected with *P. falciparum* at an oral dose of 50 mg/kg and dosed for 7 days gave robust parasite clearance and no parasitemia was detected by day 6 of treatment, along with complete inhibition of host and parasite PNP [49]. Recrudescent parasites appeared several days after treatment stopped [49]. *Aotus* monkeys, however, have approximately 40 μM circulating hypoxanthine, compared to approximately 1 μM in humans [49]. Therefore, clearing *P. falciparum* from *Aotus* is a more stringent test for the antimalaria efficacy of DADMe-ImmG than anticipated in human infections. DADMe-ImmH, the compound tested extensively in phase I and phase II clinical trials for gout, has a good safety profile in humans. DADMe-ImmH has an inhibitory potential for both *Hs*PNP and *Pf*PNPs similar to DADMe-ImmG and is a strong candidate to enter human clinical trials [50]. The efficacy of DADMe-ImmH has been established in clinical trials. A single oral dose of 0.5 mg/kg completely inhibits erythrocyte PNP with inhibition lasting for 120 days, the lifetime of the erythrocyte, making it a candidate for single-dose therapy of *P. falciparum* [132]. As inhibition of both human PNP and *Pf*PNP is required for antimalarial properties, a single dose therapy has potential as a novel antimalarial, and as described below, has a reduced potential for the induction of resistance mutations.

4.1 Antimalaria resistance to transition state analogs

P. falciparum has developed resistance to most approved antimalarials, contributing to the difficulty of disease-eradication efforts worldwide. Rapid development of resistance has led to the clinical failure of several potent antimalaria drugs early in clinical trials and has resulted in World Health Organization recommendations for combination drug therapy for malaria treatment. Chloroquine which was once the gold standard treatment for malaria was widely used until the 1950s, when widespread resistance prompted its removal from the list of approved malaria therapeutics [133, 134]. Resistance soon followed for drugs such as atovaquone, pyrimethamine, proguanil, cycloguanil, sulfadoxine and sulfadoxine-pyrimethamine (SP) [133, 134]. Recently, resistance to artemisinin, one partner of the current first line treatment has been reported in the endemic regions of Sub-Saharan Africa and the Greater Mekong region of Southeast Asia [12, 14, 135, 136].

In the field, drug resistance is characterized by delayed-clearance of parasites from the blood of infected individuals [11]. Resistant parasites often have point mutations and gene amplification which can result in decreased drug uptake, increased efflux of drugs, target overexpression, target modification that reduces drug binding, and inactivation of a drug by modification (**Figure 13**) [134]. Knowledge of these mechanisms to resistance have prompted the search for novel and unique antimalaria compounds followed by investigation of the rates and mechanisms of resistance by subjecting cultured *P. falciparum* parasites to constant pressure of the novel compounds.

One such study involving DSM265, the *Pf*DHODH inhibitor. Using a drug pressure of 3 × EC_{50} revealed a minimum inoculum for resistance (MIR) of 2 × 10^6 compared to 2 × 10^7 for atovaquone [87]. Selection of resistant parasites to DSM265 required 8 x EC_{50} of DSM265 compared to 33 × EC_{50} required to suppress atovaquone resistant parasites. The resistance mechanism in Dd2 clones (resistant to chloroquine,

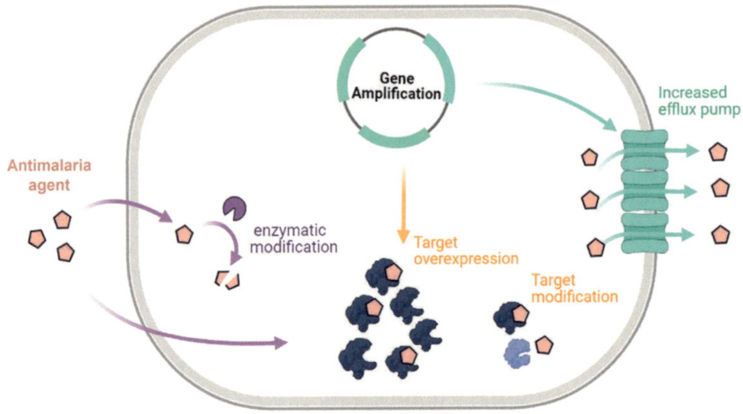

Figure 13.
Antimalarial resistance mechanism frequently employed by Plasmodium parasites to overcome drug pressure.

pyrimethamine and mefloquine) revealed both gene amplification of the DHODH gene and the G181C mutation that confers a 13-fold shift in IC_{50} of the drug compared to wild-type enzyme and 26-fold reduction of the EC_{50} in parasite growth assay. Kinetic characterization of the recombinant mutant enzyme revealed a 2-fold increase in the k_{cat}, and K_m was unchanged [87]. Resistance to DSM265 in Dd2 parasites developed rapidly with a profile similar to resistance development for atovaquone. However, resistance was not as easily generated at higher concentrations of DSM265 in other *P. falciparum* strains, questioning if resistance would develop in the field [90]. DSM265 in phase II clinical trials for malaria led to the appearance of resistance during the clinical trial phase [94].

In contrast to DSM265, resistance to transition state analogs is not easily generated. Loss of transition state features in the protein also generates severe catalytic penalties predicted to induce a fitness cost to the parasites. For example, treatment of cultured *P. falciparum* with DADMe-ImmG for 1 year in culture resulted in a 6-fold resistance (6-fold increase in IC_{50}) [44]. The resistance was caused by a 6-fold amplification of wild-type *PfPNP* gene and protein levels. After 3 years of drug pressure (over 2^{136} clonal selections) in cultured cells, increased resistance was marked by a 12-fold amplification in the target *PfPNP* gene [44]. The 12-fold gene amplification was accompanied by two point mutations in PNP occurring in separate clones (M183L and V181D) to give rise to a 500-fold increase in the IC_{50}. Interestingly, point mutations were only present in 50% of the transcripts and the remainders were wild type [44]. Recombinant expression of mutant PNP revealed that the kinetic properties were incompatible with the purine salvage function of PNP [44]. Particularly, the M183L mutation resulted in a 17,000-fold decrease in the catalytic efficiency (30-fold decrease in k_{cat}) of the enzyme and a 39,000-fold decrease in affinity for DADMe-ImmG [44]. Therefore, the mutation reduced the catalytic efficiency and DADMe-ImmG efficacy by approximately the same amount, highlighting a key feature of transition state analogs. Mutations that prevent binding of the analog are expected to decrease catalytic activity to the same degree.

Resistance to DADMe-ImmG in *P. falciparum* arises by a unique mechanism. Hybrid PNP expression of 50% mutant M183L subunits and 50% wild-type subunits is proposed to generate hybrid hexameric PNPs demonstrating a 6-fold decrease in catalytic efficiency, as three of the six subunits are native. This hybrid hexameric construct of three native and three mutant subunits displays negative cooperativity in binding to DADMe-ImmG, always leaving a fraction of the native subunits free to catalyze the formation of hypoxanthine [137]. Therefore, in addition to 12-fold target overexpression and point mutations, *P. falciparum* also employs hybrid multimeric PNP to achieve robust resistance [137]. This example emphasizes the severe catalytic costs and threat to biological function that resistance to transition state analogs produces in the parasites. This slow development of resistance to DADMe-ImmG suggests that resistance may be slow to develop in the field.

Conditions for generating laboratory DADMe-ImmG-resistant *P. falciparum* clones are stringent, requiring up to 3 years of drug pressure *on the same culture* before robust resistance appeared. In the field, effective anti-parasitics clear parasites in a matter of days, and it is unlikely that parasites would encounter conditions of continuous drug pressure. Notwithstanding, these *in vitro* resistance assays help identify mechanisms and molecular markers of resistance and resistance phenotypes that will aid in recognizing resistance development in the field. Like most antimalarials, the proposed use of DADMe-ImmG or related transition state analogs would be in drug combinations to provide an extra layer of protection against development of resistance.

5. Summary and conclusion

During the intraerythrocytic stages, *Plasmodium* parasites proliferate rapidly and require extensive nucleic acid synthesis. The building blocks are either salvaged from the human host in the form of purines or synthesized de novo (pyrimidines). There are distinct differences between the purine and pyrimidine synthesis pathways of humans and the malaria parasites. Therefore, targeting these pathways can aid in the development of novel chemotherapeutic agents to combat emerging resistance to the current first line antimalarials. Transition state analogs against various purine and pyrimidine pathway enzymes are emerging as promising candidates for antimalarial therapy. The slow development of resistance and the unusual resistance mechanism employed by the parasites to drug pressure against transition state analogs may lead to slow resistance development in the field. Finally, the recent advances made with the RTS,S vaccine in endemic African countries is promising and point in the right direction for population control of malaria. However, until an effective vaccine is approved for widespread use, chemotherapeutic agents managing the disease and vector control measures are still needed.

Acknowledgements

Preparation of this manuscript was supported by NIH research grants (AI127807 and GM041916). We thank our collaborators in Dr. Peter C. Tyler's group at Ferrier Research Institute, Victoria University of Wellington, New Zealand, for the synthesis of the Immucillins and transition state analogs.

Conflict of interest

The authors declare no conflict of interest.

Author details

Yacoba V. T. Minnow and Vern L. Schramm*
Department of Biochemistry, Albert Einstein College of Medicine, New York, USA

*Address all correspondence to: vern.schramm@einsteinmed.edu

References

[1] WHO. World Malaria Report 2021. Geneva: World Health Organization; 2021

[2] WHO. World Malaria Report 2018. Geneva: World Health Organization; 2018

[3] WHO. World Malaria Report 2020. Geneva: World Health Organization; 2020

[4] WHO. World Malaria Report. Geneva: World Health Organization; 2019

[5] Sato S. Plasmodium-a brief introduction to the parasites causing human malaria and their basic biology. Journal of Physiological Anthropology. 2021;**40**(1):1. DOI: 10.1186/s40101-020-00251-9

[6] White NJ, Pukrittayakamee S, Hien TT, Faiz MA, Mokuolu OA, Dondorp AM. Malaria. Lancet. 2014;**383**(9918):723-735. DOI: 10.1016/S0140-6736(13)60024-0

[7] Haldar K, Bhattacharjee S, Safeukui I. Drug resistance in Plasmodium. Nature Reviews. Microbiology. 2018;**16**(3):156-170. DOI: 10.1038/nrmicro.2017.161

[8] Achan J et al. Quinine, an old anti-malarial drug in a modern world: Role in the treatment of malaria. Malaria Journal. 2011;**10**:144. DOI: 10.1186/1475-2875-10-144

[9] Renslo AR. Antimalarial drug discovery: From quinine to the dream of eradication. ACS Medicinal Chemistry Letters. 2013;**4**(12):1126-1128. DOI: 10.1021/ml4004414

[10] Miller LH, Su X. Artemisinin: Discovery from the Chinese herbal garden. Cell. 2011;**146**(6):855-858. DOI: 10.1016/j.cell.2011.08.024

[11] Tilley L, Straimer J, Gnadig NF, Ralph SA, Fidock DA. Artemisinin action and resistance in plasmodium falciparum. Trends in Parasitology. 2016;**32**(9):682-696. DOI: 10.1016/j.pt.2016.05.010

[12] Dondorp AM et al. Artemisinin resistance: Current status and scenarios for containment. Nature Reviews. Microbiology. 2010;**8**(4):272-280. DOI: 10.1038/nrmicro2331

[13] Thu AM, Phyo AP, Landier J, Parker DM, Nosten FH. Combating multidrug-resistant *Plasmodium falciparum* malaria. The FEBS Journal. 2017;**284**(16):2569-2578. DOI: 10.1111/febs.14127

[14] Balikagala B et al. Evidence of Artemisinin-Resistant Malaria in Africa. The New England Journal of Medicine. 2021;**385**(13):1163-1171. DOI: 10.1056/NEJMoa2101746

[15] Imwong M et al. The spread of artemisinin-resistant plasmodium falciparum in the greater Mekong subregion: A molecular epidemiology observational study. The Lancet Infectious Diseases. 2017;**17**(5):491-497. DOI: 10.1016/S1473-3099(17)30048-8

[16] Laurens MB. RTS,S/AS01 vaccine (Mosquirix): An overview. Human Vaccines & Immunotherapeutics. 2020;**16**(3):480-489. DOI: 10.1080/21645515.2019.1669415

[17] Zavala F. RTS,S: The first malaria vaccine. Journal of Clinical Investigation. 2022;**132**(1). DOI: 10.1172/JCI156588

[18] Schramm VL. Enzymatic transition states and drug design. Chemical Reviews. 2018;**118**(22):11194-11258. DOI: 10.1021/acs.chemrev.8b00369

[19] Downie MJ, Kirk K, Mamoun CB. Purine salvage pathways in the intraerythrocytic malaria parasite *Plasmodium falciparum*. Eukaryotic Cell. 2008;7(8):1231-1237. DOI: 10.1128/EC.00159-08

[20] Hyde JE. Targeting purine and pyrimidine metabolism in human apicomplexan parasites. Current Drug Targets. 2007;**8**(1):31-47. DOI: 10.2174/138945007779315524

[21] Queen SA, Jagt DL, Reyes P. In vitro susceptibilities of *Plasmodium falciparum* to compounds which inhibit nucleotide metabolism. Antimicrobial Agents and Chemotherapy. 1990;**34**(7):1393-1398. DOI: 10.1128/AAC.34.7.1393

[22] Berman PA, Human L, Freese JA. Xanthine oxidase inhibits growth of *Plasmodium falciparum* in human erythrocytes in vitro. The Journal of Clinical Investigation. 1991;**88**(6): 1848-1855. DOI: 10.1172/JCI115506

[23] Piro F, Focaia R, Dou Z, Masci S, Smith D, Di Cristina M. An uninvited seat at the dinner table: How apicomplexan parasites scavenge nutrients from the host. Microorganisms. 2021;**9**(12):2592. DOI: 10.3390/microorganisms9122592

[24] Carter NS et al. Isolation and functional characterization of the PfNT1 nucleoside transporter gene from *Plasmodium falciparum*. The Journal of Biological Chemistry. 2000;**275**(14):10683-10691. DOI: 10.1074/jbc.275.14.10683

[25] Quashie NB, Ranford-Cartwright LC, de Koning HP. Uptake of purines in *Plasmodium falciparum*-infected human erythrocytes is mostly mediated by the human equilibrative nucleoside transporter and the human facilitative nucleobase transporter. Malaria Journal. 2010;**9**:36. DOI: 10.1186/1475-2875-9-36

[26] Frame IJ, Merino EF, Schramm VL, Cassera MB, Akabas MH. Malaria parasite type 4 equilibrative nucleoside transporters (ENT4) are purine transporters with distinct substrate specificity. Biochemical Journal. 2012;**446**(2):179-190. DOI: 10.1042/BJ20112220

[27] Kirk K, Lehane AM. Membrane transport in the malaria parasite and its host erythrocyte. Biochemical Journal. 2014;**457**(1):1-18. DOI: 10.1042/BJ20131007

[28] Downie MJ, Saliba KJ, Howitt SM, Broer S, Kirk K. Transport of nucleosides across the *Plasmodium falciparum* parasite plasma membrane has characteristics of PfENT1. Molecular Microbiology. 2006;**60**(3):738-748. DOI: 10.1111/j.1365-2958.2006.05125.x

[29] Frame IJ et al. Yeast-based high-throughput screen identifies *Plasmodium falciparum* equilibrative nucleoside transporter 1 inhibitors that kill malaria parasites. ACS Chemical Biology. 2015;**10**(3):775-783. DOI: 10.1021/cb500981y

[30] Deniskin R, Frame IJ, Sosa Y, Akabas MH. Targeting the plasmodium vivax equilibrative nucleoside transporter 1 (PvENT1) for antimalarial drug development. International Journal for Parasitology: Drugs and Drug Resistance. 2016;**6**(1):1-11. DOI: 10.1016/j.ijpddr.2015.11.003

[31] Ting LM et al. Targeting a novel *Plasmodium falciparum* purine recycling pathway with specific immucillins.

The Journal of Biological Chemistry. 2005;**280**(10):9547-9554. DOI: 10.1074/jbc.M412693200

[32] Tyler PC, Taylor EA, Frohlich RF, Schramm VL. Synthesis of 5′-methylthio coformycins: Specific inhibitors for malarial adenosine deaminase. Journal of the American Chemical Society. 2007;**129**(21):6872-6879. DOI: 10.1021/ja0708363

[33] Luo M, Singh V, Taylor EA, Schramm VL. Transition-state variation in human, bovine, and *Plasmodium falciparum* adenosine deaminases. Journal of the American Chemical Society. 2007;**129**(25):8008-8017. DOI: 10.1021/ja072122y

[34] Ho MC et al. Structural and metabolic specificity of methylthiocoformycin for malarial adenosine deaminases. Biochemistry. 2009;**48**(40):9618-9626. DOI: 10.1021/bi9012484

[35] Bzowska A, Kulikowska E, Shugar D. Purine nucleoside phosphorylases: Properties, functions, and clinical aspects. Pharmacology & Therapeutics. 2000;**88**(3):349-425. DOI: 10.1016/s0163-7258(00)00097-8

[36] Donaldson TM et al. Structural determinants of the 5′-methylthioinosine specificity of plasmodium purine nucleoside phosphorylase. PLoS ONE. 2014;**9**(1):e84384. DOI: 10.1371/journal.pone.0084384

[37] Köllisch G et al. TLR8 is activated by 5′-methylthioinosine, a Plasmodium falciparum-derived intermediate of the purine salvage pathway. Cell Reports. 2022;**39**(2):110691. DOI: 10.1016/j.celrep.2022.110691

[38] Kicska GA, Tyler PC, Evans GB, Furneaux RH, Kim K, Schramm VL. Transition state analogue inhibitors of purine nucleoside phosphorylase from *Plasmodium falciparum*. The Journal of Biological Chemistry. 2002;**277**(5):3219-3225. DOI: 10.1074/jbc.M105905200

[39] Lewandowicz A, Schramm VL. Transition state analysis for human and *Plasmodium falciparum* purine nucleoside phosphorylases. Biochemistry. 2004;**43**(6):1458-1468. DOI: 10.1021/bi0359123

[40] Ho MC et al. Four generations of transition-state analogues for human purine nucleoside phosphorylase. Proceedings of the National Academy of Sciences of the United States of America. 2010;**107**(11):4805-4812. DOI: 10.1073/pnas.0913439107

[41] Li CM et al. Transition-state analogs as inhibitors of human and malarial hypoxanthine-guanine phosphoribosyltransferases. Nature Structural Biology. 1999;**6**(6):582-587. DOI: 10.1038/9367

[42] Evans GB, Furneaux RH, Lewandowicz A, Schramm VL, Tyler PC. Synthesis of second-generation transition state analogues of human purine nucleoside phosphorylase. Journal of Medicinal Chemistry. 2003;**46**(24):5271-5276. DOI: 10.1021/jm030305z

[43] Evans GB, Furneaux RH, Tyler PC, Schramm VL. Synthesis of a transition state analogue inhibitor of purine nucleoside phosphorylase via the Mannich reaction. Organic Letters. 2003;**5**(20):3639-3640. DOI: 10.1021/ol035293q

[44] Ducati RG et al. Genetic resistance to purine nucleoside phosphorylase inhibition in *Plasmodium falciparum*. Proceedings of the National Academy of Sciences of the United States of America.

2018;**115**(9):2114-2119. DOI: 10.1073/pnas.1525670115

[45] Kicska GA, Tyler PC, Evans GB, Furneaux RH, Schramm VL, Kim K. Purine-less death in *Plasmodium falciparum* induced by immucillin-H, a transition state analogue of purine nucleoside phosphorylase. The Journal of Biological Chemistry. 2002;**277**(5):3226-3231. DOI: 10.1074/jbc.M105906200

[46] Madrid DC, Ting LM, Waller KL, Schramm VL, Kim K. *Plasmodium falciparum* purine nucleoside phosphorylase is critical for viability of malaria parasites. The Journal of Biological Chemistry. 2008;**283**(51):35899-35907. DOI: 10.1074/jbc.M807218200

[47] Bantia S, Kilpatrick JM. Purine nucleoside phosphorylase inhibitors in T-cell malignancies. Current Opinion in Drug Discovery & Development. 2004;7(2):243-247. [Online]. Available from: https://www.ncbi.nlm.nih.gov/pubmed/15603259

[48] Kicska GA et al. Immucillin H, a powerful transition-state analog inhibitor of purine nucleoside phosphorylase, selectively inhibits human T lymphocytes. Proceedings of the National Academy of Sciences of the United States of America. 2001;**98**:4593-4598, 4598. DOI: 10.1073/pnas.071050798

[49] Cassera MB et al. Plasmodium falciparum parasites are killed by a transition state analogue of purine nucleoside phosphorylase in a primate animal model. PLoS ONE. 2011;**6**(11):e26916. DOI: 10.1371/journal.pone.0026916

[50] Evans GB, Tyler PC, Schramm VL. Immucillins in infectious diseases. ACS Infectious Diseases. 2018;**4**(2):107-117. DOI: 10.1021/acsinfecdis.7b00172

[51] Cheviet T, Lefebvre-Tournier I, Wein S, Peyrottes S. Plasmodium purine metabolism and its inhibition by nucleoside and nucleotide analogues. Journal of Medicinal Chemistry. 2019;**62**(18):8365-8391. DOI: 10.1021/acs.jmedchem.9b00182

[52] Keough DT, Ng AL, Winzor DJ, Emmerson BT, de Jersey J. Purification and characterization of *Plasmodium falciparum* hypoxanthine-guanine-xanthine phosphoribosyltransferase and comparison with the human enzyme. Molecular and Biochemical Parasitology. 1999;**98**(1):29-41. DOI: 10.1016/s0166-6851(98)00139-x

[53] Moffatt BA, Ashihara H. Purine and pyrimidine nucleotide synthesis and metabolism. Arabidopsis Book. 2002;**1**:e0018. DOI: 10.1199/tab. 0018

[54] Leung HB, Schramm VL. The role of adenosine monophosphate nucleosidase in the regulation of adenine nucleotide levels in Azotobacter vinelandii during aerobic-anaerobic transitions. Archives of Biochemistry and Biophysics. 1978;**190**(1):46-56. DOI: 10.1016/0003-9861(78)90252-7

[55] Reyes P, Rathod PK, Sanchez DJ, Mrema JE, Rieckmann KH, Heidrich HG. Enzymes of purine and pyrimidine metabolism from the human malaria parasite, *Plasmodium falciparum*. Molecular and Biochemical Parasitology. 1982;**5**(5):275-290. DOI: 10.1016/0166-6851(82)90035-4

[56] Furuhashi M. New insights into purine metabolism in metabolic diseases: Role of xanthine oxidoreductase activity. American Journal of Physiology. Endocrinology and Metabolism. 2020;**319**(5):E827-E834. DOI: 10.1152/ajpendo.00378.2020

[57] Roy S, Nagappa LK, Prahladarao VS, Balaram H. Kinetic mechanism

of *Plasmodium falciparum* hypoxanthine-guanine-xanthine phosphoribosyltransferase. Molecular and Biochemical Parasitology. 2015;**204**(2):111-120. DOI: 10.1016/j.molbiopara.2016.02.006

[58] Roy S, Karmakar T, Prahlada Rao VS, Nagappa LK, Balasubramanian S, Balaram H. Slow ligand-induced conformational switch increases the catalytic rate in plasmodium falciparum hypoxanthine guanine xanthine phosphoribosyltransferase. Molecular Biosystems. 2015;**11**(5):1410-1424. DOI: 10.1039/c5mb00136f

[59] Makobongo MO et al. The purine salvage enzyme hypoxanthine guanine xanthine phosphoribosyl transferase is a major target antigen for cell-mediated immunity to malaria. Proceedings of the National Academy of Sciences of the United States of America. 2003;**100**(5):2628-2633. DOI: 10.1073/pnas.0337629100

[60] Keough DT et al. Inhibition of hypoxanthine-guanine phosphoribosyltransferase by acyclic nucleoside phosphonates: A new class of antimalarial therapeutics. Journal of Medicinal Chemistry. 2009;**52**(14): 4391-4399. DOI: 10.1021/jm900267n

[61] Ducati RG, Firestone RS, Schramm VL. Kinetic isotope effects and transition state structure for hypoxanthine-guanine-xanthine phosphoribosyltransferase from *Plasmodium falciparum*. Biochemistry. 2017;**56**(48):6368-6376. DOI: 10.1021/acs.biochem.7b01027

[62] Keough DT et al. Acyclic nucleoside phosphonates containing a second phosphonate group are potent inhibitors of 6-oxopurine phosphoribosyltransferases and have antimalarial activity. Journal of Medicinal Chemistry. 2013;**56**(6): 2513-2526. DOI: 10.1021/jm301893b

[63] Keough DT et al. Aza-acyclic nucleoside phosphonates containing a second phosphonate group as inhibitors of the human, Plasmodium falciparum and vivax 6-oxopurine phosphoribosyltransferases and their prodrugs as antimalarial agents. Journal of Medicinal Chemistry. 2015;**58**(2): 827-846. DOI: 10.1021/jm501416t

[64] Clinch K et al. Acyclic phosph(on)ate inhibitors of Plasmodium falciparum hypoxanthine-guanine-xanthine phosphoribosyltransferase. Bioorganic & Medicinal Chemistry. 2013;**21**(17):5629-5646. DOI: 10.1016/j.bmc.2013.02.016

[65] Hazleton KZ et al. Acyclic immucillin phosphonates: Second-generation inhibitors of Plasmodium falciparum hypoxanthine-guanine-xanthine phosphoribosyltransferase. Chemistry & Biology. 2012;**19**(6):721-730. DOI: 10.1016/j.chembiol.2012.04.012

[66] Hockova D et al. Antimalarial activity of prodrugs of N-branched acyclic nucleoside phosphonate inhibitors of 6-oxopurine phosphoribosyltransferases. Bioorganic & Medicinal Chemistry. 2015;**23**(17):5502-5510. DOI: 10.1016/j.bmc.2015.07.038

[67] Bhatia HK, Singh H, Grewal N, Natt NK. Sofosbuvir: A novel treatment option for chronic hepatitis C infection. Journal of Pharmacology and Pharmacotherapeutics. 2014;**5**(4): 278-284. DOI: 10.4103/0976-500X.142464

[68] Bhat JY, Shastri BG, Balaram H. Kinetic and biochemical characterization of Plasmodium falciparum GMP synthetase. Biochemical Journal. 2008;**409**(1):263-273. DOI: 10.1042/BJ20070996

[69] Hedstrom L. IMP dehydrogenase: Structure, mechanism, and inhibition. Chemical Reviews. 2009;**109**(7): 2903-2928. DOI: 10.1021/cr900021w

[70] Fotie J. Inosine 5'-monophosphate dehydrogenase (IMPDH) as a potential target for the development of a new generation of Antiprotozoan agents. Mini Reviews in Medicinal Chemistry. 2018;**18**(8):656-671. DOI: 10.2174/138955 7516666160620065558

[71] Ballut L et al. Active site coupling in Plasmodium falciparum GMP synthetase is triggered by domain rotation. Nature Communications. 2015;**6**:8930. DOI: 10.1038/ncomms9930

[72] Veletzky L et al. In vitro activity of immunosuppressive drugs against *Plasmodium falciparum*. Malaria Journal. 2014;**13**:476. DOI: 10.1186/1475-2875-13-476

[73] Mogire RM et al. Target-similarity search using *Plasmodium falciparum* proteome identifies approved drugs with anti-malarial activity and their possible targets. PLoS ONE. 2017;**12**(10):e0186364. DOI: 10.1371/ journal.pone.0186364

[74] Webster HK, Whaun JM. Antimalarial properties of bredinin. Prediction based on identification of differences in human host-parasite purine metabolism. The Journal of Clinical Investigation. 1982;**70**(2): 461-469. DOI: 10.1172/jci110636

[75] Park MH, Igarashi K. Polyamines and their metabolites as diagnostic markers of human diseases. Biomolecules & Therapeutics. 2013;**21**(1):1-9. DOI: 10.4062/biomolther.2012.097

[76] El Bissati K et al. Novel synthetic polyamines have potent antimalarial activities in vitro and in vivo by decreasing intracellular spermidine and spermine concentrations. Frontiers in Cellular and Infection Microbiology. 2019;**9**:9. DOI: 10.3389/ fcimb.2019.00009

[77] Ramya TN, Surolia N, Surolia A. Polyamine synthesis and salvage pathways in the malaria parasite *Plasmodium falciparum*. Biochemical and Biophysical Research Communications. 2006;**348**(2):579-584. DOI: 10.1016/j. bbrc.2006.07.127

[78] Krungkrai J. Malaria parasite pyrimidine nucleotide metabolism: A promising drug target. Archives of Parasitology. 2017;**1**(1):101

[79] Krungkrai SR, Krungkrai J. Insights into the pyrimidine biosynthetic pathway of human malaria parasite *Plasmodium falciparum* as chemotherapeutic target. Asian Pacific Journal of Tropical Medicine. 2016;**9**(6):525-534. DOI: 10.1016/j. apjtm.2016.04.012

[80] Hyde JE. Exploring the folate pathway in *Plasmodium falciparum*. Acta Tropica. 2005;**94**(3):191-206. DOI: 10.1016/j.actatropica.2005.04.002

[81] Moreno-MorcilloM, Grande-GarciaA, Ruiz-Ramos A, Del Cano-Ochoa F, Boskovic J, Ramon-Maiques S. Structural insight into the core of CAD, the multifunctional protein leading de novo pyrimidine biosynthesis. Structure. 2017;**25**(6):912-923 e5. DOI: 10.1016/j. str.2017.04.012

[82] Asai T, O'Sullivan WJ, Kobayashi M, Gero AM, Yokogawa M, Tatibana M. Enzymes of the de novo pyrimidine biosynthetic pathway in *Toxoplasma gondii*. Molecular and Biochemical Parasitology. 1983;**7**(2):89-100. DOI: 10.1016/0166-6851(83)90037-3

[83] Krungkrai SR et al. Human malaria parasite orotate

phosphoribosyltransferase: Functional expression, characterization of kinetic reaction mechanism and inhibition profile. Molecular and Biochemical Parasitology. 2004;**134**(2):245-255. DOI: 10.1016/j.molbiopara.2003.12.006

[84] Sykes DB. The emergence of dihydroorotate dehydrogenase (DHODH) as a therapeutic target in acute myeloid leukemia. Expert Opinion on Therapeutic Targets. 2018;**22**(11):893-898. DOI: 10.1080/14728222.2018.1536748

[85] Singh A, Maqbool M, Mobashir M, Hoda N. Dihydroorotate dehydrogenase: A drug target for the development of antimalarials. European Journal of Medicinal Chemistry. 2017;**125**:640-651. DOI: 10.1016/j.ejmech.2016.09.085

[86] White J et al. Identification and mechanistic understanding of dihydroorotate dehydrogenase point mutations in *Plasmodium falciparum* that confer in vitro resistance to the clinical candidate DSM265. ACS Infectious Diseases. 2019;**5**(1):90-101. DOI: 10.1021/acsinfecdis.8b00211

[87] Phillips MA et al. A long-duration dihydroorotate dehydrogenase inhibitor (DSM265) for prevention and treatment of malaria. Science Translational Medicine. 2015;**7**(296):296ra111. DOI: 10.1126/scitranslmed.aaa6645

[88] Gujjar R et al. Lead optimization of aryl and aralkyl amine-based triazolopyrimidine inhibitors of *Plasmodium falciparum* dihydroorotate dehydrogenase with antimalarial activity in mice. Journal of Medicinal Chemistry. 2011;**54**(11):3935-3949. DOI: 10.1021/jm200265b

[89] Baldwin J et al. High-throughput screening for potent and selective inhibitors of Plasmodium falciparum dihydroorotate dehydrogenase. The Journal of Biological Chemistry. 2005;**280**(23):21847-21853. DOI: 10.1074/jbc.M501100200

[90] Phillips MA et al. A triazolopyrimidine-based dihydroorotate dehydrogenase inhibitor with improved drug-like properties for treatment and prevention of malaria. ACS Infectious Diseases. 2016;**2**(12):945-957. DOI: 10.1021/acsinfecdis.6b00144

[91] Dickerman BK et al. Identification of inhibitors that dually target the new permeability pathway and dihydroorotate dehydrogenase in the blood stage of *Plasmodium falciparum*. Scientific Reports. 2016;**6**:37502. DOI: 10.1038/srep37502

[92] Pavadai E, El Mazouni F, Wittlin S, de Kock C, Phillips MA, Chibale K. Identification of new human malaria parasite *Plasmodium falciparum* dihydroorotate dehydrogenase inhibitors by pharmacophore and structure-based virtual screening. Journal of Chemical Information and Modeling. 2016;**56**(3):548-562. DOI: 10.1021/acs.jcim.5b00680

[93] Guler JL, White J 3rd, Phillips MA, Rathod PK. Atovaquone tolerance in *Plasmodium falciparum* parasites selected for high-level resistance to a dihydroorotate dehydrogenase inhibitor. Antimicrobial Agents and Chemotherapy. 2015;**59**(1):686-689. DOI: 10.1128/AAC.02347-14

[94] Llanos-Cuentas A et al. Antimalarial activity of single-dose DSM265, a novel plasmodium dihydroorotate dehydrogenase inhibitor, in patients with uncomplicated *Plasmodium falciparum* or *Plasmodium vivax* malaria infection: A proof-of-concept, open-label, phase 2a study. The Lancet Infectious Diseases.

2018;**18**(8):874-883. DOI: 10.1016/S1473-3099(18)30309-8

[95] Luth MR, Winzeler EA. SnapShot: Antimalarial drugs. Cell. 2020;**183**(2):554-554 e1. DOI: 10.1016/j.cell.2020.09.006

[96] Suchi M et al. Molecular cloning of the human UMP synthase gene and characterization of point mutations in two hereditary orotic aciduria families. American Journal of Human Genetics. 1997;**60**(3):525-539. [Online]. Available from: https://www.ncbi.nlm.nih.gov/pubmed/9042911; https://www.ncbi.nlm.nih.gov/pmc/articles/PMC1712531/pdf/ajhg00003-0063.pdf

[97] Paojinda P, Imprasittichai W, Krungkrai SR, Palacpac NMQ, Horii T, Krungkrai J. Bifunctional activity of fused *Plasmodium falciparum* orotate phosphoribosyltransferase and orotidine 5′-monophosphate decarboxylase. Parasitology International. 2018;**67**(1):79-84. DOI: 10.1016/j.parint.2017.04.003

[98] Krungkrai SR, Prapunwattana P, Horii T, Krungkrai J. Orotate phosphoribosyltransferase and orotidine 5′-monophosphate decarboxylase exist as multienzyme complex in human malaria parasite *Plasmodium falciparum*. Biochemical and Biophysical Research Communications. 2004;**318**(4):1012-1018. DOI: 10.1016/j.bbrc.2004.04.124

[99] Scott HV, Gero AM, O'Sullivan WJ. In vitro inhibition of *Plasmodium falciparum* by pyrazofurin, an inhibitor of pyrimidine biosynthesis de novo. Molecular and Biochemical Parasitology. 1986;**18**(1):3-15. DOI: 10.1016/0166-6851(86)90045-9

[100] Rathod PK, Khatri A, Hubbert T, Milhous WK. Selective activity of 5-fluoroorotic acid against *Plasmodium falciparum* in vitro. Antimicrobial Agents and Chemotherapy. 1989;**33**(7):1090-1094. DOI: 10.1128/AAC.33.7.1090

[101] Rathod PK, Leffers NP, Young RD. Molecular targets of 5-fluoroorotate in the human malaria parasite, *Plasmodium falciparum*. Antimicrobial Agents and Chemotherapy. 1992;**36**(4):704-711. DOI: 10.1128/AAC.36.4.704

[102] Zhang Y, Luo M, Schramm VL. Transition states of *Plasmodium falciparum* and human orotate phosphoribosyltransferases. Journal of the American Chemical Society. 2009;**131**(13):4685-4694. DOI: 10.1021/ja808346y

[103] Zhang Y et al. Transition state analogues of *Plasmodium falciparum* and human orotate phosphoribosyltransferases. The Journal of Biological Chemistry. 2013;**288**(48):34746-34754. DOI: 10.1074/jbc.M113.521955

[104] Miller BG, Wolfenden R. Catalytic proficiency: The unusual case of OMP decarboxylase. Annual Review of Biochemistry. 2002;**71**:847-885. DOI: 10.1146/annurev.biochem.71.110601.135446

[105] Callahan BP, Miller BG. OMP decarboxylase—An enigma persists. Bioorganic Chemistry. 2007;**35**(6):465-469. DOI: 10.1016/j.bioorg.2007.07.004

[106] Imprasittichail W, Roytrakul S, Krungkrai SR, Krungkrail J. A unique insertion of low complexity amino acid sequence underlies protein-protein interaction in human malaria parasite orotate phosphoribosyltransferase and orotidine 5′-monophosphate decarboxylase. Asian Pacific Journal of Tropical Medicine. 2014;**7**(3):184-192. DOI: 10.1016/S1995-7645(14)60018-3

[107] Krungkrai SR et al. A novel enzyme complex of orotate phosphoribosyltransferase and orotidine 5′-monophosphate decarboxylase in human malaria parasite *Plasmodium falciparum*: Physical association, kinetics, and inhibition characterization. Biochemistry. 2005;**44**(5):1643-1652. DOI: 10.1021/bi048439h

[108] Langley DB et al. Structure and inhibition of orotidine 5′-monophosphate decarboxylase from *Plasmodium falciparum*. Biochemistry. 2008;**47**(12):3842-3854. DOI: 10.1021/bi702390k

[109] Shuvalov O, Petukhov A, Daks A, Fedorova O, Vasileva E, Barlev NA. One-carbon metabolism and nucleotide biosynthesis as attractive targets for anticancer therapy. Oncotarget. 2017;**8**(14):23955-23977. DOI: 10.18632/oncotarget.15053

[110] Antosiewicz A et al. Human dihydrofolate reductase and thymidylate synthase form a complex in vitro and co-localize in normal and cancer cells. Journal of Biomolecular Structure & Dynamics. 2017;**35**(7):1474-1490. DOI: 10.1080/07391102.2016.1186560

[111] Meek TD, Garvey EP, Santi DV. Purification and characterization of the bifunctional thymidylate synthetase-dihydrofolate reductase from methotrexate-resistant Leishmania tropica. Biochemistry. 1985;**24**(3): 678-686. DOI: 10.1021/bi00324a021

[112] Chaianantakul N, Sirawaraporn R, Sirawaraporn W. Insights into the role of the junctional region of Plasmodium falciparum dihydrofolate reductase-thymidylate synthase. Malaria Journal. 2013;**12**(91). DOI: 10.1186/1475-2875-12-91

[113] Reynolds MG, Roos DS. A biochemical and genetic model for parasite resistance to antifolates. *Toxoplasma gondii* provides insights into pyrimethamine and cycloguanil resistance in *Plasmodium falciparum*. The Journal of Biological Chemistry. 1998;**273**(6):3461-3469. DOI: 10.1074/jbc.273.6.3461

[114] Chulay JD, Watkins WM, Sixsmith DG. Synergistic antimalarial activity of pyrimethamine and sulfadoxine against *Plasmodium falciparum* in vitro. The American Journal of Tropical Medicine and Hygiene. 1984;**33**(3):325-330. DOI: 10.4269/ajtmh.1984.33.325

[115] Deloron P, Bertin G, Briand V, Massougbodji A, Cot M. Sulfadoxine/pyrimethamine intermittent preventive treatment for malaria during pregnancy. Emerging Infectious Diseases. 2010;**16**(11):1666-1670. DOI: 10.3201/eid1611.101064

[116] Sibley CH et al. Pyrimethamine-sulfadoxine resistance in *Plasmodium falciparum*: What next? Trends in Parasitology. 2001;**17**(12):582-588. DOI: 10.1016/s1471-4922(01)02085-2

[117] Srivastava IK, Vaidya AB. A mechanism for the synergistic antimalarial action of atovaquone and proguanil. Antimicrobial Agents and Chemotherapy. 1999;**43**(6):1334-1339. DOI: 10.1128/AAC.43.6.1334

[118] Bilsland E et al. Plasmodium dihydrofolate reductase is a second enzyme target for the antimalarial action of triclosan. Scientific Reports. 2018;**8**(1):1038. DOI: 10.1038/s41598-018-19549-x

[119] Tarnchompoo B et al. Hybrid inhibitors of malarial dihydrofolate reductase with dual binding modes that can forestall resistance. ACS Medicinal

Chemistry Letters. 2018;**9**(12):1235-1240. DOI: 10.1021/acsmedchemlett.8b00389

[120] Kamchonwongpaisan S et al. Flexible diaminodihydrotriazine inhibitors of *Plasmodium falciparum* dihydrofolate reductase: Binding strengths, modes of binding and their antimalarial activities. European Journal of Medicinal Chemistry. 2020;**195**:112263. DOI: 10.1016/j.ejmech.2020.112263

[121] Hoarau M, Vanichtananankul J, Srimongkolpithak N, Vitsupakorn D, Yuthavong Y, Kamchonwongpaisan S. Discovery of new non-pyrimidine scaffolds as *Plasmodium falciparum* DHFR inhibitors by fragment-based screening. Journal of Enzyme Inhibition and Medicinal Chemistry. 2021;**36**(1):198-206. DOI: 10.1080/14756366.2020.1854244

[122] Chaianantakul N, Sungkapong T, Supatip J, Kingsang P, Kamlaithong S, Suwanakitti N. Antimalarial effect of cell penetrating peptides derived from the junctional region of *Plasmodium falciparum* dihydrofolate reductase-thymidylate synthase. Peptides. 2020;**131**:170372. DOI: 10.1016/j.peptides.2020.170372

[123] Schramm VL, Horenstein BA, Kline PC. Transition state analysis and inhibitor design for enzymatic reactions. Journal of Biological Chemistry. 1994;**269**(28):18259-18262. [Online]. Available from: https://www.ncbi.nlm.nih.gov/pubmed/8034566; http://www.jbc.org/content/269/28/18259.full.pdf

[124] Schramm VL. Enzymatic transition states and transition state analog design. Annual Review of Biochemistry. 1998;**67**:693-720. DOI: 10.1146/annurev.biochem.67.1.693

[125] Schramm VL. Enzymatic transition states and transition state analogues. Current Opinion in Structural Biology. 2005;**15**(6):604-613. DOI: 10.1016/j.sbi.2005.10.017

[126] Schramm VL. Enzymatic transition states: Thermodynamics, dynamics and analogue design. Archives of Biochemistry and Biophysics. 2005;**433**(1):13-26. DOI: 10.1016/j.abb.2004.08.035

[127] Schramm VL. Transition states and transition state analogue interactions with enzymes. Accounts of Chemical Research. 2015;**48**(4):1032-1039. DOI: 10.1021/acs.accounts.5b00002

[128] Schramm VL. Transition states, analogues, and drug development. ACS Chemical Biology. 2013;**8**(1):71-81. DOI: 10.1021/cb300631k

[129] Schramm VL. Enzymatic transition state theory and transition state analogue design. The Journal of Biological Chemistry. 2007;**282**(39):28297-28300. DOI: 10.1074/jbc.R700018200

[130] Julander JG et al. An update on the progress of galidesivir (BCX4430), a broad-spectrum antiviral. Antiviral Research. 2021;**195**:105180. DOI: 10.1016/j.antiviral.2021.105180

[131] Thomson JM, Lamont IL. Nucleoside analogues as antibacterial agents. Frontiers in Microbiology. 2019;**10**:952. DOI: 10.3389/fmicb.2019.00952

[132] Gebre ST, Cameron SA, Li L, Babu YS, Schramm VL. Intracellular rebinding of transition-state analogues provides extended in vivo inhibition lifetimes on human purine nucleoside phosphorylase. The Journal of Biological Chemistry. 2017;**292**(38):15907-15915. DOI: 10.1074/jbc.M117.801779

[133] Tse EG, Korsik M, Todd MH. The past, present and future of

anti-malarial medicines. Malaria Journal. 2019;**18**(1):93. DOI: 10.1186/s12936-019-2724-z

[134] Klein EY. Antimalarial drug resistance: A review of the biology and strategies to delay emergence and spread. International Journal of Antimicrobial Agents. 2013;**41**(4):311-317. DOI: 10.1016/j.ijantimicag.2012.12.007

[135] Dondorp AM et al. Artemisinin resistance in *Plasmodium falciparum* malaria. The New England Journal of Medicine. 2009;**361**(5):455-467. DOI: 10.1056/NEJMoa0808859

[136] Taylor SM, Juliano JJ, Meshnick SR. Artemisinin resistance in *Plasmodium falciparum* malaria. The New England Journal of Medicine. 2009;**361**(18):1807. DOI: 10.1056/NEJMc091737. author reply 1808

[137] Minnow YVT, Harijan RK, Schramm VL. A resistant mutant of plasmodium falciparum purine nucleoside phosphorylase uses wild-type neighbors to maintain parasite survival. The Journal of Biological Chemistry. 2021;**296**:100342. DOI: 10.1016/j.jbc.2021.100342

Chapter 12

Antioxidant Efficacy of Selected Plant Extracts Debilitates the *Plasmodium* Invasion through Erythrocytic Membrane Stabilisation - An *In Vitro* Study

Urja Joshi, Dhara Jani, Linz-Bouy George and Hyacinth Highland

Abstract

Most dangerous and prevalent form of malaria is caused by the *Plasmodium falciparum* mediated malaria and poses the greatest threat to the humans. Emergence of multi drug resistant parasite hindered the prevention of malaria burden worldwide. This study is mainly focused on the erythrocytic membrane stabilisation using regionally available medicinal plant extracts and its corelation with the oxidative stress generated during the intracellular erythrocytic stages development of *Plasmodia*. The results disclosed that antioxidant potential of the medicinal plants can diminish the reactive oxygen species generation leads to restrict the plasmodial invasion into erythrocytes ultimately decreases the parasitic load. Hence, the evidence of the effective phytochemicals present in the selected medicinal plants can be the promising anti-plasmodial drug candidates as a future perspective.

Keywords: *Plasmodium falciparum*, erythrocytic membrane stabilisation, antioxidant activity, anti-plasmodial activity, oxidative stress

1. Introduction

The burden of malaria is still felt worldwide and caused by Apicomplexa parasite *Plasmodium* spp., in which, *Plasmodium falciparum (P. falciparum)* primarily causes severe malaria and remains the leading cause of morbidity and mortality worldwide. According to World Health Organisation (WHO), 241 million cases of malaria and 627,000 deaths were reported globally in 2022 [1] in which the WHO African Region has consistently reported a significant portion of the worldwide malaria burden. Moreover, Malaria cases in the WHO South-East Asia Region dropped significantly and made up roughly 2% (5 million cases in 2020) of all malaria cases worldwide [1]. Still, more than 4,00,000 people around the world killed due to malaria every year [2, 3]. It mostly occurs due to the delay in treating *P. falciparum* caused malaria.

Plasmodia requires at least two hosts a) Female *Anopheles* mosquitoes – for sexual cycle b) Human beings – for asexual cycle, to accomplish its life cycle. It infects in form of sporozoites via female *Anopheles* mosquitoes' bites enters the human being, within 60 mins it invades hepatocytes via circulatory system [4]. Eventually sporozoites matures and complete its pre erythrocytic stages into 6–15 days, which is clinically remains silent, and leave the liver in form of merozoites and enters the circulation to invade erythrocytes [4]. During erythrocytic stages, merozoites develop into (trophozoites – ring stages – schizonts - merozoites) in <48 hrs and on the time of maturation thousand of merozoites leave that erythrocyte to infect new erythrocytes. Bursting of erythrocytes into circulation onset the progression of symptoms including chills, fever, headache, etc. associated with malaria [5]. Severe malaria includes the series of complications include cytoadherence, and sequestration found in *Plasmodium falciparum* infected erythrocytes (*Pf*-iEs) leads to unregulated inflammatory processes, sequestration, coma, severe anaemia, multiple organ dysfunctionality and cerebral malaria like complications in vital organs [5]. In addition, mortality rates in *P. falciparum* caused malaria remained elevated mainly in pregnant women, young children >5 years, etc. [6]. Although the availability of wide spectrum of anti-malarial drugs in the markets, emergence of drug resistant of malaria parasite especially of *P. falciparum* has created an urgent demand for newer, more efficacious, anti-plasmodial agents, with minimal side effects. The search for a safe, efficient treatment agent for the control and management of this dreadful disease may perhaps now have an answer thanks to several plant extracts and formulations that are highly concentrated in powerful phytochemicals. According to estimates from the WHO, 80% of people rely on herbal remedies as their primary form of healthcare. Around 21,000 plant species have the potential to be used as medical plants, according to the WHO [7]. The prophylactic anti-malarial medication derived from medicinal plants is one possible source since certain secondary plant compounds have a significant potential for cell-cell and cell-molecular interactions [8]. Natural products have been essential in the discovery and development of new medications for a long time since plant primary and secondary metabolites have significant biological functions [9].

Here, two medicinal plants:

1. *Lantana camara* L. (*L. camara*), generally known as wild or red sage has been extensively studied for its phytochemical composition in last few decades and belongs to the Verbenaceae family [10]. It is used in the treatment of cancer, chicken pox, measles, asthma, ulcers, swellings, high blood pressure, rheumatism, and other conditions due to its active phytochemicals and components [11, 12]. The plant is traditionally used to treat tetanus, epilepsy, diarrhoea, gastropathy, and metabolic process infections and disorders (cough, cold, and bronchitis) [12]. It is also used as a diaphoretic, carminative, antispasmodic agent, tonic, and antiemetic. Infusions of the leaves are used for bilious fever, eczema, and eruptions. Pulverised leaves are used for cuts, wounds, ulcers, and swellings. Protozoal infections, rheumatism, skin rashes, dermatitis, eczema, mycotic infections, tract infections, grippe, and T.B. are all treated with the foundation [13].

2. *Calotropis procera* L (*C. procera*) is a medium-sized tree or spreading shrub belong to the family Apocynaceae. It can be found in areas with excessively drained soil where yearly precipitation can reach up to 2000 mm and in arid

habitats where rainfall is restricted to 150 to 1000 mm, as well it found in typical habitats including roadside sand dunes, seashore dunes, and heavily populated urban areas [14]. *C. procera* possess a wide range of pharmacological activity. Plant part such as root bark, stem bark, leaf, flower, and latex and their extracts, fraction, and isolated compound proved larvicidal, anticancer, acaricidal, schizonticidal, antibacterial, anthelmintic, insecticidal, anti-inflammatory and antidiarrheal special effects [15, 16]. Numerous cardenolides, alkaloids, flavonoids, sterols, organic carbonates, norditerpenic esters, cysteine protease procerain and other chemicals have made this plant a popular subject of study for many years. Although, due to the existence of cardenolides, plants have the potential to be poisonous (cardiac glycosides). Cardenolides were discovered to be most abundant in the latex [17]. According to research, the leaf of this plant consists of cardenolides 162 mg/g at dry weight and 2 mg/g [18].

Recent research indicates that during malarial infections, the concentration of reactive oxygen species (such as superoxide and hydroxyl radicals) rises [19], due to haemoglobin digestion, parasite metabolism and host defense mechanism of the *Pf*-iEs. Reactive oxygen species plays a crucial role in various physiological processes for both host and parasite, as well as overproduction of intracellular ROS attack and damage lipids, proteins, nucleic acids, and integrity of cell membrane, which affects the survival of the cell and induce, the gradual apoptosis by suppressing the specific gene expressions [20]. To maintain the intracellular redox homeostasis parasite activates the machinery includes enzymes like iron-superoxide synthetase (Fe-SOD), glutathione-S-transferase (GST), glutathione synthetase (GS), γ-glutamylcysteine synthetase (γ-GCS), thioredoxin reductase (TrxR), and peroxiredoxins (nPrx) but, it lacks the catalase and glutathione peroxidase [21]. Therefore, it is understood that oxidative stress has a significant clinical and pathological role in malaria infection [22]. In addition, oxidative stress factor is also an effective therapeutic tool for example quinolines and artemisinin act chiefly via the production of ROS but, resistance development against Quinoline and Artemisinin- Based Combination Therapies (ACTs) in Southeast Asia and various regions of Africa over a long-term usage adds more complications in treating *P. falciparum* infected patients [21].

The goal of the current study is to evaluate the antioxidant activity and potential anti-plasmodial activity of the hydro-alcoholic extract of *L. camara* and *C. procera* leaves as well as to investigate how it affects the stabilisation of the erythrocyte membrane and in reducing the oxidative damage that this parasite onslaught caused in erythrocytes.

2. Methods

Traditional antimalarial drugs use Reactive Oxygen Species (ROS), which eventually causes their parasiticidal effects. However, the antimalarial activity mediated by ROS is something that *Plasmodium's* evolutionary dynamism actively works to displace [21]. In light of this, current studies have focused on developing natural medicines to reduce *Plasmodium* infections. The inclusion of several secondary phytochemicals endows *L. camara* L. and *C. procera* L. plant extracts with strong therapeutic capabilities.

To perform the phytochemical extraction from the selected plants (*L. camara* and *C. procera),* the following method has been implemented.

2.1 Plant collection and extraction

Leaves of *L. camara* and *C. procera* were collected from the Gujarat University campus, Ahmedabad, Gujarat. Samples of plant material were authenticated by the Botany Department, Gujarat University, Ahmedabad, India. The plant material was thoroughly cleansed with distilled water, shade dried at ambient temperatures (27–37°C), then manually powdered using a commercial electrical stainless-steel blender. For defattation step, powder was treated with petroleum ether and continuously stirred on a magnetic stirrer for 48 hours. Using a Soxhlet extractor, 20 grammes of defatted powdered plant material were extracted for 72 hours with 200 ml of solvent (hydro-alcoholic: 70:30). At low pressure, the diluted crude solvent that had accumulated in the flask was concentrated. The yield that was obtained after drying was stored at 4°C until use [23].

2.2 *In vitro* cultivation of chloroquine (CQ)-sensitive strain 3D7 of *Plasmodium falciparum*

It is obtained from National Institute Malaria Research (NIMR), New Delhi. Erythrocytic stages were developed to determine the correlation between the anti-plasmodial efficacy of the plant extracts and the reactive oxygen species generated. Asynchronized *P. falciparum* culture was maintained according to the method described by Trager and Jensen [24] with minor modifications.

2.3 Determination of antioxidant activity of the plant extracts by DPPH assay

Both the plant extracts were assessed by the 2, 2-diphenyl-1-picrylhydrazyl (DPPH) to determine its antioxidant activity by scavenging the free radicles as per the method reported by Gyamfi *et al.* [25]. EC50 value of the plant extract was evaluated by the dose response curve using Microsoft Excel.

2.4 *In vitro* study of erythrocyte membrane stabilisation and % inhibition of parasite entry

In many underdeveloped nations today, medicinal plants represent an important part of the traditional healthcare infrastructure. The bioactive chemicals found in these medicinal plants have been used to create several medications since antiquity [26, 27]. This study also suggests that the extract may alter the erythrocyte membrane in a way that renders red blood cells hostile and incompatible as parasite host cells or that it may prevent the parasite from entering the erythrocyte even when extract is not present in the growing media. *L. camara* and *C. procera* extracts are rich in phenolic and flavonoid components [12, 28].

Erythrocyte membrane stabilisation efficacy of the two plant extracts were assessed using the haemolysis method mentioned by Jansen *et al.* [29] and Linz-Buoy *et al.* [28]. In which, control O^{+ve} erythrocytes were resuspended in 10% PBS (v/v) and incubated with crude plant extracts consisting of the range (1000 μg/ml with serial dilution up to 7.18 μg/ml concentration) under agitation for 24 hours at room temperature, this mixture then subjected to centrifugation for 5 minutes at 10,000 x g followed by the absorbance of the supernatants was measured at 550 nm with a microplate reader.

*2.4.1 **In vitro** % inhibition of parasite entry into RBCs*

In vitro percent inhibition of parasite entry into RBCs was calculated as mentioned in Linz-Buoy *et al.*, [12]. For each concentration, growth inhibition was calculated as a percentage of the number of schizonts compared to five untreated controls. Dose-response curves were used to get the mean IC50 values (percentage of schizonts vs. logarithm of drug concentration).

2.5 Oxidative stress parameters

By preventing the emergence of new free radical species, stopping radical chain reactions, changing existing free radicals into less dangerous molecules, and repairing oxidative damage, antioxidants work through protective processes at various levels within cells [30].

2.5.1 Cellular sample preparation

Intracellular ROS: Cells were harvested after 48 hours of incubation at 37°C. Cultured cells were harvested and centrifuged to remove the culture media at 500 g for 10 minutes at 4°C. The pelleted cells were haemolysed in four times volume of ice-cold injection water/1x RBC lysis buffer and centrifuged again at 4°C. This cell lysate was then used to measure intracellular ROS by Metta *et al.* [31] with minor modifications.

2.6 Parameters

2.6.1 Lipid peroxidation (LPO)

The method of Okhawa *et al.* [32] was used to measure the quantities of thiobarbutiric acid reactive species (TBARS) in Control erythrocytes, *Pf*-iEs, and Pre-treated Control erythrocytes with the plant extract.

2.6.2 Superoxide dismutase (SOD)

The NADH-phenazinemethosulphate-nitroblue tetrazolium formazon is the foundation of the superoxide dismutase (SOD) test. The activity of SOD in Control erythrocytes, *Pf*-iEs, and Pre-treated Control erythrocytes with the plant extracts by the method of [33].

2.6.3 Catalase

As hydrogen peroxide is broken down by the enzyme catalase, its UV absorbance at 240 nm can be used in this method to evaluate enzyme activity. The method of Sinha [34] was employed to determine the activity of catalase enzyme in control erythrocytes, *Pf*-iEs, and Pre-treated Control erythrocytes with the plant extracts. By decrease in absorbance, the activity of an enzyme can be calculated.

2.6.4 Reduced glutathione (GSH)

The method outlined by Ellaman *et al.* [35] was used to measure the reduced glutathione (GSH) level. When GSH reacts with DTNB (5, 5′-dithiobis nitro benzoic acid), a yellow compound formed. Control erythrocytes, *Pf*-iEs, and Pre-treated Control erythrocytes with the plant extracts were taken as samples.

2.6.5 Glutathione peroxidase (GPx)

The Rotruck *et al.* [36] method was used to measure the glutathione peroxidase (GPx) enzyme activity in control erythrocytes, *Pf*-iEs, and pre-treated control erythrocytes A cytosolic enzyme called GPx catalyses the conversion of peroxide radicals to alcohols and oxygen as well as the conversion of hydrogen peroxide to water and oxygen.

2.7 %Inhibition of growth proliferation (MTT) assay

3- (4, 5-dimethyl thiazol-2-yl)-2, 5-diphenyl tetrazolium bromide (MTT) Assay is based on the capacity of Mitochondria succinate dehydrogenase dimethyl thiazol-2-yl)-2, 5-diphenyl tetrazolium bromide (MTT) into an insoluble, coloured formazan product which is measured spectrophotometrically at 540 nm [37, 38]. Since reduction of MTT can only occur in metabolically active cells, the level of activity is a measure of the viability/cytotoxicity of the cells.

In vitro confirmations of the toxic effect of the phytocomponents have measured on the HeLa cell lines with 6 serial dilutions from 250 to 0.0156 μg/ml. The formazan crystals were formed, following the reduction of MTT by metabolically active (viable) cells.

2.8 Haemoglobin (Hb) determination

Haemoglobin determination was carried out using a Sahli's hemoglobinometer with standard colour comparator and the final value was recorded as g/dl Haemoglobin content [39]. The amount of Hb of control, *Pf*-iEs and pre-treated erythrocytes is given in **Figure 8**.

3. Results

3.1 Antioxidant activity of the plant extracts by DPPH assay

Antioxidant activity demonstrates the plant extract's ability to scavenge Reactive Oxygen Species (ROS) in a dose-dependent manner. The antioxidant potency of two plant extracts is revealed in this study. Ascorbic acid is used as the standard here (**Figure 1**).

As antioxidants are required to protect cells from oxidative stress, the *L. camara and Calotropis Procera* extracts tested in this study were found to be high in antioxidants *L camara* showed the higher antioxidant activity compared to *C. procera* plant extract, with 85.23% at the highest concentration of 250 g/ml. Linz-Buoy *et al.* [28] demonstrated *in vitro* that this effective antioxidant capability is beneficial in this control.

3.2 *In vitro* erythrocyte membrane stabilisation and % inhibition of parasite entry

The % erythrocyte membrane stabilisation assay with haemolysis (osmotic fragility test) is shown in **Figure 2**. The property of erythrocyte membrane stabilisation is performed in dose dependent manner i.e., from the highest concentration (250 μg/ml to 7.81 μg/ml).

DOI: http://dx.doi.org/10.5772/intechopen.106844

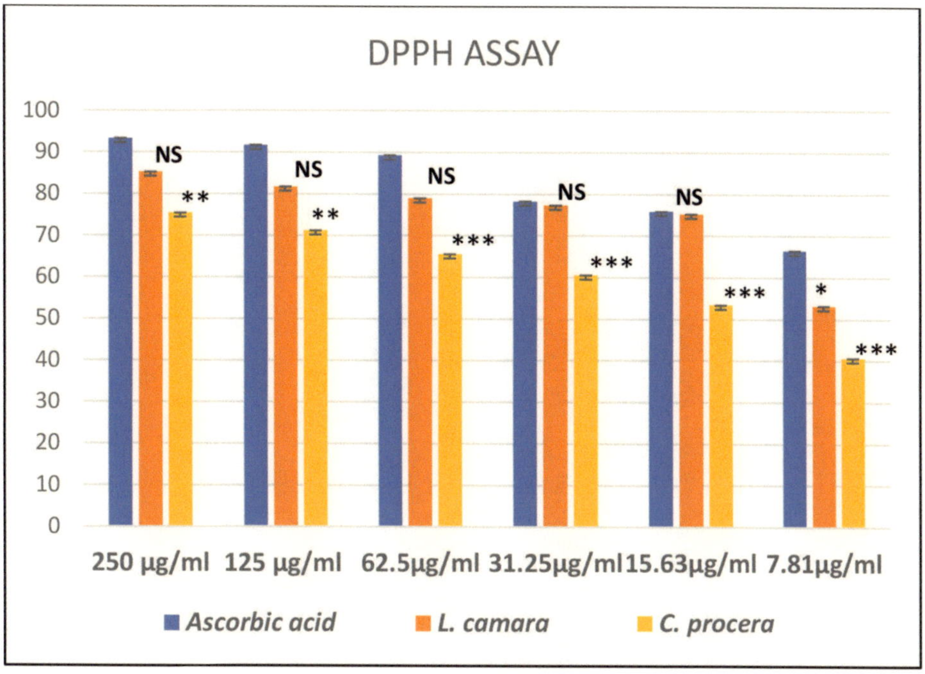

Figure 1.
Bar graph presentation of antioxidant activity of two selected plant's hydro-alcoholic extracts, compared with the standard ascorbic acid. Values are Mean ± S.E. n = 6. ($p<0.01$, ** $p < 0.001$, *** $p <0.0001$).*

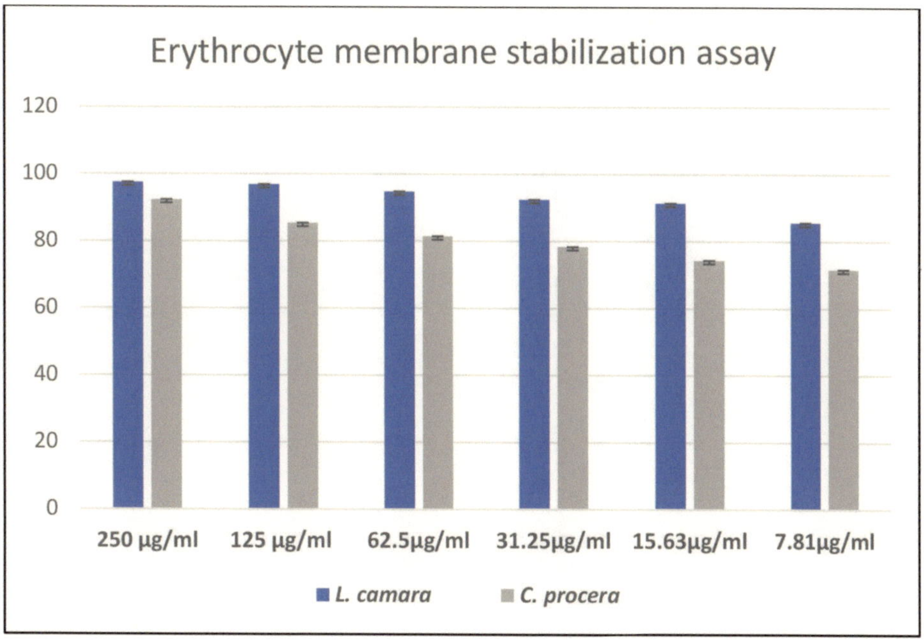

Figure 2.
The % erythrocyte membrane stabilization with haemolytic assay reported via bar graph presentation of selected hydroalcoholic extracts of the two plants (L. camara and C. procera).

MRC-2	Concentration	1.95 µg/ml	3.91 µg/ml	7.81 µg/ml	15.63 µg/ml	31.25 µg/ml	62.5 µg/ml	125 µg/ml	250 µg/ml
% Inhibition	*L. camara* (HA)	41.5 ± 0.09	43 ± 0.12	48 ± 0.05	51.5 ± 0.07	63 ± 0.28	75.5 ± 0.16	86 ± 0.04	86.5 ± 0.21
	C. procera (HA)	26.02 ± 0.23	30.09 ± 0.47	35.65 ± 0.59	45.65 ± 0.63	59.1 ± 1.21	68.23 ± 0.08	81 ± 0.45	83.45 ± 0.23

Table 1.
% Inhibition of entry of P. falciparum MRC-2 strain in pre-treated erythrocytes with hydro-alcoholic extract of L. camara and C. procera. This shows the hydro-alcoholic extract of L. camara and C. procera were assessed for their anti-plasmodial activity. Here, asynchronized culture of P. falciparum MRC-2 were subjected to pre-treated control erythrocytes for 24 hours.

RKL-9	Concentration	1.95 µg/ml	3.91 µg/ml	7.81 µg/ml	15.63 µg/ml	31.25 µg/ml	62.5 µg/ml	125 µg/ml	250 µg/ml
% Inhibition	*L. camara* (HA)	26.02 ± 0.23	30.09 ± 0.47	35.65 ± 0.59	45.65 ± 0.63	59.1 ± 1.21	68.23 ± 0.08	81 ± 0.45	83.45 ± 0.23
	C. procera (HA)	29.5 ± 1.09	35.0 ± 0.19	40.0 ± 0.06	50.0 ± 0.11	52.5 ± 0.21	65.0 ± 0.19	70 ± 0.05	73.5 ± 0.17

Table 2.
% Inhibition of entry of P. falciparum RKL-9 strain in pre-treated erythrocytes with hydro-alcoholic extract of L. camara and C. procera. This shows the hydro-alcoholic extract of L. camara and C. procera were assessed for their anti-plasmodial activity. Here, asynchronized culture of P. falciparum RKL-9 were subjected to pre-treated control erythrocytes for 24 hours.

Only 2.48 percent of the erythrocytes were hemolyzed when treated with the hydroalcoholic extract of *L. camara* at the highest concentration (250 g/ml) used in the study. Pretreatment with *C. procera* hydroalcoholic extracts yielded 7.66 percent at the concentration (250 g/ml).

In the pretreatment of control erythrocytes, haemolysis increases as the crude extract concentration decreases.

3.2.1 % Inhibition of parasite entry

The experimental results of this study showed that pre-treatment of the hydroalcoholic extracts of selected two plants showed anti-plasmodial efficacy for an asynchronized culture of *P. falciparum* MRC2 and RKL-9 (**Tables 1** and **2**).

Among these two plants *L. camara* is found more effective in killing 50% of malaria parasites in the appropriate course of incubation time (24 hours) of the asynchronized parasite of strain MRC-2 and RKL-9 according to the experimental evidence obtained in our study. Among the two plants *L. camara* reported highest antioxidant activity and thus same result reflected in the % erythrocyte membrane stabilisation assays and proves its potent anti-plasmodial activity.

3.3 Oxidative stress parameters

3.3.1 Lipid peroxidation (LPO)

When *Pf*-iEs were compared to control erythrocytes, lipid peroxidation was significantly increased (**Figure 3**). The results also revealed that, when compared to the negative control, pre-treated erythrocytes with the plant extracts had significantly lower levels of lipid peroxidation, as evidenced by higher MDA values.

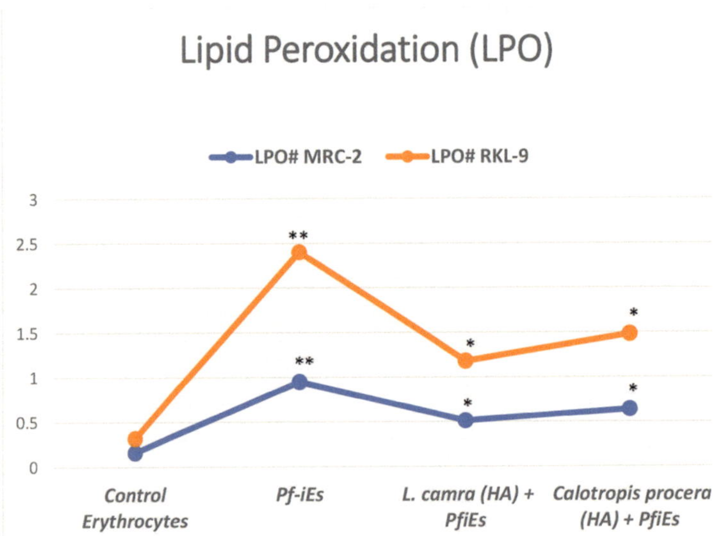

Figure 3.
Showing the lipid peroxidation (TBARS) level in control, infected and pre-treated erythrocytes with the hydroalcoholic extracts of L. camara and C. procera. extract. Values are mean ± S.E. # (×10^4 nmoles of MDA/100mg cells wt/60min).

The results also indicated that there was a significant reduction (** p < 0.001) in lipid peroxidation as indicated by the elevated MDA values, for the control erythrocytes when compared to negative control, were treated with both the extracts when subjected to *Pf-MRC2* and *Pf-RKL9* for 24 hours.

3.3.2 Superoxide dismutase (SOD)

While *Pf*-iEs were compared to control erythrocytes, the activity of superoxide dismutase was found to be significantly lower (p < 0.001). Once control erythrocytes were pre-treated with hydroalcoholic extracts of *L. camara* and *C. procera* and then subjected to *Plasmodium* infection (MRC-2 and RKL-9) for 24 hours, SOD activity increased significantly (**Figure 4**).

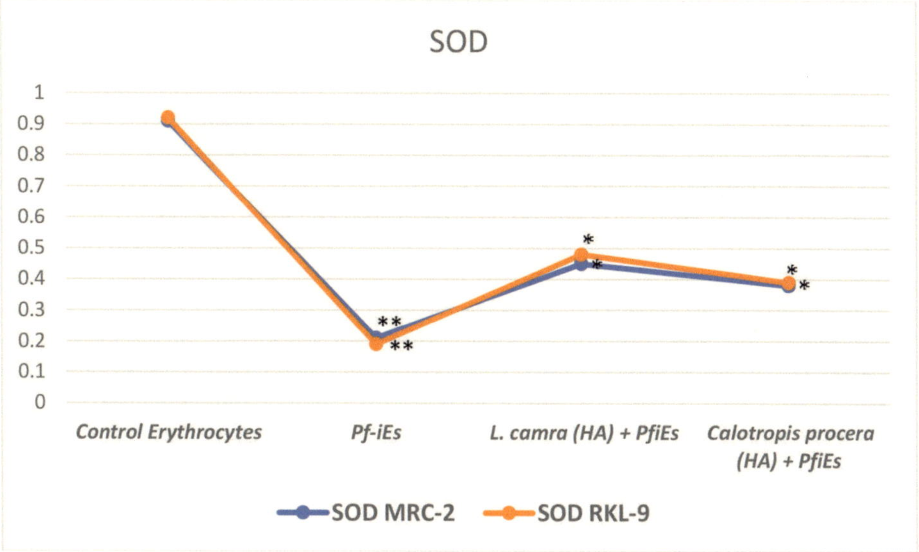

Figure 4.
*SOD enzyme activity in control and Pf-iEs, compared with the pre-treated control erythrocytes with the hydroalcoholic extracts of L. camara and C. procera. The unit of SOD is SOD (units/mg protein). Values are mean ± S.E. ** p < 0.001; * p < 0.01.*

3.3.3 Catalase

The results obtained show that catalase activity significantly decreases with *Plasmodium* infection but, it is significantly improved with the use of plant extracts (**Figure 5**).

3.3.4 Reduced glutathione (GSH)

The study revealed a significant (p < 0.01) increase in reduced glutathione level in the *Pf*-iEs. After pre-treatment with the hydroalcoholic extracts of both the plants, decrease in the GSH level was observed (**Figure 6**).

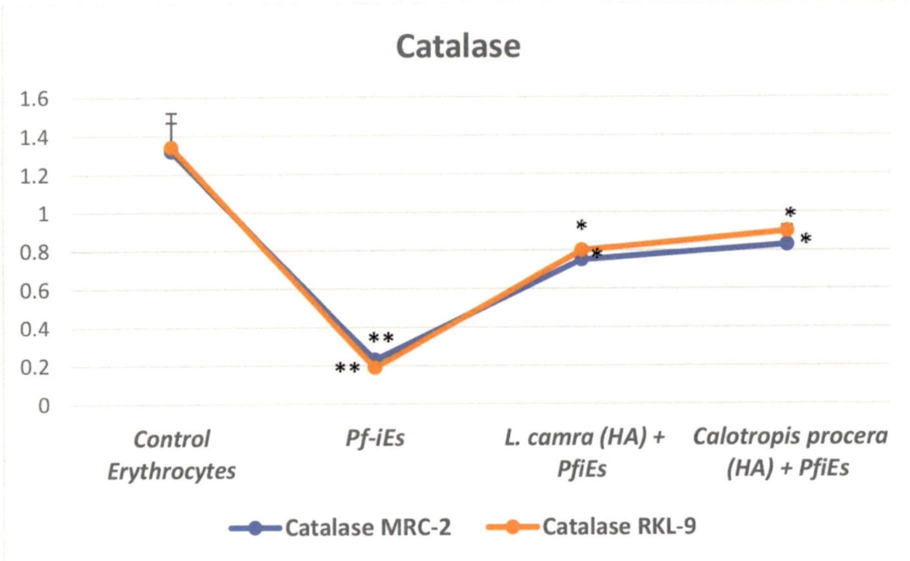

Figure 5.
*Shows the catalase enzyme activity in control erythrocytes, PfMRC-2 and PfRKL-9 infected and treated control erythrocytes with the hydroalcoholic extracts of L. camara and C. procera. Values are mean ± S.E. Unit of catalase activity measured: mmol of H_2O_2 consumed/min/mg protein) ** p < 0.001; * p < 0.01.*

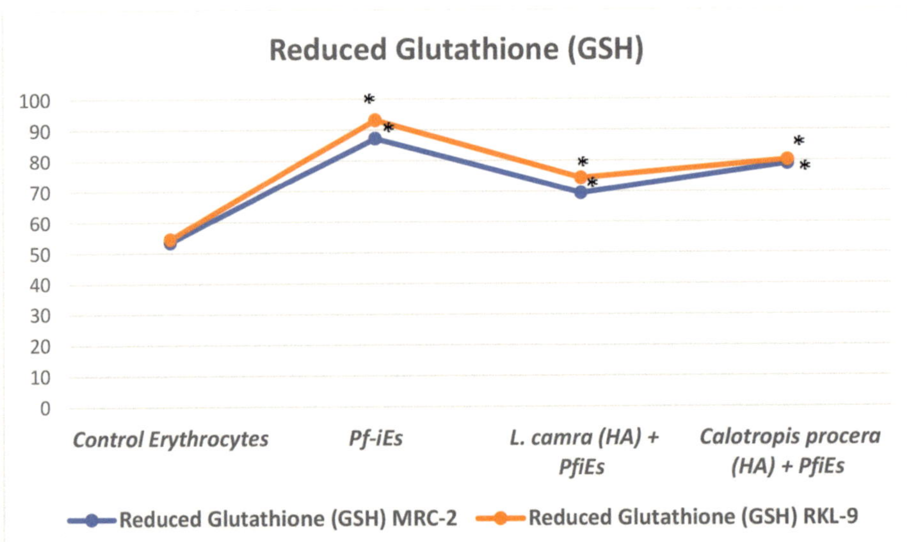

Figure 6.
*Shows the reduced Glutathione content differs during the Plasmodium infection as it increases compared to control erythrocytes but, when pre-treated with hydroalcoholic extracts, decreases the glutathione level. Among two plants L. camara hydroalcoholic extract shows most effective decline. Values are mean ± S.E. * p < 0.01. The unit of GSH measurement (µg/100mg cells weight).*

3.3.5 Glutathione peroxidase (GPx)

The study revealed that the *Plasmodium* infection resulted in a considerable decline in GPx activity. Following the application of the plant extracts via pre-treatment to control erythrocytes, there were noticeable increase seen in the Glutathione peroxidase activity (**Figure 7**).

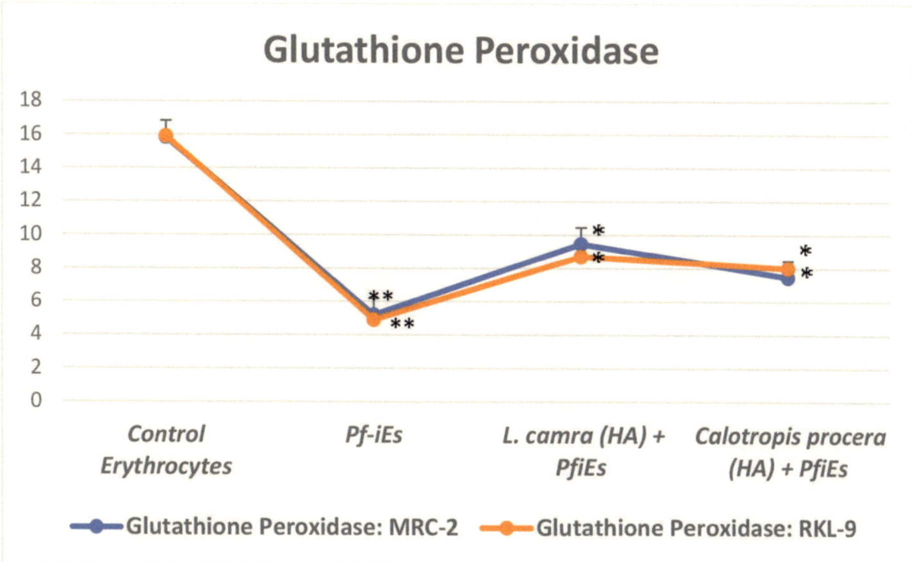

Figure 7.
*Showing GPx enzyme activity in control erythrocytes, Pf-iEs and pre-treated erythrocytes with hydroalcoholic extracts of L. camara and C. procera. Values are mean ± S.E. ** $p < 0.001$.*

3.4 % Inhibition of growth proliferation (MTT) assay

The result decreases of % growth proliferation after pre-treatment with both extracts has tabulated in **Table 3**.

	Concentration of the crude extract of the plants (µg/ml)					
	7.81 µg/ml	15.63 µg/ml	31.25 µg/ml	62.5 µg/ml	125 µg/ml	250 µg/ml
L. camara (HA)	98.12 ± 0.51	96.90 ± 1.24	97.56 ± 0.90	97.88 ± 0.43	97.79 ± 1.09	98.46 ± 0.90
C. procera (HA)	98.08 ± 0.54	97.53 ± 0.77	97.08 ± 1.15	97.17 ± 0.41	97.24 ± 0.67	96.86 ± 1.2

Table 3.
Showing the results of MTT assay in which % growth inhibition of extracts of both L. camara and C. procera on the HeLa cells. In vitro confirmation of the toxic effect of the phytocomponents has measured on the HeLa cell lines with 6 dilutions from 250 to 7.81 µg/ml. The formazan crystals were formed, following the reduction of MTT by metabolically active (viable) cells.

3.5 Haemoglobin (Hb) determination

The highly significant decrease of Hb content has been observed in the infected erythrocytes (iEs). Compared with the control erythrocytes much significant changes in the amount of Hb has not been observed in the pre-treated erythrocytes (**Figure 8**).

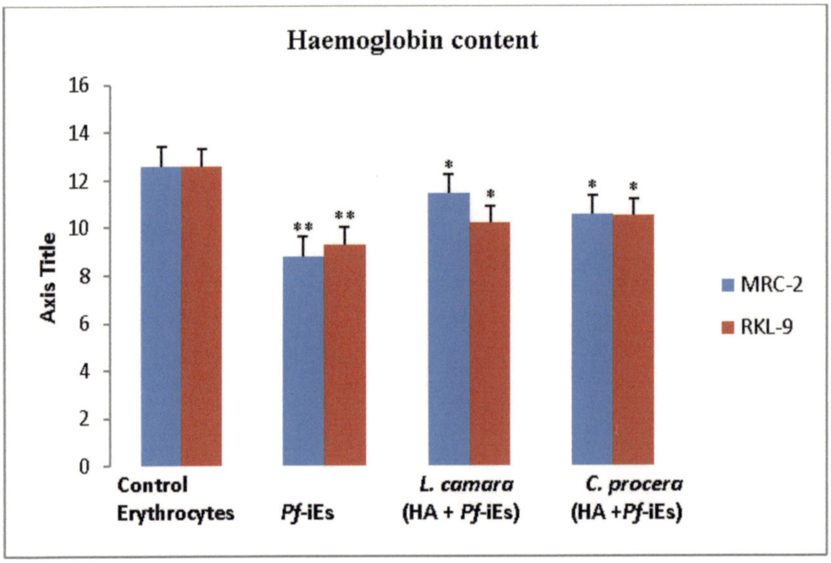

Figure 8.
Showing the haemoglobin content in control, Pf-iEs and pre-treated erythrocytes with plant extracts. Values are Mean ± S.E. $^{*}p<0.01$ $^{**}p<0.001$.

4. Discussion

Membrane stabilising profiles of various extracts of *L. camara* on bovine red blood cells exposed to both heat and hypotonic induced lysis were reported previously [40]. Earlier studies have shown that various herbal drugs can stabilise the red blood cell membrane [41]. The mode of action of the extracts could relate to binding to the erythrocyte membranes with subsequent alteration of the surface charges of the cells. This might have prevented physical interaction with aggregating agents or promote dispersal by mutual repulsion of like charges which are involved in the haemolysis of red blood cells. It has been reported that certain saponins and flavonoids exerted profound stabilising effect on lysosomal membrane both *in vivo* and *in vitro*, while tannins and saponins possess ability to bind cations, there by stabilising erythrocyte membrane and other biological macro molecules [41]. It is not surprising that *P. falciparum* develops resistance to antimalarial medications whose mode of action is dependent on the production of ROS in a shorter amount of time. This shows a common pathway of resistance to the K13 propeller gene mutation, which is supported by the development of artemisinin resistance to novel endoperoxide-based hybrid molecules [42].

The ROS-managing machinery of the parasite could be disrupted to preserve and improve the actions of the antimalarials, ensuring the ongoing relevance of ROS-producing antimalarials [21]. Moreover, aromatic and therapeutic plants make up much of India's natural resources. According to reports, phenolic and flavonoid compounds function as antioxidants to exert anti-allergic, anti-inflammatory, antidiabetic, antimicrobial, antiviral, antithrombotic, and vasodilatory effects. As a result, they may prevent diseases like cancer, cardio-vascular disease, cataract, eye disorders, and Alzheimer's [43, 44].

Free radicals are vital to many metabolic processes and play a crucial role in aerobic metabolism and life. Reactive oxygen species (ROS) have been implicated in mediating oxidative damage to macromolecules such lipids, proteins, and DNA.

Antioxidants protect cells at multiple levels by inhibiting the formation of free radical species, interfering with radical chain reactions, converting existing free radicals into less harmful molecules, and repairing oxidative damage [30]. Flavonoids and phenolic compounds are abundant in *L. camara* extracts [28]. Flavonoids and tannins are most likely responsible for the free radical scavenging effect. Plant phenolic compounds also serve as primary antioxidants.

Becker *et al.* [45] have shown an increase in the lipid peroxidation of *Plasmodium* infected RBCs. Moreover Erel *et al.* [46] have demonstrated that *plasmodia* succeed in accumulating free radical scavenging enzymes within their own cells but deplete them in red blood cells of the host. Polyphenols (flavonoids) have been known to effectively restrict free radical induced peroxidation of lipid. According to [47] in addition to their protein binding and direct scavenging activity, these potent antioxidants interact with membrane lipids and prevent the access of deleterious molecules across the cell membrane. Thus, the infected erythrocytes, treated with the extracts showed decreased lipid peroxidation, due to the potent antioxidant activity of these extracts.

The current study found a highly significant decrease in the erythrocyte antioxidant machinery, superoxide dismutase (SOD), catalase (CAT), and glutathione peroxidase (GPx), indicating the presence of a high amount of ROS. *Plasmodium* erythrocytic stages are subjected to a variety of oxidative stress-inducing events, such as haemoglobin metabolism [48]. *P. falciparum* generates H_2O_2 within RBCs during haemoglobin degradation [45]. Furthermore, the Fenton reaction exposes intra-erythrocytic parasite stages to increased ROS formation [49, 50]. *P. falciparum*-infected erythrocytes produced significantly more hydroxyl (OH) radicals and H_2O_2 than uninfected erythrocytes, according to Atamna and Ginsburg [51]. *Plasmodium* infection was found to cause a significant increase in lipid peroxidation in red blood cells; however, when treated with a hydro-alcoholic extract of *L. camara*, a significant decrease in LPO in infected RBCs was obtained.

SOD activity in *plasmodium*-infected RBCs was significantly lower than in normal RBCs. Several other studies have found a decrease in SOD activities in erythrocytes in malaria patients [52, 53], which supports the findings. This supports its role as an antioxidant, where levels decreased to counteract oxidative stress. The main characteristics of these changes are changes in erythrocyte GSH content, lipid peroxidation levels, and oxidative stress enzymes like SOD, CAT, and GPx. *L. camara and C. procera* extracts were found to be effective enough to overcome this change and return the cell to normalcy as a result, the *L. camara and C. procera* extracts exhibit enormous potential and promise in controlling *Plasmodium* ingress into the host erythrocytes and further reducing the subsequent oxidative stress.

5. Conclusion

Herbal products are well thought-out to be symbols of safeguard in comparison to the synthetic product that are regarded as unsafe to human life and environment. Phytochemical and pharmacological studies are conducted on *L. camara* and *C. procera*. Based on the results obtained in the study, it can be inferred that the leaves of *L. camara* are rich sources of lot of secondary metabolites/phytocomponents which can be used as a prophylactic drug against malaria.

Finally, the current investigation's experimental work was focused on using membrane stabilisation to assess the anti-plasmodial activity of *L. camara* hydro-alcoholic crude extract. This extract did show evidence of potent phytochemicals with erythrocyte membrane stabilising activity. Furthermore, this study found that *L. camara* has better anti-plasmodial activity than *C. procera* against MRC2 and RKL9 *Plasmodium falciparum* strains, in contrast to synthetic products, which frequently have side effects and are dangerous to human life. This plant extract's potent antioxidant phytochemicals are both effective and relatively safe.

Both extracts of *L. camara* leaves had shown positive results on the effect on erythrocyte membrane stabilisation. They could inhibit the entry of parasites, also show effective antioxidant property, and has no toxic effect due to certain unknown compounds in the crude extracts on the normal cells which is proved by the MTT assay.

Acknowledgements

The data acquisition and analysis: Miss. Urja Joshi.

Participate in drafting or revising the work: Dr. Dhara Jani.

Contribute to the conception or design of the work:Dr. Linz-Buoy George.

Interpretation of data for the work& approve the final version of the work to be published: Dr. Hyacinth Highland.

Conflict of interest

"The authors declare no conflict of interest."

Abbreviations

DPPH	2, 2-diphenyl-1-picrylhydrazyl
MTT	3- (4, 5-dimethyl thiazol-2-yl)-2, 5-diphenyl tetrazolium bromide
ACTs	Artemisinin- Based Combination Therapies
C. procera	*C. procera* L
CAT	Catalase
DTNB	5, 5′-dithiobis nitro benzoic acid
GPx	Glutathione peroxidase
Hb	Haemoglobin
L. camara	*L. camara* L.
LPO	Lipid Peroxidation
MDA	malondialdehyde
P. falciparum	*Plasmodium falciparum*
Pf-iEs	*Plasmodium falciparum* infected erythrocytes
ROS	Reactive Oxygen Species
GSH	Reduced Glutathione
SOD	Superoxide Dismutase
TBARS	thiobarbutiric acid reactive species
WHO	World Health Organisation

Author details

Urja Joshi[1,2]*, Dhara Jani[2], Linz-Bouy George[2] and Hyacinth Highland[2]

1 Department of Biochemistry, School of Sciences, Gujarat University, Ahmedabad, Gujarat, India

2 Department of Zoology, BMTC, and Human Genetics, School of Sciences, Gujarat University, Ahmedabad, Gujarat, India

*Address all correspondence to: urjajoshi@gujaratuniversity.ac.in

References

[1] World Health Organization. World Malaria Report 2021. World malaria report. Geneva: World Health Organization; 2021

[2] Centre of Disease Control and prevention (CDC) report 2021. 2021. https://www.cdc.gov/malaria/features/world_malaria_day_2021.html. [Accessed: May 30, 2022]

[3] Grinev A, Fokina N, Bogomolov D, Berechikidze I, Lazareva Y. Prediction of gene expression regulation by human microRNAs in Plasmodium falciparum. Genes and Environment. 2021;**43**(1):1-9

[4] Phillips MA, Burrows JN, Manyando C. Nature reviews disease primers. Malaria. 2017;**3**:17050

[5] Gupta H, Rubio M, Sitoe A, Varo R, Cisteró P, Madrid L, et al. Plasma MicroRNA profiling of plasmodium falciparum biomass and association with severity of malaria disease. Emerging Infectious Diseases. 2021;**27**(2):430

[6] Oleinikov AV. Malaria parasite plasmodium falciparum proteins on the surface of infected erythrocytes as targets for novel drug discovery. Biochemistry (Moscow). 2022;**87**(1):S192-S2022

[7] Kadam ST, Pawar AD. Conservation of medicinal plants: A review. International Ayurvedic Medical Journal. 2020;**8**:3890-3895

[8] Cock IE, Selesho MI, Van Vuuren SF. A review of the traditional use of southern African medicinal plants for the treatment of malaria. Journal of Ethnopharmacology. 2019;**5**(245):112176

[9] Velu G, Palanichamy V, Rajan AP. Phytochemical and pharmacological importance of plant secondary metabolites in modern medicine. In Bio organic Phase in Natural Food: An Overview. Cham: Springer; 2018. pp. 135-156

[10] Thorat VH, Tamboli FA, Jadhav AS, Chavan R. Phytochemical analysis and antimicrobial activity of Lantana camara. International Journal of Pharmaceutical Chemistry and Analysis. 2021;**8**(4):171-173

[11] Rahma NA, Rohman A. UPLC MS/MS profile and antioxidant activities from nonpolar fraction of Patiwala (Lantana camara) leaves extract. Separations. 2022;**9**(3):75

[12] Dhara J, Shivali G, Urja J, Linz-buoy G and Hyacinth H. Hydroalcoholic extract of Alstonia scholaris arrests invasion of plasmodium falciparum by effective RBC membrane stabilization. Journal of Advances in Medical and Pharmaceutical Sciences. 2016;**9**(2):1-9

[13] Chaitali A, Rao P, Vikhe SR. Phytochemical and pharmacological activities of lantana camara-review. Research Journal of Pharmacognosy and Phytochemistry. 2022;**14**(2):128-131

[14] Mohebi Z. The important medicinal and industrial properties of Calotropis procera (Aiton) WT. Journal of Medicinal Plants Biotechnology. 2021;**7**(1):16-29

[15] Kaur A, Batish DR, Kaur S, Chauhan BS. An overview of the characteristics and potential of Calotropis procera from botanical, ecological, and economic perspectives. Frontiers in Plant Science. 2021;**17**(12):1188

[16] Ogundola AF, Yekeen TA, Arotayo RA, Akintola AO, Ibrahim AO, Adedosu HO,

et al. Evaluation of nutrients in leaves and seeds of calotropis procera (linn): A multipurpose plant. Journal of Pharmacy and Nutrition Sciences. 2021;**2**(11):33-39

[17] Ibrahim SR, Mohamed GA, Shaala LA, Moreno L, Banuls Y, Kiss R, et al. Proceraside A, a new cardiac glycoside from the root barks of Calotropis procera with in vitro anticancer effects. Natural Product Research. 2014;**28**(17):1322-1327

[18] Alzaidi SA. Genetic Assessment of Streptococcus spp. Group B and their susceptibility against *Calotropis procera* extract. Abasyn Journal of Life Sciences. 2020;**3**(1):24-30

[19] Gomes ARQ, Cunha N, Varela ELP, Brígido HPC, Vale VV, Dolabela MF, et al. Oxidative stress in Malaria: Potential benefits of antioxidant therapy. International Journal of Molecular Sciences. 2022;**23**(11):5949

[20] Hancock JT, Desikan R, Neill SJ. Role of reactive oxygen species in cell signalling pathways. Biochemical Society Transactions. 2001;**29**(2):345-349

[21] Egwu CO, Augereau JM, Reybier K, Benoit-Vical F. Reactive oxygen species as the brainbox in malaria treatment. Antioxidants. 2021;**10**(12):1872

[22] Tripathy S, Roy S. Redox sensing and signaling by malaria parasite in vertebrate host. Journal of Basic Microbiology. 2015;**55**(9):1053-1063

[23] Harborne JB. Textbook of phytochemical methods, 1st Edn, Champraan and Hall Ltd. London. pp. 1973:110-113

[24] Trager W, Jensen JB. Human malaria parasites in continuous culture. Science. 1976;**193**(4254):673-675

[25] Gyamfi MA, Yonamine M, Aniya Y. Free-radical scavenging action of medicinal herbs from Ghana: Thonningia sanguinea on experimentally-induced liver injuries. General Pharmacology: The Vascular System. 1999;**32**(6):661-667

[26] Rahmati H, Salehi S, Malekpour A, Farhangi F. Antimicrobial activity of castor oil plant (Ricinus communis) seeds extract against gram positive bacteria, gram negative bacteria and yeast. International Journal of Molecular Medicine and Advance Sciences. 2015;**11**(1):9-12

[27] Ahmad W, Singh S, Kumar S. Phytochemical screening and antimicrobial study of Euphorbia hirta extracts. Journal of Medicinal Plants Studies. 2017;**5**(2):183-186

[28] George LB, Mathew S, Jani D, Patel S, Highland H. Tylophora indica extracts manifest potent in vitro anti-plasmodium activity. International Journal of Pharma Sciences. 2015;**5**(6):1297-1306

[29] Jansen O, Tits M, Angenot L, Nicolas JP, De Mol P, Nikiema JB, et al. Anti-plasmodial activity of Dicoma tomentosa (Asteraceae) and identification of urospermal A-15-O-acetate as the main active compound. Malaria Journal. 2012;**11**(1):1-9

[30] Kumar S, Sandhir R, Ojha S. Evaluation of antioxidant activity and total phenol in different varieties of Lantana camara leaves. BMC Research Notes. 2014;**7**(1):1-9

[31] Metta S, Uppala S, Basalingappa DR, Badeti SR, Gunti SS. Impact of smoking on erythrocyte indices and oxidative stress in acute myocardial infarction. Journal of Dr. NTR University of Health Sciences. 2015;**4**(3):159

[32] Ohkawa H, Ohishi N, Yagi K. Assay for lipid peroxides in animal tissues by thiobarbituric acid reaction. Analytical Biochemistry. 1979;**95**(2):351-358

[33] Kakkar P, Das B, Viswanathan PN. A modified spectrophotometric assay of superoxide dismutase. Indian J Biochem Biophys. 1984 Apr;**21**(2):130-132. PMID: 6490072

[34] Sinha AK. Colorimetric assay of catalase. Analytical Biochemistry. 1972;**47**(2):389-394

[35] Ellman M. A spectrophotometric method for determination of reduced glutathione in tissues. Analytical Biochemistry. 1959;**74**(1):214-216

[36] Rotruck JT, Pope AL, Ganther HE, Swanson AB, Hafeman DG, Hoekstra W. Selenium: Biochemical role as a component of glutathione peroxidase. Science. 1973;**179**(4073):588-590

[37] Mosmann T. Rapid colorimetric assay for cellular growth and survival: Application to proliferation and cytotoxicity assays. Journal of Immunological Methods. 1983;**65**(1-2):55-63

[38] Wilson AP. Cytotoxicity and viability assays. Animal Cell Culture: A Practical Approach. 2000;**29**(1):175-219

[39] Mulcahy MF. Blood values in the pike Esoxlucius L. Journal of Fish Biology. 1970;**2**(3):203-209

[40] Oyedapo OO, Akinpelu BA, Akinwunmi KF, Adeyinka MO, Sipeolu FO. Red blood cell membrane stabilizing potentials of extracts of Lantana camara and its fractions. International Journal of Plant Physiology and Biochemistry. 2010;**2**(4):46-51

[41] Thenmozhi V, Elango V, Sadique J. Anti-inflamatory activity of some Indian medicinal plants. Ancient Science of Life. 1989;**8**(3-4):258

[42] Paloque L, Witkowski B, Lelièvre J, Ouji M, Ben Haddou T, Ariey F, et al. Endoperoxide-based compounds: cross-resistance with artemisinins and selection of a Plasmodium falciparum lineage with a K13 non-synonymous polymorphism. Journal of Antimicrobial Chemotherapy. 2018;**73**(2):395-403

[43] Comunian TA, Ravanfar R, de Castro IA, Dando R, Favaro-Trindade CS, Abbaspourrad A. Improving oxidative stability of echium oil emulsions fabricated by Microfluidics: Effect of ionic gelation and phenolic compounds. Food Chemistry. 2017;**15**(233):125-134

[44] Shahidi F, Ambigaipalan P. Phenolics and polyphenolics in foods, beverages and spices: Antioxidant activity and health effects–A review. Journal of Functional Foods. 2015;**1**(18):820-897

[45] Becker K, Tilley L, Vennerstrom JL, Roberts D, Rogerson S, Ginsburg H. Oxidative stress in malaria parasite-infected erythrocytes: host–parasite interactions. International Journal for Parasitology. 2004;**34**(2):163-189

[46] Erel O, Kocyigit A, Avci S, Aktepe N, Bulut V. Oxidative stress and antioxidative status of plasma and erythrocytes in patients with vivax malaria. Clinical Biochemistry. 1997;**30**(8):631-639

[47] Verstraeten SV, Keen CL, Schmitz HH, Fraga CG, Oteiza PI. Flavan-3-ols and procyanidins protect liposomes against lipid oxidation and disruption of the bilayer structure. Free Radical Biology and Medicine. 2003;**34**(1):84-92

[48] Duran-Bedolla J, Rodriguez MH, Saldana-Navor V, Rivas-Arancibia S, Cerbon M, Rodriguez MC. Oxidative stress: Production in several processes and organelles during Plasmodium sp development. Oxidants and Antioxidants in Medical Science. 2013;**2**(2):93-100

[49] Müller S. Thioredoxin reductase and glutathione synthesis in Plasmodium falciparum. Redox report. 2003;**8**(5):251-255

[50] Rahbari M, Rahlfs S, Jortzik E, Bogeski I, Becker K. H2O2 dynamics in the malaria parasite Plasmodium falciparum. PLoS One. 2017;**12**(4):e0174837

[51] Atamna H, Ginsburg H. Origin of reactive oxygen species in erythrocytes infected with Plasmodium falciparum. Molecular and Biochemical Parasitology. 1993;**61**(2):231-241

[52] Tyagi A, Tyagi R, Vekariya R, Ahuja A. Study of Antioxidant Enzymes. MDA and Lipid Profile in Cerebral Malaria. Indian J Clin Pract. 2013;**23**(12):823-825

[53] Ezzi AA, Salahy MB, Shnawa BH, Abed GH, Mandour AM. Changes in levels of antioxidant markers and status of some enzyme activities among falciparum malaria patients in Yemen. Journal of Microbiology & Experimentation. 2017;**4**(6):00131